DIABETES, OBESITY, AND VASCULAR DISEASE

Advances in Modern Nutrition

Series Editor
Myron A. Mehlman

Advances in Modern Nutrition

VOLUME 2

DIABETES, OBESITY, AND VASCULAR DISEASE

Metabolic and Molecular Interrelationships
Part 1

EDITORS

HOWARD M. KATZEN
MERCK INSTITUTE FOR THERAPEUTIC RESEARCH

RICHARD J. MAHLER
EISENHOWER MEDICAL CENTER

**HEMISPHERE
PUBLISHING CORPORATION**

Washington   London

A HALSTED PRESS BOOK

JOHN WILEY & SONS

New York   London   Sydney   Toronto

Hemisphere Publishing Corporation
1025 Vermont Ave., N.W., Washington, D.C. 20005

Distributed solely by Halsted Press, a Division of John Wiley & Sons, Inc.,
New York.

1 2 3 4 5 6 7 8 9 0   D O D O   7 8 3 2 1 0 9 8

Library of Congress Cataloging in Publication Data

Main entry under title:

Diabetes, obesity, and vascular disease.

      (Advances in modern nutrition; v. 2)
      Includes indexes.
      1. Diabetes—Nutritional aspects. 2. Obesity—
Nutritional aspects. 3. Arteriosclerosis—
Nutritional aspects. 4. Metabolism, Disorders of.
I. Katzen, Howard M. II. Mahler, Richard J.,
1934–   III. Series. [DNLM: 1. Diabetes
mellitus—Complications. 2. Diabetes mellitus—
Metabolism. 3. Obesity—Complications. 4. Obesity
—Metabolism. 5. Vascular diseases—Complications.
6. Vascular diseases—Metabolism W1 AD682M v. 2 /
WK810 D5394]
RC660.D543   616.3'9   77-24993
ISBN 0 470-99360-X

Printed in the United States of America

CONTENTS

v

PREFACE

In this monograph we have attempted to encompass the key metabolic and hormonal events currently under study in the field of diabetes mellitus, as well as to focus on these events more closely at a molecular level. Additionally, we have also asked the contributors to provide, where applicable, a clinical and nutritional orientation to these considerations of the disease. Special emphasis is placed upon how these events may be implicated in the obese state, while a considerable portion of the volume has been allocated to the vascular sequelae that often accompany and complicate this disease. Although much has previously been reported on diabetes, obesity, and vascular disease as separate and distinct subjects, there have been few texts primarily concerned with how these disorders relate to each other. It is our intention to describe these interrelationships with their particular orientation to diabetes.

No more appropriate introductory chapter could have been written than that provided by the distinguished authority Dr. Rachmiel Levine, who has eloquently reviewed the historical background of the role of modern nutrition in diabetes mellitus. Every individual from medical student to clinician to basic scientist will find this chapter a rewarding experience.

Following this are chapters specifically reviewing the basic principles of the intermediary metabolism of the carbohydrates and the lipids as they may pertain to diabetes, obesity, and the vascular diseases. We believe that these chapters will provide convenient reference sources for the reader to review these principles and to gain a better understanding of the significance of the subsequent subject matter. Included in this regard are the classifications and basic characteristics of the lipoprotein abnormalities.

With this foundation, the reader can turn to considerations of the factors themselves that are directly involved in the diseased states and in their interrelationships. In those chapters linking obesity to diabetes, such factors as the size and number of adipocytes, their metabolic character, membrane insulin receptors and transport mechanisms, key intracellular enzyme reactions, regulation of appetite, and neuroendocrine, nutritional, and psychological factors are emphasized.

The roles of hormones, insulin and glucagon in particular, in the development and maintenance of obesity, diabetes, and the concomitant state of insulin resistance provide an additional perspective on how these disease entities relate to each other. The often overlooked role of energy intake and balance is also reviewed and evaluated.

In a consideration of the vascular complications of diabetes, special attention is directed to various aspects of the development of atherosclerosis as well as to the factors concerned with, and implications of, the lipoprotein abnormalities associated with the hyperlipemias.

No treatise oriented toward diabetes would be complete without a discussion of the implications of insulin secretion. Of equal importance is a chapter extending the discussion beyond the membrane and cellular level to the level of the intact organs wherein the interplay among such key tissues as muscle, liver, and adipose is of fundamental importance in the utilization of the metabolic intermediates. In addition, one should not overlook the developing role of minerals and trace elements, particularly in diabetes and its vascular complications. In view of its importance, the diagnosis and treatment of diabetes in the pediatric population is given separate consideration, and finally, detailed sections on diet and insulin therapy are also provided.

It is hoped that the provision of a monograph linking the key elements of obesity and vascular disease to the many facets of diabetes at biochemical, physiological, nutritional, and clinical levels will provide both the scientist and physician with a fertile reference source as well as a comprehensive review and evaluation of our knowledge in these fields of current interest.

Howard M. Katzen
Richard J. Mahler

DIABETES, OBESITY, AND VASCULAR DISEASE

Chapter 1

INTRODUCTION:
MODERN DEVELOPMENT OF
THE PRINCIPLES OF NUTRITION

Rachmiel Levine
City of Hope Medical Center
Duarte, California

Lavoisier's dictum that life is a chemical function ("la vie est une fonction chimique") ended a long era of mysticism in the approach to the study of living beings (Levoisier and Laplace, 1780). It was the beginning of our understanding of the similarities in structure and function among plants, animals, and humans. It also marks the origin of the science of nutrition, because Lavoisier's work established clearly that exhaled CO_2 was derived from the carbon of bodily constituents, reacting with inhaled O_2. This process accounted as well for bodily heat. It became evident then that "burning" of nutrient carbon provided energy in a manner similar to the production of light and heat by a burning candle. It was eminently logical, in the face of the then prevailing knowledge, to place the site of energy production in the lungs. Techniques for the measurement of regional temperature led first to the concept that the site of oxidation was really the blood and not the lungs, and finally to individual tissues and the cells composing them as the loci of energy production, the seat of oxidation.

From prehistoric times on it was evident to humans that food provided the basis for growth, maintenance, and energetic expression of human and animal bodies. How was food incorporated—that is, how did it become part of the corpus? And in what state did it reach the loci of energy production? Reaumur and Spallanzani noted that gastric juice "dissolved" meat. Kirchhoff and Schweigger (1815) pointed out that barley seeds contained a material that converted the starch of the seeds into sugars, and in 1833 Payen and Persoz isolated from malt a substance that "possesses the remarkable power of quickly separating the envelopes [of starch granules] from the transformed interior substance, the dextrin...." They gave this substance the name diastase from the Greek word for separation. From that time on it was realized that diastases or enzymes were agents that "solubilized" or broke

1

down foodstuffs, not only in plants but also in the gut of animals (ptyalin, pepsin, amylase, trypsin, invertase, and so on). The first effect of the body itself on ingested foodstuffs was seen to be cleavage of the raw material by specific hydrolytic enzymes.

Concurrently, it was realized that the many varieties of food available could be classified into three chemically defined groups: carbohydrates, fats, and proteins.

We must realize that the development of the concepts of intermediary metabolism of foodstuffs—that is, the step-by-step conversion of materials to the ultimate products, water and CO_2, with liberation of energy—was a slow intellectual process and had to await the accretion of knowledge of organic chemistry and, above all, the realization of the catalytic nature of the enzymes and their infinite variety. It was Berzelius, in 1837, who set forth these principles in clear and prescient fashion. He wrote,

> We have justifiable reasons to suppose that, in living plants and animals, thousands of catalytic processes take place between the tissues and liquids and result in the formation of the great number of dissimilar chemical compounds, for whose formation out of the common raw material, plant juice or blood, no probable cause could be assigned. The cause will perhaps in the future be discovered in the catalytic power in the organic tissues of which the organs of the living body consist.

The term "enzyme" was introduced in 1878. It was proposed by Kühne. He linked two Greek words, "en zyme" or "in yeast," to suggest that, as regards the fermentative process, the "complex organisms from which the enzymes, pepsin, trypsin, etc. can be obtained are not so fundamentally different from the unicellular organisms as some people would have us believe."

As a matter of fact, our knowledge of cell metabolism since Kühne's time was in the main derived from the needs of industry and of medicine. The brewer required a better knowledge of the process of yeast fermentation. The army and industry in general stimulated the acquisition of data concerning the physiology of work—the fuel and mechanics of muscular contraction. And the inquiring physicians were seeking to understand the chemical diseases, such as diabetes. These "applied areas" stimulated research and made possible our basic understanding of protein chemistry and functions, of the control of bodily growth and maintenance, and of the pathways and mechanisms by which food builds and maintains the machinery of the cell. It was only later that more complex questions were being asked: How is chemical bond energy translated into bodily motion? into cell secretion? into neural impulse propagation and sense perception?

Although the amazing and complex details of intermediary metabolism were still to be filled in by the turn of the 20th century, the basic principles of the modern science of nutrition were laid down by that time.

The free sugars and their polymeric derivatives comprised the broad category of the carbohydrates. The glucose derived from this food category was shown to be a ready fuel for bodily functions, especially for muscular work. Excess carbohydrate led to its storage, partly as glycogen but mainly as fat.

The fats in food were known to furnish energy, especially during periods of fasting; that is, fats formed the reserve fuel supply.

By the 1870s the basic importance of proteins or albuminoids was recognized sufficiently to evoke the dictum by Engels that "life was the expression of the behavior of albumens." Many of the constituent amino acids were soon discovered and their structures were being elucidated. Protein as a food was seen to serve as the basic element for growth and tissue replacement. It was also realized that the liver was capable of converting the nonnitrogenous portions of some amino acids to glucose, and that this process—gluconeogenesis—served to maintain normal blood sugar levels between meals.

In 1881, Lunin published a paper on the importance of inorganic salts for animal nutrition. In it he stated

> Since as shown by the above experiments they [rats] were not able to survive on albuminates, fat, sugar, salts and water, it follows that in milk (which was added) there must be other substances besides casein, lactose and salt that are essential for nutrition. It would be of great interest to track them down and to study their significance in nutrition.

This prophetic statement soon became a reality through the work of Eijkman, Hopkins, Osborne and Mendel, McCallum, and others and led to the vitamin concept.

As the details of intracellular metabolic reactions began to unfold (in the first three decades of the present century) it was soon realized that the vitamins and the minerals were constituent parts of the enzymatic apparatus, serving as coenzymes and activators in both anabolic and catabolic reactions—for growth, maintenance, and the regulated delivery of energy that served the various functions of the organism.

The newest of the biological disciplines underlying the rational principles of nutrition is endocrinology, since many of the hormones were found to regulate directly and indirectly the disposal, storage, mobilization, and rates of turnover of the foodstuffs (e.g., insulin, glucagon, thyroxine, glucocorticoids, and somatotropin).

There is a nutritional aspect in the etiology as well as in the treatment of virtually all diseases. Consider the effect of caloric overfeeding on the growth and spread of tumors, or the relation of an adequate protein intake to the immunological reactions of microbial diseases, or the need for protein restriction in impending renal failure. But the impact of nutrition is most dramatic in the constellation of disorders that affect us most heavily when we reach middle age, when we have attained the stage of food abundance and the leisure time to enjoy the fruits of our labor. We have just emerged from the pitfalls of infancy and adolescence and have successfully fought off the devastating effects of microorganisms. The array of chronic morbid intruders operative in the second half of our life-span consists of obesity, diabetes, and hypertension, and their several or joint vascular sequelae subsumed under the term arteriosclerosis.

It is therefore right that the editors of this volume have called on a goodly company of experts in the relevant disciplines for a thorough exposition and understanding of nutrition as it applies to the care and prevention of diabetes and atherosclerosis. And it is quite proper that the expert contributors present their conclusions together with the basic scientific data that underlie them. This volume should serve both the practitioner and the student well. It has much that is important and useful to tell them. If patients were counseled by their physicians in accord with the principles and measures herein detailed and if they then adhered to these nutritional prescriptions, much morbidity could be avoided and lessened mortality would be expected. What stands in the way, however, is the silent course of these disorders. One often wishes that rises in blood pressure or blood sugar produced some harmless but annoying symptoms—an itch perhaps, or a feeling of heat or a visible discoloration—and that compliance with diet and hygienic habits removed the symptoms promptly and satisfyingly. Unfortunately, only the "complications" produce symptoms, and only after many years.

Even more helpful would be a clearer understanding of the neuro-hormonal control of appetite, especially the precise reason for the seemingly addictive nature of overeating. A deep understanding of these mechanisms, one that could lead to control of intake over the years, would certainly prevent the development of and the invidious progress of hyperglycemia, hyperglyceridemia, hyperuricemia, and hypertension to the end-stages of arteriorsclerotic disease of vital arterial conduits. However, it is not likely that simple harmless chemical intervention will prove to be possible. This is because natural selection has evidently found lipogenesis to be a most useful and advantageous process during early growth and the reproductive period. Biological evolution is not concerned with what may happen to the middle-aged burgher of today with a lot of large and hungry fat cells. The only hope would seem to be to influence the whole process by the power of cultural evolution—that is, by the transmission of accurate knowledge. Hence, the book.

REFERENCES

Berzelius, J. J., 1837. *Lehrb. Chem.* 6:22.
Kirchhoff, C., and Schweigger, J. 1815. *Chem. Phys.* 14:385.
Kühne, W., 1878. *Untersuch. Physiol. Inst. Heidelberg* 1:291.
Lavoisier, A. L. and Laplace, P. S. 1780. *Mem. Acad. Sci.,* p. 379.
Lunin, N. 1881. *Z. Physiol. Chem.* 5:31.
Payen, C. and Persoz. 1833. *Ann. Chim. Phys.* 53:73.

BIBLIOGRAPHY

Bayliss, W. M. 1924. *Principles of general physiology,* 4th. ed. London: Longmans, Green.

Fruton, J. 1972. *Molecules and life.* New York: Wiley-Interscience.

Lust, G. 1928. *The elements of the science of nutrition,* 4th ed. Philadelphia: Saunders.

Chapter 2

CARBOHYDRATE METABOLISM AND ITS IMPLICATIONS

Earl Shrago and Robin B. Lockhart Ewart
Departments of Medicine and Nutritional Sciences
University of Wisconsin
Madison, Wisconsin

INTRODUCTION

Carbohydrates have fulfilled a critical role in the evolutionary history of biological systems. Possibly the most important metabolic cycle in the development of our planet as we know it is represented by the scheme shown in Fig. 1. Animal life on earth originated when green plants developed the ability to absorb and utilize certain wavelengths from the energy spectrum of the sun for the biosynthesis of carbohydrates, with oxygen being liberated as a by-product. The carbon dioxide and water required as substrates for this glyconeogenic process are, in turn, regenerated by the degradative metabolic reactions characteristic of animal species. As concern grows over our progressive interference with the qualities of our environment, it is all too apparent that whether life continues depends crucially on the maintenance of this steady-state carbon cycle.

So far as carbohydrate metabolism in humans is concerned, our understanding has proceeded historically from the identification of individual enzyme-catalyzed reactions through the determination of detailed enzyme kinetics and the recognition of entire metabolic pathways. More recently, an appreciation of the related allosteric controls has defined the physiological mechanism by which carbon flux through various alternative pathways is regulated. To review all of the complexities of carbohydrate metabolism is beyond the scope of the present review, and this chapter will be restricted to a discussion of those aspects of intermediary metabolism which seem to be most important for the analysis and understanding of such clinical disorders as diabetes mellitus, obesity, and vascular disease. The nutritional significance of carbohydrate as well as its potential importance as a factor in disease states can best be appreciated when it is realized that more than 50% of the caloric requirement of Western humans is satisfied by this nutrient.

This work was supported by U.S. Public Health Service grant AM 15893.

7

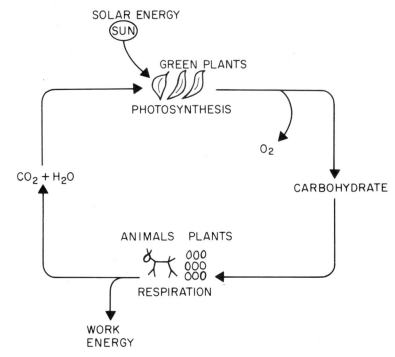

FIGURE 1 Life cycle of carbon.

PLASMA GLUCOSE AND ITS REGULATION

Glucose Assimilation by the Liver

The concentration of plasma glucose in normal humans is maintained within limits of 3–7 millimolar (mM) in widely differing nutritional states. During absorption of a glucose load or immediately following a carbohydrate-rich meal, the portal venous glucose concentration is elevated to levels that may reach 15 mM or more. Since the hepatocyte plasma membrane is freely permeable to glucose, rapid uptake of the sugar by the liver occurs, reducing the glucose load delivered to the periphery. The glucose cleared in this way is employed mainly for replenishing glycogen stores, but in part is metabolized by the glycolytic and pentose phosphate pathways. Rapid partial clearing of absorbed glucose by the liver normally ensures that the peripheral plasma glucose concentration rises only to around 7 mM in the period immediately after a carbohydrate load, thus avoiding renal losses, which would become apparent if plasma glucose levels of 10 mM or more were attained (Mortimore, 1972).

Effect of Insulin

Like the hepatocytes, the B-cells of the pancreatic islet possess plasma membranes that permit almost instantaneous equilibration of intra- and extracellular glucose concentrations. Without attempting to speculate on the nature of the stimulus-secretion coupling mechanism of the B-cell, it is clear that this arrangement provides the insulin secretory mechanism with information concerning minute-to-minute variations in plasma glucose concentration. A rise in plasma glucose from 4–7 mM is associated with a striking increase in the rate of insulin delivery to the circulation, and it is of interest to note that the concentration of glucose leading to half-maximal stimulation of insulin release is approximately the maximum circulating glucose concentration attained after a carbohydrate load.

The primary effect of the insulin is to activate, by mechanisms as yet unknown, the glucose transport systems of tissues that, unlike liver and B-cells, are relatively impermeable to glucose in the absence of the hormone (Levine and Goldstein, 1955). In addition, there is evidence for a direct effect of insulin in inhibiting hepatic glucose output (Madison et al., 1959). Insulin thus leads to a reduction in circulating glucose concentration and permits the distribution of substrate to the peripheral tissues for immediate energy production or storage, for example, as muscle glycogen (Neely, 1973).

Contributions of Glycogenolysis and Gluconeogenesis

If, after such a carbohydrate load, a period of fasting supervenes, there is a continuing tendency for the plasma glucose concentration to fall. Under these circumstances, the insulin secretion rate also declines, leading among other consequences to a reduction in the availability of glucose as a substrate for the insulin-dependent peripheral tissues. Reduction in the circulating insulin concentration also permits accelerated lipolysis with the provision of nonesterified fatty acids to meet tissue energy requirements. Some tissues, however, such as brain, red cells, renal medulla, and testes, are glucose-dependent but insulin-independent. Although in prolonged fasting it appears that brain can derive up to 75% of its caloric requirement from ketone bodies (Owen et al., 1967), a rapid major reduction in the level of plasma glucose would threaten the functional integrity of these tissues.

To prevent the deleterious effects of hypoglycemia during fasting, the liver in the absence of insulin releases free glucose, produced by the hydrolytic cleavage of glucose 6-phosphate, into the circulation. The primary source of glucose 6-phosphate for this process is liver glycogen, the major storage form of carbohydrate. When the caloric equivalent of the carbohydrate stores of normal humans (Table 1) is compared with the daily glucose requirement of certain important tissues (Table 2), it is readily apparent that the carbohydrate reserves would last for only a short time and that glucose must be continuously replenished from exogenous or endogenous sources. Thus, with prolonged fasting, when a glycogen is depleted, liver glucose 6-phosphate must be derived from such alternative substrates as lactate, alanine, glutamine, and glycerol by the process of gluconeogenesis.

It should be stressed that the liver and, during prolonged fasting, the

TABLE 1 Carbohydrate Content of Normal Humans[a]

Carbohydrate	Amount (g)
Muscle glycogen	120–245
Liver glycogen	70–108
Blood and extracellular glucose	17–20

[a]Data from Soskin and Levine (1952) and Newsholme and Start (1973).

TABLE 2 Tissue Glucose Requirement[a]

Tissue	Glucose (g/day)
Brain	120
Muscle	30–100
Erythrocytes Renal medulla Testes	40

[a]Data from Newsholme and Start (1973).

kidney fulfill a unique role in maintaining the plasma glucose concentration by reason of their possession of the key gluconeogenic enzyme glucose-6-phosphatase. Thus, for example, muscle glycogen can contribute glucose 6-phosphate to the muscle substrate pool for immediate energy production, but the glucosyl residue cannot be released into the circulation as free glucose because of the absence of a muscle glucose-6-phosphatase (Ruderman et al., 1976).

GLUCOSE TRANSPORT INTO CELLS

Hepatocytes are freely permeable to glucose, and the rate of uptake of the sugar into these cells is determined primarily by the rate of its further intracellular metabolism. All other body cells possess specific membrane carriers for glucose transport. In the case of glucose-dependent tissues such as brain and erythrocytes, these glucose carriers operate independently of insulin, a fact that has clear survival value. In contrast, tissues such as muscle and adipocytes, which constitute the main body mass, take up glucose poorly from the extracellular pool in the absence of insulin. The effect of insulin on glucose transport into cells was elegantly demonstrated by Levine and co-workers (1949, 1950) in a classical experiment based on the knowledge that in the eviscerated dog, galactose, unlike glucose, is a nonmetabolizable sugar (Fig. 2). With this preparation, a galactose load was given and the blood concentration of sugar allowed to stabilize over a period of 3 hr. At this time the administration of insulin was shown to be associated with an approximately 50% reduction in blood galactose over a period of 30 min. This significant increase in galactose space was clearly interpreted as the result of an insulin-induced passage of galactose into the intracellular compartment of the extrahepatic tissues. Although this particular experiment cannot be reproduced with glucose because of the rapid further metabolism of this sugar, subsequent investigations (Ross, 1956) indicated that glucose transport is similarly enhanced by insulin.

INTRACELLULAR METABOLISM OF CARBOHYDRATES

Phosphorylation of Glucose

There is relatively little free glucose in cells. Having gained access to the intracellular compartment, glucose rapidly undergoes phosphorylation by ATP in a nonequilibrium reaction catalyzed by glucokinase and a group of three isozymes collectively called hexokinase, with the formation of glucose 6-phosphate.

The hexokinases. The hexokinases differ from glucokinase in several important respects. They are much the more widely distributed of the two classes of enzymes and catalyze the phosphorylation not only of D-glucose but also of many other hexoses and hexose derivatives (Katzen, 1967). The apparent K_m of the hexokinases for glucose is in the range of 1.0 μM to 0.1 mM. The hexokinase reaction is highly regulated, being inhibited by its own product, glucose 6-phosphate. Whenever the cell has a high concentration of glucose 6-phosphate and requires no more for its energy demands, the hexokinases are inhibited, thus preventing the formation of additional glucose 6-phosphate (Rose et al., 1974).

Glucokinase. Earlier in this chapter, reference was made to the uptake of glucose by the hepatocytes when the portal venous glucose concentration is elevated—for example, following an alimentary carbohydrate load. This property of liver cells is explained by their possession of the enzyme glucokinase first demonstrated by Sharma et al. (1963) and Vinuela et al. (1963). The glucokinase isozyme that predominates in liver shows much greater specificity for glucose than do the hexokinases. The K_m for its preferred substrate is higher by two orders of magnitude, being of the order of 10 mM. It is not

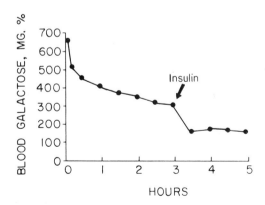

FIGURE 2 Effect of insulin on the transport of galactose from the extracellular to the intracellular space in muscle (Levine et al., 1950).

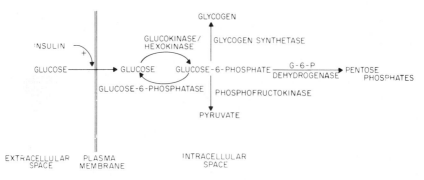

FIGURE 3 Diagram illustrating the formation of glucose 6-phosphate and its role as a
branch point in the intracellular metabolism of glucose.

inhibited by its product, glucose 6-phosphate, and its maximal activity is some
15-fold greater than that of the hexokinases.

Consideration of these properties together with the free permeability of
the hepatocyte plasma membrane to glucose makes it clear that glucokinase is
uniquely suited to effect the conversion of portal venous glucose to glucose
6-phosphate in the liver cell. Thus, for example, a change of the portal venous
glucose concentration from 4 to 15 mM, which would have little effect on the
activities of the hexokinases, greatly accelerates glucose phosphorylation in
liver by glucokinase. Glucose 6-phosphate, to which the cell membrane is
completely impermeable and which therefore cannot leave the cell, is a key
branch point in the metabolism of carbohydrate, as shown in Fig. 3. The
direction of carbon flow from glucose 6-phosphate depends on the nutritional
and hormonal status of the animal and on the regulation of enzymes
catalyzing key reactions in the subsequent degradative and synthetic pathways
(Newsholme and Start, 1973).

Glycogen Synthesis and Degradation

Glycogen is a highly branched polymer of molecular weight 10^6-10^8
composed of glucose residues linked by -1, 4-glycosidic bonds to form chains
that are branched by the formation of 1,6-linkages (Stetten and Stetten,
1960). Glycogen can be detected in almost every tissue but assumes particular
importance in liver, where it functions to provide a store of glucosyl units for
the maintenance of the plasma glucose concentration, and in muscle, where it
represents a fuel respository for muscle contraction. In a well-nourished man,
liver and muscle glycogen stores amount to 70 and 120 g, respectively.

The first step in glycogen synthesis is the phosphoglucomutase-catalyzed
conversion of glucose 6-phosphate to glucose 1-phosphate, which then reacts
with uridine triphosphate under the influence of uridine diphosphoglucose
pyrophosphorylase to form uridine diphosphoglucose. The latter intermediate
then acts as a glucosyl donor, adding a glucose residue to an outer chain of

the glycogen molecule. When repetition of this process results in the formation of outer chains 12 to 18 residues in length, the branching enzyme, 1,4-α-glucan: 1,4-glucan 6-glycosyltransferase acts to transfer a glucosyl residue from a 1,4 to a 1,6 linkage.

In terms of the overall regulation of glycogen metabolism, it is convenient at this point also to consider glycogen degradation (Villar-Palasi and Larner, 1970). The enzyme responsible for glycogen breakdown, phosphorylase, catalyzes the formation of glucose 1-phosphate from glycogen in the presence of inorganic phosphate. Thus, the enzymatic pathways for glycogen synthesis and degradation are entirely distinct and, in this circumstance, a control mechanism must exist to prevent the establishment of a "futile cycle" with consequent dissipation of energy (Villar-Palasi and Larner, 1970). This possibility is avoided because both glycogen synthetase and phosphorylase exist in active and inactive forms, the proportions of which are regulated by intricately coordinated control devices involving phosphorylation of the enzyme proteins by protein kinases, whose activities are determined primarily by the concentration of cyclic AMP within the cell. Thus, as shown in Fig. 4, cyclic AMP leads to dissociation of the regulatory and catalytic subunits of protein kinase, resulting in activation of the latter. The active protein kinase then simultaneously catalyzes the phosphorylation of glycogen synthetase, leading to its inactivation, and the phosphorylation of phosphorylase kinase, which is inactive in its dephosphorylated form. The now active phosphorylase kinase then catalyzes the phosphorylation of inactive phosphorylase *b* to yield phosphorylase *a*, which in turn acts on glycogen to form glucose 1-phosphate, which can then yield glucose 6-phosphate under the influence of phosphoglucomutase.

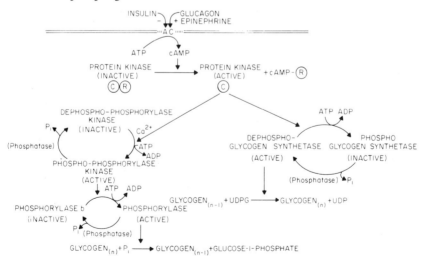

FIGURE 4   Interrelationships of glycogen synthetase and phosphorylase in the synthesis and degradation of glucose.

This sequence of reactions represents the well-characterized cascade phenomenon of glycogenolysis (Newsholme and Start, 1973). Thus, in the presence of high intracellular concentrations of cyclic AMP, induced by the interaction of glucagon or epinephrine with their specific membrane receptors, glycogen synthetase is inactivated and phosphorylase is simultaneously activated, leading to the degradation of glycogen. With discontinuance of the hormonal stimuli, the enzyme proteins are dephosphorylated by the action of a protein phosphatase. In cases of carbohydrate repletion, when insulin levels are high, it is reasonable to suppose that in liver this hormone lowers intracellular concentrations of cyclic AMP, leading to reduced activity of protein kinase and unopposed protein phosphatase activity. This would ensure activation of glycogen synthetase and inactivation of phosphorylase. However, although insulin-stimulated glycogen synthesis is associated with a reduced intracellular concentration of cyclic AMP in liver, this is not the case in muscle tissue. A possible explanation for this incongruity is provided by the observation that two forms of protein kinase exist in muscle, one cyclic AMP-dependent and the other not (Villar-Palasi and Wegner, 1967). It appears that insulin increases the proportion of the cyclic AMP-dependent form of the enzyme, so that in the presence of this hormone (which does not alter the muscle concentration of cyclic AMP) the overall activity of protein kinase is decreased, favoring glycogen deposition.

Glycolysis

The second pathway available to glucose 6-phosphate is the glycolytic series of reactions, which can be recognized as comprising two major sequences. The first of these is the conversion of glucose 6-phosphate to glyceraldehyde 3-phosphate, and the second the onward metabolism of this intermediate to pyruvate or lactate. The individual reactions of the glycolytic pathway that occur in the cytosol compartment are well known and are presented in summary form in Fig. 5.

Functions of glycolysis. The functions of glycolysis vary in different tissues. Thus, in liver a major role of glycolysis is to provide pyruvate for conversion to acetyl CoA, the substrate for fatty acid biosynthesis (see Chap. 3). By contrast, extra hepatic tissues depend to a great extent on glycolysis for energy production. In tissues possessing sufficient numbers of mitochondria and operating under aerobic conditions, the pyruvate formed during glycolysis is converted to acetyl CoA, whose further complete oxidation to carbon dioxide and water is coupled to ATP synthesis. However, in tissues with few or no mitochondria, such as white muscle and the red cell, or in situations of anaerobiosis, the glycolytic pathway is an end in itself, the final product being not pyruvate but lactate.

The energetic yield of the glycolytic pathway depends on the precise substrate involved. Thus, conversion of 1 mol of free glucose to pyruvate or lactate leads to formation of 2 mol of ATP, whereas when glucosyl units of

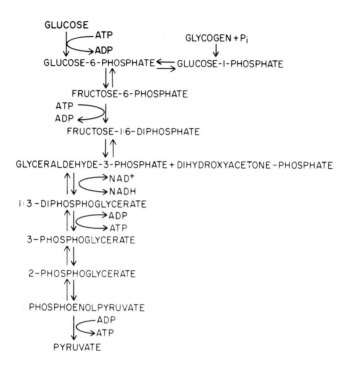

GLUCOSE

GLUCOSE-6-PHOSPHATE ⇌ GLUCOSE-1-PHOSPHATE

GLYCOGEN + Pᵢ

FRUCTOSE-6-PHOSPHATE

FRUCTOSE-1·6-DIPHOSPHATE

GLYCERALDEHYDE-3-PHOSPHATE + DIHYDROXYACETONE-PHOSPHATE

1·3-DIPHOSPHOGLYCERATE

3-PHOSPHOGLYCERATE

2-PHOSPHOGLYCERATE

PHOSPHOENOLPYRUVATE

PYRUVATE

FIGURE 5 The glycolytic pathway. Physiologically irreversible reactions are designated with a single arrow.

glycogen are employed as the substrate, avoidance of hexokinase or gluco-kinase-catalyzed phosphorylation allows for the formation of 3 mol of ATP from each 1 mol of glucose.

Regulation of glycolysis. The energy requirements that must be fulfilled by the glycolytic pathway are quite variable from moment to moment. In no tissue is this more apparent than in skeletal muscle where, in the absence of ATP regeneration, the available energy store would be exhausted within seconds of initiation of active contraction. Thus, the transition from rest to muscle work requires a major and rapid increase in glycolytic flux. Whereas for this reason most of the investigations into the mechanisms of glycolytic control have utilized muscle tissue, there is evidence to support the generality of the regulatory systems thus identified (Lowry and Passonneau, 1964). Four regulatory steps are emphasized below.

The Hexokinases. Earlier in this chapter the transmembrane passage of glucose and its phosphorylation catalyzed by the hexokinases were discussed as determinants of the intracellular concentration of glucose 6-phosphate (Walker, 1966; Purich et al., 1973). While there are circumstances in which these processes may limit rates of glycolysis, it is clear that control of the glycolytic pathway at this level alone would be inappropriate, since glucose

6-phosphate is the initial substrate of pathways other than glycolysis. Thus, for example, inhibition exerted primarily at the level of hexokinase-catalyzed phosphorylation of glucose would interfere with the activities of metabolic sequences such as glycogen synthesis and the pentose phosphate pathway.

Phosphofructokinase. For the reason discussed above, a regulatory site for glycolysis is required at some point in the pathway distal to glucose 6-phosphate. The phosphofructokinase-catalyzed conversion of fructose 6-phosphate to fructose 1,6-diphosphate is now considered to be the most important control point in glycolysis and appears to be the step that primarily fulfills this function (Passonneau and Lowry, 1962; Chance et al., 1964).

In general, the steps of a biochemical pathway at which regulatory influences can be brought to bear are catalyzed by enzymes whose activities are insufficient to bring substrates and products to the theoretical equilibrium state and which can be shown to be modified by factors other than substrate concentration. Phosphofructokinase can be shown to fulfill these conditions by a number of criteria (Newsholme and Start, 1973). First, in skeletal muscle phosphofructokinase has been shown to have the lowest activity of any enzyme catalyzing reactions between glucose 6-phosphate and pyruvate. In addition, the apparent equilibrium constant for the enzyme, calculated by standard thermodynamic means, differs markedly from the mass action ratio experimentally determined. Since for an equilibrium reaction the mass action ratio should approximate the equilibrium constant, the phosphofructokinase-catalyzed reaction is clearly displaced far from equilibirum. Finally, when glycolysis is stimulated by an uncoupler of oxidative phosphorylation or by anaerobiosis, the concentration of fructose 6-phosphate can be shown to be reduced. A similar, though reversed, dissociation between phosphofructokinase activity and substrate concentration can be demonstrated under conditions where muscle tissue is provided with alternative energy substrates such as pyruvate.

From these facts, phosphofructokinase clearly meets the requirements for a regulatory enzyme. It remains to be demonstrated how this potential regulatory function is exploited in the cell. The observation that the activity of phosphofructokinase has a biphasic response to increasing concentrations of ATP, being initially enhanced and then, above an optimal concentration of the nucleotide, showing progressive inhibition, appears to provide a means by which control might be exercised. Thus, in situations characterized by an abundant supply of ATP phosphofructokinase would be inhibited, while a reduced availability of ATP would activate the enzyme, increasing glycolytic flux and thus ATP generation. Experimentally, however, variations in ATP concentration between resting and contracting muscles are entirely too small to allow regulation of phosphofructokinase on this basis alone. The finding that AMP reverses the inhibition of phosphofructokinase by ATP provides the basis for a mechanism by which the effects on the enzyme of small alterations in ATP concentration can be amplified. Thus, as cellular ATP is consumed the concentration of ADP rises. This ADP is acted on by the enzyme adenylate kinase, which catalyzes the reaction

$$2 \text{ ADP} \rightleftharpoons \text{ATP} + \text{AMP}$$

Since in the cell the concentration of ATP is much higher than that of AMP, it can be predicted that even small reductions in the concentration of cellular ATP will, through the amplification provided by the adenylate kinase, lead to larger proportional increases in the concentration of AMP (Newsholme and Start, 1973).

Other substances that modify phosphofructokinase activity *in vitro* include inorganic phosphate and fructose 1,6-diphosphate, which, like AMP, relieve inhibition of the enzyme by ATP, and citrate, which inhibits the enzyme by potentiating the ATP effect. The value of such controls is self-evident. Thus, in muscle, ATP utilization leads to the net breakdown of creatine phosphate with liberation of inorganic phosphate, which will tend to relieve phosphofructokinase inhibition and accelerate glycolysis (Sacktor and Hurlbut, 1966). Activation of phosphofructokinase by its own product represents a further amplification mechanism since increased glycolytic flux initiated by AMP or inorganic phosphate is augmented by an autocatalytic process (Regen et al., 1964). Conversely, accumulation of citrate and ATP, which occurs when alternative substrates such as fatty acids are available, leads to inhibition of glycolytic flux and reduced pyruvate production.

The overall modulation of phosphofructokinase activity, particularly by the concentrations of the adenine nucleotides and inorganic phosphate, offers the most logical explanation for the regulation of glycolytic flux and can account for the inhibition of aerobic glycolysis by mitochondrial respiration (Krebs, 1972). Commonly referred to as the "Pasteur effect," this regulation at the level of phosphofructokinase represents a classical example of biological control.

Glyceraldehyde-3-phosphate Dehydrogenase. The conversion of 1 mol of glucose 6-phosphate to 2 mol of pyruvate is associated with the reduction of 2 mol of NAD^+ to NADH by a glyceraldehyde-3-phosphate dehydrogenase. In the sense that reoxidation of this NADH is required for the maintenance of glycolysis, glyceraldehyde-3-phosphate dehydrogenase, an equilibrium reaction, has a control function. Reducing equivalents are removed from the cytosol by the hydrogen shuttle systems (see section Hydrogen Shuttle Systems). However, in the absence of mitochondria or of available molecular oxygen, a regeneration of NAD^+ is provided by the reaction catalyzed by lactate dehydrogenase, and the concerted action of glyceraldehyde-3-phosphate dehydrogenase and lactate dehydrogenase is therefore essential for optimum anaerobic glycolysis.

$$\text{Glyceraldehyde 3-phosphate} \xrightleftharpoons[\text{NAD}^+\quad\text{NADH}]{} \text{1,3-diphosphoglycerate}$$

$$\text{Pyruvate} \xrightleftharpoons[\text{NADH}\quad\text{NAD}^+]{} \text{lactate}$$

The lactate produced is released into the circulation and transported to the liver, where it can be reconverted to glucose.

Pyruvate kinase. The final important regulatory site in glycolysis is the formation of pyruvate from phosphoenolpyruvate, yielding ATP. This non-equilibrium reaction is highly exergonic and has been found to be irreversible under normal physiologic conditions (Sacktor and Wormser-Shavit, 1966). The enzyme requires alkali metal cations, of which potassium may be the normal activator. The regulatory aspects of pyruvate kinase depend on the isozymes that exist in various tissues. The liver isozyme is activated by fructose 1,6-diphosphate and high concentration of phosphoenolpyruvate, which increases glycolytic flux beyond phosphofructokinase.

Metabolism of sugars other than glucose. Hexoses other than glucose enter the liver glycolytic pathway by specific kinases and are further metabolized to pyruvate or reconverted to glucose by gluconeogenesis (Fig. 6). For this reason, the preferential use of fructose and galactose rather than glucose in the diabetic has no biochemical rationale. Of some possible significance, as will be discussed subsequently, is the specific pathway for the metabolism of fructose. The enzyme fructokinase forms fructose 1-phosphate, which is a substrate for liver aldolase. The products of this reaction, glyceraldehyde and dihydroxyacetone phosphate, bypass the important regulatory step catalyzed by phosphofructokinase. This lack of control at the level of phosphofructokinase could result in the formation of excess acetyl units from the glycolysis of fructose, which would then be available for fatty acid synthesis by the liver.

Pentose Phosphate Pathway

Also known as the hexose monophosphate shunt, this complex metabolic sequence (Axelrod, 1967), shown in Fig. 7, is widely but not uniformly distributed in tissues, being essentially absent in muscle. The pathway is concerned not primarily with the provision of energy, but rather with the production of pentose phosphates for DNA and RNA biosynthesis and with the generation of reducing equivalents for pathways, such as fatty acid synthesis, that require NADPH rather than NADH as an essential cofactor.

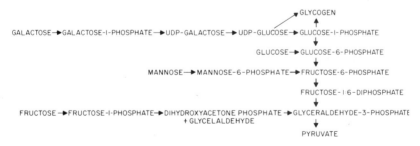

FIGURE 6 Metabolism of hexoses other than glucose.

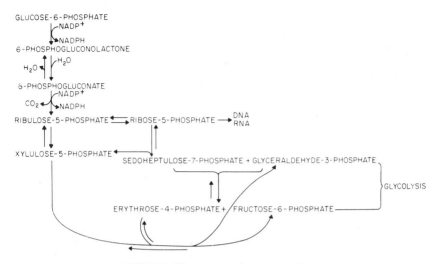

FIGURE 7 The pentose phosphate pathway.

This pathway is initiated by the $NADP^+$-linked dehydrogenation of glucose 6-phosphate to form the acid lactone, which is then acted on by a lactonase with the production of 6-phosphogluconate. This, in turn, is dehydrogenated with the formation of ribulose 5-phosphate and CO_2, $NADP^+$ being again the specific cofactor. Thus, each mol of glucose 6-phosphate converted to ribulose 5-phosphate leads to the generation of 2 mol of NADPH.

By the action of ribose phosphate isomerase, ribulose 5-phosphate can be converted to ribose 5-phosphate, which acts as a precursor for nucleotide synthesis. However, in liver, mammary gland, and adrenal cortex the observed flux of glucose 6-phosphate through the pentose phosphate pathway greatly exceeds that required for DNA and RNA synthesis, and the cycle is geared primarily for generation of NADPH. In these tissues, pentose 5-phosphate undergoes further transformations catalyzed by the following enzymes:

1. Ribulose-5-phosphate epimerase, which converts ribulose 5-phosphate to xylulose 5-phosphate.
2. Transketolase, which transfers a glycoaldehyde group from xylulose 5-phosphate to ribose 5-phosphate to form sedoheptulose 7-phosphate and glyceraldehyde 3-phosphate.
3. Transaldolase, which acts initially on the products of the transketolase reaction, forming fructose 6-phosphate and erythrose 4-phosphate. A second transaldolase-catalyzed reaction then converts erythrose 4-phosphate and xylulose 5-phosphate to fructose 6-phosphate and glyceraldehyde 3-phosphate.

These multiple interconversions of sugar phosphates clearly provide a high degree of metabolic flexibility, and it should be remembered that certain of the products formed—for example, fructose 6-phosphate and glyceraldehyde 3-phosphate—are capable of further metabolism through the glycolytic pathway or reconversion to glucose 6-phosphate. The complete oxidation of 1 mol of glucose 6-phosphate by the pentose phosphate pathway is described by the equation:

$$6 \text{ glucose 6-phosphate} + 12 \text{ NADP}^+ + 7 \text{ H}_2\text{O} \rightarrow$$

$$5 \text{ glucose 6-phosphate} + 6 \text{ CO}_2 + 12 \text{ NADPH} + 12 \text{ H}^+ + \text{P}_i$$

The high yield of NADPH, 12 mol per mol of glucose 6-phosphate oxidized, is explained by the fact that NADPH formed in the initial steps of the pathway is not required for the resynthesis of glucose 6-phosphate from the pentose phosphates.

An isotopic technique based on the differential initial rates of $^{14}\text{CO}_2$ generation from glucose labeled in the C-1 and C-6 positions has been widely employed to estimate the fractions of the glucose 6-phosphate pool metabolized by the glycolytic and pentose phosphate pathways (Katz and Wood, 1960). This method depends on the fact that in glycolysis the initial rates of $^{14}\text{CO}_2$ generation from both carbons of the glucose molecule are equal, while in the pentose phosphate pathway $^{14}\text{CO}_2$ arises initially only from the C-1 carbon. Using this method, it has been shown that up to 25% of the total $^{14}\text{CO}_2$ liberated from rat liver may derive from the pentose pathway, while in adipose tissue and lactating mammary gland, where active fatty acid synthesis is the major metabolic activity, a considerably higher fraction is attributable to this route.

HYDROGEN SHUTTLE SYSTEMS

The reducing equivalents of NADH formed by glyceraldehyde-3-phosphate dehydrogenase, which must be reoxidized to prevent cessation of glycolysis, can be transported into the mitochondria by hydrogen shuttle systems (Borst 1963; Bücher and Klingenberg, 1958).

Malate-Aspartate Shuttle

The malate-aspartate cycle (Fig. 8) is considered to be the major pathway for the transport of reducing equivalents generated in the cytosol to the mitochondria for further oxidation (Safer and Williamson, 1973). In addition to the mitochondrial and cytosolic isozymes of glutamate oxalacetate transaminase and malate dehydrogenase, the system involves two mitochondrial carriers. One of these catalyzes a one-for-one exchange of glutamate for aspartate, while the other exchanges malate for α-ketoglutarate. In the cytosol, malate dehydrogenase catalyzes the NADH-dependent reduction of oxalacetate to malate, which is transported into the mitochondria, where the NADH is reformed and oxidized by the electron transport system. In addition to

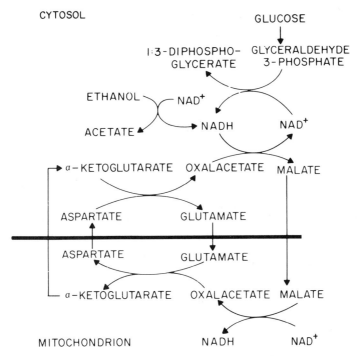

FIGURE 8 The malate-aspartate shuttle. NADH from glycolysis or ethanol oxidation is transported as malate into the mitochondria, where it is reoxidized by the electron transport system.

removing reducing equivalents from the cytosol, this shuttle system permits the generation of an addition 6 mol of ATP per glucosyl unit by the pathway of oxidative phosphorylation, thus significantly increasing the energetic yield of glycolysis under aerobic conditions.

Glycerolphosphate Shuttle

Of less significance as a hydrogen carrier is the α-glycerolphosphate shuttle. In this system the reducing equivalents in α-glycerolphosphate arising from the reduction of dihydroxyacetone phosphate by the cytosolic α-glycerol phosphate dehydrogenase enzyme are reoxidized in the mitochondria by the flavoprotein isozyme. Only 4 mol of ATP per glucosyl unit are synthesized through this shuttle system. Alternatively, the α-glycerolphosphate formed can be utilized in the cytosol for synthesis of triglyceride.

Clearly these shuttle systems can operate only in tissues with high rates of aerobic metabolism. As discussed previously, in cells that lack mitochondria or during anaerobiosis, reoxidation of NADH by lactate dehydrogenase is the mechanism for preventing the accumulation of hydrogen ions (see the section on glycolysis).

PYRUVATE METABOLISM

Energy Production

Pyruvate, the principal three-carbon fragment derived from glycolysis, can be further metabolized through a series of alternative pathways leading to lipid and protein synthesis as well as to energy production. One of the most important series of metabolic sequences in terms of the economy of the organism is the energy-yielding Krebs or tricarboxylic acid cycle (Fig. 9). In aerobic tissue, the complete oxidation of 2 mol of pyruvate derived from each mol of glucose leads to the production of 30 mol of ATP; this is added to the yield of 6–8 mol of ATP derived from glycolysis (Lehninger, 1975). The formation of ATP from pyruvate, which takes place in the mitochondria by oxidative phosphorylation, is the most important source of energy for tissues such as brain, heart, and red skeletal muscle and, to a lesser extent, liver and kidney cortex. By contrast, tissues such as red blood cells, renal medulla, and white skeletal muscle, which possess few or no mitochondria, convert the pyruvate formed from glucose directly to lactate, which then diffuses into the venous system to be transported to the liver for subsequent metabolism.

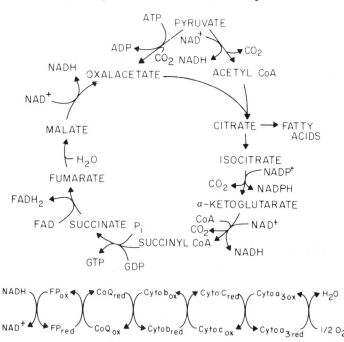

FIGURE 9 The tricarboxylic acid cycle and the electron transport chain. NADH and NADPH generated by the cycle within the mitochondria are reoxidized by the electron transport system, which serves as the major source of synthesis of ATP.

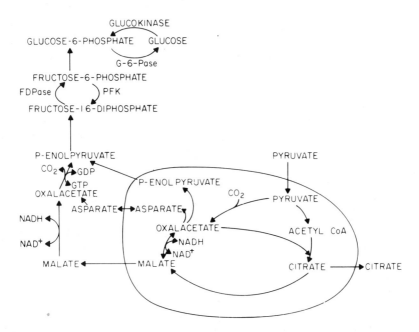

FIGURE 10 Interrelationship of enzyme reactions in the mitochondria and cytosol that account for the metabolism of pyruvate and its conversion of glucose. Although many of the cytosolic reactions are reversible, the figure is intended to show the direction of carbon flow from pyruvate to glucose.

Intramitochondrial Metabolism and Regulation

In liver, intramitochondrial pyruvate is predominantly converted either to acetyl CoA and citrate for fatty acid biosynthesis or to oxalacetate for resynthesis of glucose (Fig. 10). This branch point in intermediary metabolism—where pyruvate enters the mitochondrial tricarboxylic acid cycle, undergoing either decarboxylation to acetyl CoA through pyruvate dehydrogenase or carboxylation to oxalacetate through pyruvate carboxylase—is considered to be one of the more important regulatory sites in cell metabolism. Although there are distinct differences, the coordination of pyruvate dehydrogenase and pyruvate carboxylase is analogous to that of the glycogen synthetase and phosphorylase enzymes. Thus, it has been demonstrated by Linn et al. (1969) that pyruvate dehydrogenase can exist in an inactive (phosphorylated) or active (dephosphorylated) form. In contrast to the glycogen synthetase and phosphorylase regulatory system, however, the protein kinase responsible for phosphorylation and inactivation of the pyruvate dehydrogenase complex is not cyclic AMP-dependent. A fine control mechanism for determining the ratio between the active and inactive forms of the enzyme does exist, however, in that the protein kinase and phosphatase involved are susceptible to modulation by the concentrations of the intramitochondrial nucleotides and other reactants. Thus, elevated concentrations of ATP, NADH, and acetyl CoA promote phosphorylation and inactivation of pyruvate dehydrogenase (Pettit et al., 1975; Batenburg and Olson, 1975). In addition, calcium ions may play a role in promoting the dephosphorylation and activation of the enzyme by pyruvate dehydrogenase phosphatase (Denton et al., 1972).

Whereas a typical phosphorylation/dephosphorylation mechanism does not apply to the pyruvate carboxylase enzyme, extensive studies have clearly demonstrated that, in addition to acetyl CoA acting as an obligatory cofactor for catalytic activity, ADP inhibits formation of oxalacetate (Utter and Scrutton, 1969; Stuki et al., 1972). Thus the regulation of both pyruvate dehydrogenase and pyruvate carboxylase, in a reciprocal manner, is dependent on the ATP/ADP, NADH/NAD$^+$, and acetyl CoA/CoA ratios in the mitochondrial matrix. In well-fed insulinized animals these ratios are so set that the flux of pyruvate is predominantly through pyruvate dehydrogenase and the tricarboxylic acid cycle, whereas during fasting and in uncontrolled diabetes the ratios favor entry of pyruvate carbon into the gluconeogenic pathway through pyruvate carboxylase to oxalacetate and phosphoenolpyruvate (Utter 1963; Lardy, 1965). However, under all metabolic conditions, sufficient oxalacetate must still be formed through pyruvate carboxylase to replenish the tricarboxylic acid cycle intermediates lost during the synthesis of macromolecules such as fatty acids in order to maintain the activity of the cycle.

Compartmentation of Enzymes and Metabolites

One of the more important and only recently appreciated determinants of carbon flux is the subcellular localization of key enzymes and metabolites of the lipogenic and gluconeogenic carbon pathways (Srere and Bhaduri, 1962; Spencer and Lowenstein, 1964; Lardy, 1965; Greenbaum et al., 1971). In both liver and adipose tissue, the specific compartmentation of key enzymes in either the cytosol or the mitochondria requires appropriate carrier systems to transport critical metabolites. A typical example is shown in Fig. 11. The enzymes for fatty acid biosynthesis from acetyl CoA are located in the cytosol of the cell. Acetyl CoA, which is formed in the mitochondrial matrix, cannot directly penetrate the inner mitochondrial membrane and therefore its transport to the cytosol must be indirect.

It is now recognized that the citrate formed from acetyl CoA in the mitochondria can be transported on the citrate or tricarboxylate carrier system across the inner mitochondrial membrane to the cytosol (Chappell, 1968). Subsequent reconversion of citrate to acetyl CoA in the cytosol occurs through the specific ATP-citrate lyase or citrate cleavage enzyme. Oxalacetate, the other product of the reaction, is reduced to malate and malate-covered pyruvate, which can then reenter the mitochondria to complete the cycle. This cycle, in addition to generating acetyl CoA units in the cytosol, also produces NADPH necessary for fatty acid biosynthesis by a transhydrogena-

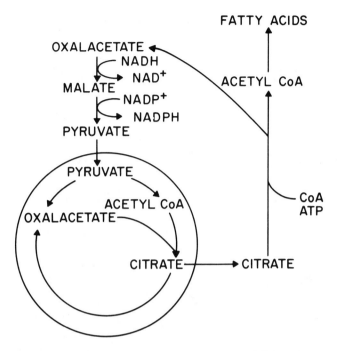

FIGURE 11 Pathway of intramitochondrial acetyl CoA transport to the cytosol for fatty acid synthesis. Reprinted with permission from Young et al. (1964). Copyright by the American Chemical Society.

tion mechanism utilizing the NAD^+ malate dehydrogenase and $NADP^+$-linked malic enzyme (Young et al., 1964; Wise and Ball, 1964). In both liver and adipose tissue important but incompletely understood control mechanisms must exist to regulate the activities of these key enzymes and to maintain appropriate rates of carbohydrate conversion to lipid.

GLUCONEOGENESIS

The liver, which is enzymatically programmed to carry out a variety of synthetic processes, presents a more complicated metabolic picture than other tissues. Depending on the nutritional and hormonal balance of the animal, not only is carbohydrate stored as glycogen, converted to lipid, and used for energy purposes, but also, under certain physiological and pathophysiological conditions, the synthesis of new glucose from amino acids and other precursors such as glycerol and lactate becomes an important function of the liver cell.

Lactate, produced as the final product of glycolysis in tissues lacking mitochondria (as well as in other tissues under anaerobic conditions), is

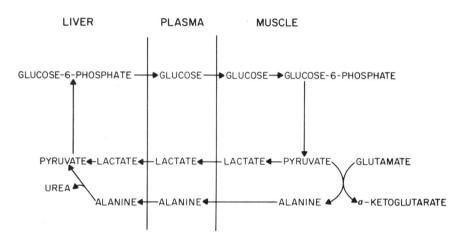

FIGURE 12 The Cori cycle.

transported to the liver, where it is converted to glucose, the entire pathway being known as the Cori cycle (Fig. 12). More recently, it has been demonstrated that in muscle, pyruvate (in addition to being reduced to lactate) is transaminated to alanine (Cahill, 1970). This glucose-alanine cycle permits the transport of nitrogen as well as carbon from muscle to liver, where they are converted respectively to urea and glucose.

It is apparent that the gluconeogenic pathway, which is basically a reversal of glycolysis, requires additional enzymes to overcome the rate-limiting nonequilibrium steps in the glycolytic sequence—namely those catalyzed by pyruvate kinase, phosphofructokinase, and the hexokinases including glucokinase.

Formation of Phosphoenolpyruvate from Pyruvate

The enzymatic sequence leading from pyruvate back to phosphoenolpyruvate is one of the more complicated and important steps in the gluconeogenic pathway.

Pyruvate carboxylase. Pyruvate cannot form phosphoenolpyruvate directly because of the unfavorable equilibrium of the pyruvate kinase reaction. To circumvent this irreversibility, pyruvate is converted to a dicarboxylic acid intermediate as the initial step in the gluconeogenic process (Topper and Hastings, 1949). Oxalacetate formed from pyruvate and CO_2 in a reaction catalyzed by pyruvate carboxylase is now recognized to be the key dicarboxylic acid intermediate involved (Utter and Scrutton, 1969). It should be remembered that while pyruvate carboxylase is considered a gluconeogenic enzyme, it in fact serves a more general purpose by forming the necessary oxalacetate to replete and maintain the tricarboxylic acid cycle.

Phosphoenolpyruvate carboxykinase. The energetically favorable formation of phosphoenolpyruvate from oxalacetate by phosphoenolpyruvate carboxykinase is dependent on a number of factors, not the least of which are the regulation and subcellular distribution of this enzyme. Unlike pyruvate carboxylase, phosphoenolpyruvate carboxykinase responds dramatically to changes in nutritional and hormonal balance. Enzyme levels are high during fasting and uncontrolled diabetes when gluconeogenesis is maximum, and low following refeeding and insulin replacement (Shrago et al., 1963). From studies carried out in rat liver it has been determined that pyruvate carboxylase is localized in the mitochondrial matrix (Brech et al., 1970), whereas phosphoenolpyruvate carboxykinase exists predominantly in the cytosol of the cell (Nordlie and Lardy, 1963). In a situation analogous to the acetyl CoA compartmentation problem discussed previously, the inner mitochondrial membrane is impermeable to oxalacetate, which therefore requires alternative means for its transport to the cytosol.

Malate-aspartate shuttle. To account for the transport of oxalacetate required by the subcellular distribution pattern of pyruvate carboxylase and phosphoenolpyruvate carboxykinase, a dicarboxylic acid shuttle system, similar to that described previously (Fig. 8) but operating in the reverse direction, was proposed as a mechanism for transferring both carbon and reducing equivalents needed for gluconeogenesis from the mitochondria to the cytosol (Lardy, 1965). Depending on the availability of NADH in the cytosol (Rognstad and Katz, 1970), oxalacetate synthesized intramitochondrially by pyruvate carboxylase is either transaminated to aspartate or reduced to malate. In contrast to oxalacetate, these two metabolites are transported by carrier systems across the inner mitochondrial membrane into the cytosol, where they are reconverted to phosphoenolpyruvate by the appropriate enzymes. Whereas this series of reactions clearly delineates the direction of carbon flow in rat liver (Williamson, 1976), the situation is more complex in other animals, including humans, where the subcellular distribution of phosphoenolpyruvate carboxykinase is bimodal, the enzyme being distributed in both the cytosol and mitochondria (Hanson and Garber, 1972).

Thus, in most animals phosphoenolpyruvate may be synthesized either directly in the mitochondria, indirectly in the cytosol, or in both compartments. Although a considerable amount of valuable information has been accumulated (Hanson and Garber, 1972), neither the specific controls nor the preferred intracellular compartment for the formation of phosphenolpyruvate during gluconeogenesis in humans has been clearly elucidated.

Cytosolic Pathway from Phosphoenolpyruvate to Glucose

To avoid the conversion of phosphoenolpyruvate back to pyruvate, thereby establishing an energy-wasting or futile cycle, the activity of pyruvate kinase must be inhibited or effectively reduced during active gluconeogenesis (Gancedo et al., 1967). In addition, the subsequent gluconeogenic conversion of phosphoenolpyruvate to glucose in the cytosol of the liver is not simply a reversal of glycolysis. Two enzymes, fructose-1,6-diphosphatase and glucose-6-

phosphatase are required to circumvent the thermodynamically unfavorable equilibria of the phosphofructokinase and glucokinase reactions. Coordination of fructose-1,6-diphosphatase with phosphofructokinase (Taketa and Pogell, 1965) and of glucose-6-phosphatase with glucokinase (Newsholme and Start, 1973) in the liver requires important allosteric regulatory mechanisms, which in turn minimize futile cycling at these sites and determine the direction of carbon flux. When gluconeogenesis predominates, the activities of glucokinase and phosphofructokinase are decreased, allowing the flow of carbon from fructose 1,6-diphosphate to glucose 6-phosphate and finally to free glucose. During glycolysis, the opposite control process predominates with a decrease in activity of fructose-1,6-diphosphatase and glucose-6-phosphatase relative to phosphofructokinase and glucokinase.

MECHANISMS OF REGULATION OF RATE-LIMITING ENZYMES

Enzyme Adaptation

It is recognized from studies with various normal and diabetic animal models (Exton et al., 1970; Tepperman and Tepperman, 1970) that conditions of fasting or of insulin deficiency initiate a series of metabolic events that result in decreased tissue carbohydrate utilization for energy production, accompanied by reduced conversion of carbohydrate to lipid and of amino acids to protein. In particular, the activities of certain key enzymes in glycolysis and in the glucose-dependent lipogenic pathway in both liver and adipose tissue are decreased significantly below normal in these states (Tepperman and Tepperman, 1970). Equally important is the observation that refeeding of the fasting animal or correction of insulin deficiency results in an overshoot above normal in the rate of conversion of carbohydrate to lipid (Tepperman and Tepperman, 1970). This acceleration in lipogenesis is accompanied by an adaptive increase in the previously reduced levels of glycolytic and lipogenic enzymes. In liver, a reciprocal relationship exists between the concentrations of certain gluconeogenic and lipogenic enzymes. During fasting and in uncontrolled diabetes, levels of the regulatory enzymes of the gluconeogenic pathway are increased. Following replacement therapy, these enhanced activities fall toward normal as a reciprocal increase in the lipogenic capacity of the liver occurs. A typical example (Fig. 13) is the relationship between the gluconeogenic enzyme phosphoenolpyruvate carboxykinase and the lipogenic malic enzyme during insulin deficiency and following its correction. These adaptive changes in enzyme activity, which for the most part represent altered rates of enzyme protein synthesis *de novo* (Schimke, 1973), provide the mechanism for the sustained flux of metabolites through the respective carbon pathways at appropriate rates.

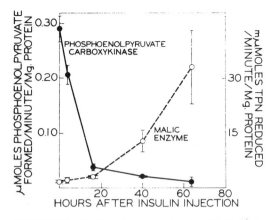

FIGURE 13 Reciprocal response of phosphoenol-pyruvate carboxykinase and malic enzyme to timed injections of insulin in alloxan diabetic rats (Shrago et al., 1963).

Allosteric Modulation

Adaptive enzyme changes, which are most likely due to the combined effects of hormones and substrate concentrations, occur too late in time to be considered initiating factors in the coordination of carbon flux. It is more likely that allosteric modifiers of rate-limiting enzymes account for the fine control necessary for minute-to-minute regulation of metabolic pathways (Stadtman, 1966). In terms of metabolic regulation, the most intricate control systems occur at sites along the pathways which are either branch points or where two enzymes have the capacity to act on the same substrate. As previously discussed, two of the most noteworthy examples are the multiple allosteric factors coordinating the activity of phosphofructokinase with that of fructose diphosphatase, and of pyruvate dehydrogenase with pyruvate carboxylase. There is now substantial evidence that certain enzymes such as pyruvate kinase, fructose diphosphatase, and phosphofructokinase may be sensitive to cyclic AMP modification (Taunton et al., 1972; Rognstad, 1975; Veneziale, 1976). This in turn suggests that insulin and glucagon may play a role in the allosteric regulation of enzyme activity as well as in leading to adaptive changes in enzyme concentration (Pitot and Dyatvin, 1973).

RELATIONSHIP OF CARBOHYDRATE NUTRITION AND METABOLISM TO CLINICAL DISORDERS

Hyperlipoproteinemia

Following a standard meal, the flux of carbon in most tissues of well-insulinized animals is through glycolysis and the tricarboxylic acid cycle, resulting in the production of ATP required for energy-utilizing reactions. However, as is usually the case in Western society, more calories are consumed than are necessary to meet immediate energy demands. In terms of carbohydrate intake, this requires either storage of calories as glycogen in the liver and muscle, which is limited, or conversion of glucose to fatty acids that are subsequently esterified to triglycerides in the liver, which is more important quantitatively. The triglycerides in turn are released into the bloodstream in the form of very low density lipoproteins, to be metabolized in peripheral tissues or stored again as triglycerides in adipocytes (see also Chap. 4).

Fructose metabolism. It has been repeatedly demonstrated in experimental animals and in humans that the ingestion of sucrose or fructose leads to a greater synthesis of glycogen and lipids than does that of glucose (Fallon and Kemp, 1968; Zakim et al., 1969; Nilsson and Hultman, 1974). In humans, a high-sucrose diet has been associated with elevated concentrations of serum triglycerides (MacDonald and Braithwaite, 1964), an effect that is attributed to enhanced hepatic lipogenesis (Wu et al., 1974). As previously discussed (Fig. 6), the liver, which is the predominant site of fructose uptake, metabolizes this sugar in a unique manner. Not only is the important regulatory site at the level of phosphofructokinase bypassed during the metabolism of fructose, but in addition, rapid assimilation of the sugar occurs because the activity of fructokinase is higher than that of the glucose phosphorylating enzymes (Heinz et al., 1968). For these reasons, under conditions of high sucrose intake, excessive conversion of fructose to acetyl CoA in the liver could occur with stimulation of lipogenesis and consequent hypertriglyceridemia.

Feeding frequency. From observations made in lower animals, as previously discussed, it can be appreciated that the homeostatic mechanisms for the regulation of intermediary metabolism are delicately set. Even differences in feeding frequency impose sufficient stress on the adaptive mechanisms to influence greatly the direction of carbon flow, particularly the conversion of carbohydrate to lipid (Cohn and Joseph, 1960). It is very probable that a similar condition exists in humans in whom unphysiological feeding habits—for example, consumption of single large meals of high carbohydrate content—may result in a predisposition to hyperlipoproteinemia as well as obesity, diabetes, and atherosclerosis.

Carbohydrate metabolism and human adipose tissue. The rat, as an animal model, appears to be unusual in that its adipose tissue has an extremely high capacity for synthesis of fatty acids from glucose *de novo*. There is evidence that in humans the liver is the predominant site for fatty acid biosynthesis from carbohydrate, with negligible rates of lipogenesis occurring in adipose tissue (Shrago et al., 1971; Patel et al., 1975). This preferred metabolic pathway for lipogenesis in humans may have important nutritional implications, since excess carbohydrate calories consumed would be expected to be converted to lipid almost exclusively in the liver, thus predisposing the human to elevated levels of serum low-density lipo-proteins.

Ethanol Metabolism

Ethyl alcohol, which provides 7 kcal/g, is able to meet a considerable proportion of the body's energy demands. However, the ill effects of alcohol consumed in large quantities obviously preclude any significant nutritional role. Over 90% of the ethanol ingested is oxidized in the liver by an alcohol dehydrogenase, which acts on ethanol and NAD^+ to produce acetaldehyde and NADH. An acetaldehyde dehydrogenase then converts the aldehyde into acetate, which can enter the tricarboxylic acid cycle as acetyl CoA. More recently, a microsomal oxygenase system has been identified which may account for approximately 10–20% of ethanol metabolism (Lieber, 1970).

The effects of ethanol on intermediary metabolism are in the main due to the generation of large quantities of NADH (Lieber, 1969). Since the alcohol dehydrogenase reaction occurs in the cytosol, the reducing equivalents must be transferred to the mitochondria for further oxidation. The transfer of NADH by the malate-aspartate cycle (Fig. 8) may be rate-limiting for ethanol oxidation. High levels of NADH in the cytosol resulting from ethanol metabolism inhibit gluconeogenesis by driving pyruvate to lactate and, together with the formation of acetate, stimulate the synthesis of triglycerides in the liver. This latter metabolic phenomenon may play a role in alcohol-induced hyperlipoproteinemia.

Formation of Sugar Alcohols—Sorbitol

Most mammalian tissues contain a complement of enzymes that catalyze the conversion of glucose to fructose. In this pathway, an $NADP^+$-specific hexitol dehydrogenase or aldose reductase forms sorbitol from glucose; the sorbitol is then converted to fructose by an NAD^+-linked hexitol dehydrogenase.

$$\text{Glucose} \underset{\longrightarrow}{\overset{NADPH \quad NADP^+}{\rightleftharpoons}} \text{sorbitol} \underset{\longrightarrow}{\overset{NAD^+ \quad NADH}{\rightleftharpoons}} \text{fructose}$$

These enzymes are not sensitive to insulin and their activities are totally dependent on substrate concentration. Thus, under conditions of elevated blood glucose, there is an increase in sorbitol and fructose formation from glucose. More important, since the NAD^+-linked sorbitol dehydrogenase is the rate-limiting step in the two sequential reactions, preferential accumulation of sorbitol occurs. The sorbitol, although in itself innocuous, at high concentrations exerts important osmotic effects, drawing water into the cells and thereby damaging the tissue.

It has been postulated that such a metabolic abnormality occurring in certain tissues, particularly neurons and the lens of the eye, might, in poorly controlled diabetics, account for the development of retinopathy and cataract formation (Gabbay, 1973). In addition, the cerebral edema which may occur in the course of rehydration of patients during treatment of diabetic ketoacidosis or nonketotic hyperosmolar coma is thought to be due to an osmotic disequilibrium to which elevated sorbitol concentrations within brain cells may make an important contribution (Clements et al., 1968).

Glycoproteins

A number of important proteins, particularly those associated with membranes, contain characteristic carbohydrate molecules in a covalent attachment. The glycosylation of proteins by simple sugars and amino sugars occurs by way of the uridine diphosphate pathway (Fig. 6).

(1) Nucleotide triphosphate + sugar 1-phosphate →

nucleotide diphosphate-sugar + PP_i

(2) Nucleotide diphosphate-sugar + protein →

glycoprotein + nucleotide diphosphate

The entry of glucose into this pathway in the retinal and renal microvascular system is, like sorbitol formation, independent of insulin and favored by a high extracellular glucose concentration. The possibility that increased synthesis of membrane glycoprotein in the small vessels of the eye and glomeruli is the biochemical basis for diabetic retinopathy and glomerulopathy is under active consideration (Spiro, 1973).

In this chapter, we have attempted to provide a brief account of the aspects of carbohydrate metabolism that are believed to have significance in the consideration of obesity, vascular disease, and diabetes. The interrelationships between carbohydrate, protein, and lipid metabolism and their regulation and integration will be developed further in other chapters of this book.

REFERENCES

Axelrod, B. 1967. Other pathways of carbohydrate metabolism. In *Metabolic pathways*, ed. D. M. Greenberg, vol. 1., pp. 272–308. New York: Academic Press.

Batenburg, J. J. and Olson, M. S. 1975. The inactivation of pyruvate dehydrogenase by fatty acid in isolated rat liver mitochondria. *Biochem. Biophys. Res. Commun.* 66:533–540.

Borst, P. 1963. III. A korrelationen zwischen zellkompartmenten: Hydrogen transport and transport metabolites. In *Functionelle und Morphologische Organization der Zelle*, ed. P. Karlson, pp. 137–162. Berlin: Springer-Verlag.

Brech, W., Shrago, E. and Wilken, D. 1970. Studies on pyruvate carboxylase in rat and human liver. *Biochim. Biophys. Acta* 201:145–154.

Bücher, T. and Klingenberg, M. 1958. Wege des Wasserstoffs in der lebendigen organisation. *Angew Chem.* 70:552–570.

Cahill, G. F., Jr. 1970. Starvation in man. *N. Engl. J. Med.* 282:668–675.

Chance, B., Estabrook, R. W. and Gosh, A. 1964. Damped sinusoidal oscillations of cytoplasmic reduced pyridine nucleotides in yeast cells. *Proc. Natl. Acad. Sci. U.S.A.* 51:1244–1251.

Chappell, J. B. 1968. Systems used for the transport of substrates into mitochondria. *Br. Med. Bull.* 24:150–157.

Clements, R. S., Jr., Prockop, L. D. and Winegrad, A. 1968. Acute cerebral edema during treatment of hyperglycemia. An experimental model. *Lancet* 2:384–386.

Cohn, C. and Joseph, F. D. 1960. Effects on metabolism produced by the rate of ingestion of the diet. *Am. J. Clin. Nutr.* 8:682–690.

Denton, R. M., Randle, P. J. and Martin, B. R. 1972. Stimulation by calcium of pyruvate dehydrogenase phosphate phosphatase. *Biochem. J.* 128:161–163.

Exton, J. H., Mallette, L. E., Jefferson, L. S., Wong, E. A., Friedmann, N., Miller, T., Jr. and Park, C. R. 1970. The hormonal control of hepatic gluconeogenesis. *Rec. Prog. Horm. Res.* 26:411–461.

Fallon, H. J. and Kemp, E. L. 1968. Effects of diet on hepatic triglyceride synthesis. *J. Clin. Invest.* 47:712–719.

Gabbay, K. H. 1973. The sorbitol pathway and the complications of diabetes. *N. Engl. J. Med.* 288:831–836.

Gancedo, J. M., Gancedo, C. and Sols, A. 1967. Regulation of the concentration or activity of pyruvate kinase in yeasts and its relationship to gluconeogenesis. *Biochem. J.* 102:23c–25c.

Greenbaum, A. L., Gumaa, K. A. and McLean, P. 1971. The distribution of hepatic metabolites and the control of pathways of carbohydrate metabolism of animals of different dietary and hormonal status. *Arch. Biochem. Biophys.* 143:617–663.

Hanson, R. W. and Garber, A. J. 1972. Phosphoenolpyruvate carboxykinase. 1. Its role in gluconeogenesis. *Am. J. Clin. Nutr.* 25:1010–1021.

Heinz, F., Lamprecht, W. and Kirsch, J. 1968. Enzymes of fructose metabolism in human liver. *J. Clin. Invest.* 47:1826–1832.

Katz, J. and Wood, H. G. 1960. The use of glucose-C^{14} in the evaluation of pathways of glucose metabolism. *J. Biol. Chem.* 235:2165–2177.

Katzen, H. M. 1967. Multiple forms of mammalian hexokinase and their significance to insulin. *Adv. Enzyme Regul.* 5:335–350.

Krebs, H. A. 1972. The Pasteur effect and the relation between respiration and fermentation. *Essays Biochem.* 8:1–34.

Lardy, H. A. 1965. Gluconeogenesis: Pathways and hormonal regulation. *Harvey Lect.* 60:261–278.

Lehninger, A. L. 1975. *Biochemistry,* pp. 417–512. New York: Worth.

Levine, R. and Goldstein, M. S. 1955. On the mechanism of action of insulin. *Recent Prog. Horm. Res.* 11:350–380.

Levine, R., Goldstein, M. S., Klein, S. P. and Huddleston, B. 1949. The action of insulin on the distribution of galactose in eviscerated nephrectomized dogs. *J. Biol. Chem.* 179:985–986.

Levine, R., Goldstein, M. S., Huddleston, B. and Klein, S. P. 1950. Action of insulin on the "permeability" of cells to free hexoses as studied by its effect on the distribution of galactose. *Am. J. Physiol.* 163:70–76.

Lieber, C. 1969. Alcohol and the liver. In *Biological basis of medicine,* eds. E. E. Bittar and N. Bittar, vol. 5, pp. 317–344. London: Academic Press.

Lieber, C. 1970. New pathway of ethanol metabolism in the liver. *Gastroenterology* 59:930–937.

Linn, T. C., Pettit, F. H. and Reed, L. J. 1969. Comparative studies of regulatory properties of the pyruvate dehydrogenase complex from beef kidney mitochondria by phosphorylation and dephosphorylation. *Proc. Natl. Acad. Sci. U.S.A.* 62:234–241.

Lowry, O. H. and Passonneau, J. V. 1964. The relationship between substrates and enzymes of glycolysis in brain. *J. Biol. Chem.* 239:31–42.

MacDonald, I. and Braithwaite, D. M. 1964. The influence of dietary carbohydrates on the lipid pattern in serum and adipose tissue. *Clin. Sci.* 27:23–30.

Madison, L. L., Combs, B., Strickland, W., Unger, R. and Adams, R. 1959. Evidence for the direct effect of insulin on hepatic glucose output. *Metabolism* 8:469–471.

Mortimore, G. E. 1972. Influence of insulin hepatic uptake and release of glucose and amino acids. In *Handbook of physiology*, Sect. 7: *Endocrinology*, eds. D. Steiner and N. Freinkel, pp. 495–504. Washington, D.C.: American Physiological Society.

Neely, J. R. 1973. Control of carbohydrate metabolism in muscle. In *Best and Taylor's physiological basis of medical practice:* Sect. M, *Endocrine control*, ed. H. E. Morgan, pp. 112–122. Baltimore: Williams & Wilkins.

Newsholme, E. A. and Start, C. 1973. *Regulation in metabolism*, pp. 88–292. New York: Wiley.

Nilsson, L. H. and Hultman, E. 1974. Liver and muscle glycogen in man after glucose and fructose infusion. *Scand. J. Clin. Invest.* 33:5–10.

Nordlie, R. C. and Lardy, H. A. 1963. The mammalian phosphoenolpyruvate carboxykinase activities. *J. Biol. Chem.* 238:2259–2263.

Owen, O. E., Morgan, A. P., Kemp, H. G., Sullivan, J. M., Herrera, M. G. and Cahill, G. F., Jr. 1967. Brain metabolism during fasting. *J. Clin. Invest.* 46:1589–1595.

Passonneau, J. V. and Lowry, O. H. 1962. Phosphofructokinase and the control of the citric acid cycle. *Biochem. Biophys. Res. Commun.* 13:373–379.

Patel, M. S., Oland, O. E., Goldman, L. I. and Hanson, R. W. 1975. Fatty acid synthesis by human adipose tissue. *Metabolism* 24:161–168.

Pettit, F. H., Pelley, J. W. and Reed, L. J. 1975. Regulation of pyruvate dehydrogenase kinase and phosphatase by acetyl CoA/CoA and NADH/NAD ratios. *Biochem. Biophys. Res. Commun.* 65:575–582.

Pitot, H. C. and Yatvin, M. D. 1973. Interrelationships of mammalian hormones and enzyme levels *in vivo*. *Physiol. Rev.* 53:228–235.

Purich, D. L., Fromm, H. J. and Rudolf, F. D. 1973. The hexokinases: Kinetic, physical and regulatory properties. *Adv. Enzymol.* 39:249–326.

Regen, D. M., Dawes, W. W., Morgan, H. E. and Park, C. R. 1964. The regulation of hexokinase and phosphofructokinase activity in heart muscle. Effects of alloxan diabetes, growth hormone control and anoxia. *J. Biol. Chem.* 239:43–49.

Rognstad, R. 1975. Cyclic AMP induced inhibition of pyruvate kinase flux in the intact liver cell. *Biochem. Biophys. Res. Commun.* 63:900–905.

Rognstad, R. and Katz, J. 1970. Gluconeogenesis in the kidney cortex. Effects of D-malate and amino-oxyacetate. *Biochem. J.* 116:483–491.

Rose, I. A., Warms, J. V. B. and Kosow, D. P. 1974. Specificity for the glucose-6-P inhibition site of the hexokinases. *Arch. Biochem. Biophys.* 164:729–735.

Ross, E. J. 1956. The "permeability hypothesis" of the action of insulin. *Medicine* 35:355–388.

Ruderman, N. B., Aoki, T. T. and Cahill, G. F., Jr. 1976. Gluconeogenesis and its disorders in man. In *Gluconeogenesis: Its regulation in mammalian species*, eds. R. W. Hanson and M. A. Mehlman, pp. 515–532. New York: Wiley.

Sacktor, B. and Hurlbut, E. C. 1966. Regulation of metabolism in working muscle *in vivo*. II. Concentrations of adenine nucleotides, arginine phosphate and inorganic phosphate in insect flight muscle during flight. *J. Biol. Chem.* 241:632–638.

Sacktor, B. and Wormser-Shavit, E. 1966. Regulation of metabolism in working muscle *in vivo*. I. Concentrations of some glycolytic, tricarboxylic acid cycle and amino acid intermediates in insect flight muscle during flight. *J. Biol. Chem.* 241:624–631.

Safer, D. and Williamson, J. R. 1973. Mitochondrial-cytosolic interaction in perfused rat heart. Role of coupled transamination and repletion of citric acid cycle intermediates. *J. Biol. Chem.* 248:2570–2579.

Schimke, R. T. 1973. Control of enzyme levels in mammalian tissues. *Adv. Enzymol.* 37:135–187.

Sharma, C., Manjeshwar, R. and Weinhouse, S. 1963. Effects of diet and insulin on glucose-adenosine diphosphate phosphotransferases in rat liver. *J. Biol. Chem.* 238:3840–3845.

Shrago, E., Lardy, H. A., Nordlie, R. C. and Foster, D. O. 1963. Metabolic and hormonal control of phosphoenolpyruvate carboxykinase and malic enzyme in rat liver. *J. Biol. Chem.* 238:3188–3192.

Shrago, E., Glennon, J. A. and Gordon, E. C. 1971. Comparative aspects of lipogenesis in mammalian tissues. *Metabolism* 20:54–62.

Soskin, S. and Levine, R. 1952. *Carbohydrate metabolism*, p. 10. Chicago: Univ. of Chicago Press.

Spencer, A. F. and Lowenstein, J. M. 1964. The supply of precursors for the synthesis of fatty acids. *J. Biol. Chem.* 237:3640–3657.

Spiro, R. G. 1973. Biochemistry of the renal glomerular basement membrane and its alteration and diabetes mellitus. *N. Engl. J. Med.* 288:1338–1342.

Srere, T. A. and Bhaduri, A. 1962. Incorporation of radioactive citrate into fatty acids. *Biochim. Biophys. Acta* 59:487–489.

Stadtman, E. R. 1966. Allosteric regulation of enzyme activity. *Adv. Enzymol.* 28:42–154.

Stetten, D., Jr. and Stetten, M. 1960. Glycogen metabolism. *Physiol. Rev.* 40:505–537.

Stuki, J. W., Brawand, F. and Walter, P. 1972. Regulation of pyruvate metabolism in rat liver mitochondria by adenine nucleotides and fatty acids. *Eur. J. Biochem.* 27:181–191.

Taketa, K. and Pogell, B. M. 1965. The inhibition of rat liver fructose 1,6-diphosphatase by adenosine 5'-monophosphate. *J. Biol. Chem.* 240:651–662.

Taunton, O. D., Stifel, F. D., Greene, H. L. and Herman, R. H. 1972. Rapid reciprocal changes of rat hepatic glycolytic enzymes and fructose 1,6-diphosphatase following glucagon and insulin injection *in vivo*. *Biochem. Biophys. Res. Commun.* 48:1663–1670.

Tepperman, J. and Tepperman, H. M. 1970. Gluconeogenesis, lipogenesis and the Sherrington metaphor. *Fed. Proc.* 29:1284–1293.

Topper, Y. J. and Hastings, A. B. 1949. A study of the chemical origins of glycogen by use of C^{14} labelled carbon dioxide, acetate and pyruvate. *J. Biol. Chem.* 179:1255–1264.

Utter, M. F. 1963. Pathways of phosphoenolpyruvate synthesis in glycogenesis. *Iowa State J. Sci.* 38:97–113.

Utter, M. F. and Scrutton, M. S. 1969. Pyruvate carboxylase. *Curr. Top. Cell. Regul.* 1:253–296.

Veneziale, C. M. 1976. Influence of glucagon on the metabolism of fructose D-glyceraldehyde and dihydroxyacetone in rat liver. In *Gluconeogenesis: Its regulation in mammalian species,* eds. R. W. Hanson and M. A. Mehlman, pp. 463–480. New York: Wiley.

Villar-Palasi, C. and Larner, J. 1970. Glycogen metabolism and glycolytic enzymes. *Annu. Rev. Biochem.* 39:639–672.

Villar-Palasi, C. and Wegner, J. I. 1967. *In vivo* effect of insulin on muscle glycogen synthetase. Identification of the action pathway. *Fed. Proc.* 26:563.

Vinuela, E., Salas, M. and Sols, A. 1963. Glucokinase and hexokinase in liver in relation to glycogen synthesis. *J. Biol. Chem.* 238:1175–1177.

Walker, D. G. 1966. The nature and function of hexokinases in animal tissue. *Essays Biochem.* 2:33–67.

Williamson, J. R. 1976. Role of anion transport in the regulation of metabolism in gluconeogenesis. In *Gluconeogenesis: Its regulation in mammalian species,* eds. R. W. Hanson and M. A. Mehlman, pp. 165–220. New York: Wiley.

Wise, E. M., Jr. and Ball, E. G. 1964. Malic enzyme and lipogenesis. *Proc. Natl. Acad. Sci. U.S.A.* 52:1255–1263.

Wu, C. H., Hoshi, M. and Shreeve, W. W. 1974. Human plasma triglyceride labelling after high sucrose feeding. 1. Incorporation of sucrose-U-^{14}C. *Metabolism* 23:1125–1140.

Young, J. W., Shrago, E. and Lardy, H. A. 1964. Metabolic control of enzymes involved in lipogenesis and gluconeogenesis. *Biochemistry* 3:1687–1692.

Zakim, D., Herman, R. H. and Gordon, W. D. 1969. Conversion of glucose and fructose to fatty acids in the human liver. *Biochem. Med.* 2:427–437.

Chapter 3

LIPID METABOLISM: FATTY ACID AND CHOLESTEROL BIOSYNTHESIS

Joseph J. Volpe

Washington University School of Medicine
St. Louis Children's Hospital
St. Louis, Missouri

SCOPE

This discussion of lipid metabolism will be restricted to the biosynthesis of fatty acids (*de novo*) and cholesterol. The synthesis of these two categories of lipids is of critical importance, in part because the immediate products generated constitute a major portion of cellular lipids in health and disease. Of considerable importance also, however, is the fact that the biosynthesis of cholesterol and fatty acids by the *de novo* pathway is an essential starting point in the generation of virtually all of the more complex lipid forms in animal cells. The following review will emphasize the *enzymatic* aspects of *de novo* fatty acid and cholesterol synthesis and will consider studies carried out *in vivo* as well as in cultured cells.

DE NOVO FATTY ACID BIOSYNTHESIS

Introduction

De novo fatty acid biosynthesis in a wide variety of biological systems is catalyzed by two enzyme systems, which function sequentially: acetyl-CoA carboxylase and fatty acid synthetase. Acetyl CoA is the source of all of the carbon atoms of the fatty acids produced, and in most biosynthetic systems palmitate is the major fatty acid produced. The stoichiometry for the synthesis of palmitate from acetyl CoA is

$$8 \text{ Acetyl CoA} + 7 \text{ ATP} + 14 \text{ NADPH} + 14 \text{ H}^+ \rightarrow \text{palmitic acid}$$

$$+ 8 \text{ CoA-SH} + 7 \text{ ADP} + 7 \text{ P}_i + 14 \text{ NADP}^+ + 6 \text{ H}_2\text{O} \quad (1)$$

From palmitate the other long-chain fatty acids—saturated, unsaturated, and hydroxy—can be derived, with the exception of some important polyunsaturated fatty acids.

This section of the review will be confined to studies of acetyl-CoA carboxylase and fatty acid synthetase. Because of space limitations, we will not review the processes of chain elongation, desaturation, or α-hydroxylation that lead to the formation of very long chain, unsaturated, hydroxy, and odd-numbered fatty acids, respectively. Acetyl-CoA carboxylase and fatty acid synthetase will be considered not only in terms of their molecular properties and subunit functions, but also in terms of their control.

Acetyl-CoA Carboxylase

Acetyl-CoA carboxylase catalyzes the first committed step in the synthesis of fatty acids from acetyl CoA, namely the biotin-dependent carboxylation of acetyl CoA to form malonyl CoA in a two-stage reaction:

$$\text{ATP} + \text{HCO}_3^- + \text{biotin-E} \xrightarrow{\text{Me}^{2+}} \text{CO}_2^--\text{biotin-E} + \text{ADP} + \text{P}_i \tag{2}$$

$$\text{CO}_2^--\text{biotin-E} + \text{CH}_3\text{CO-SCoA} \rightarrow {}^-\text{OOCCH}_2\text{CO-SCoA} + \text{biotin-E} \tag{3}$$

$$\text{Sum: ATP} + \text{HCO}_3^- + \text{CH}_3\text{CO-SCoA} \xrightarrow{\text{Me}^{2+}/\text{biotin-E}} {}^-\text{OOCCH}_2\text{CO-SCoA}$$
$$+ \text{ADP} + \text{P}_i \tag{4}$$

(Me^{2+} refers to Mg^{2+} or Mn^{2+}, which are utilized by the carboxylase with specificities that vary with the source of the enzyme and pH of the assay.)

Acetyl-CoA carboxylase has been purified from a variety of animal tissues (Kleinschmidt et al., 1969; Matsuhashi et al., 1964b; Miller and Levy, 1969; Nakanishi and Numa, 1970; Numa et al., 1966; Vagelos et al., 1963; Waite and Wakil, 1962), yeast (Matsuhashi et al., 1964a), wheat germ (Hatch and Stumpf, 1961), and several microorganisms (Alberts and Vagelos, 1968; 1972; Birnbaum, 1969; Kusunose et al., 1959). In homogenized animal cells the enzyme is located in the cytoplasm, although an association with the microsomal fraction of pigeon liver (Margolis and Baum, 1966) and lactating rabbit mammary gland (Easter and Dils, 1968) has been suggested. However, under various conditions of pH and tricarboxylic acid concentrations the carboxylase aggregates, and thus it is difficult to draw any definite conclusions about an association with subcellular particles on the basis of current information. It is interesting in this regard that in green plants acetyl-CoA carboxylase is localized in the chloroplast (Brooks and Stumpf, 1966) and the biotin carboxyl carrier protein component (BCCP) is membrane-bound (Kanangara and Stumpf, 1972).

Molecular properties. Homogeneous acetyl-CoA carboxylase from avian liver (Goto et al., 1967; Gregolin et al., 1966a, 1966b, 1968a, 1968b), bovine adipose tissue (Kleinschmidt et al., 1969; Moss et al., 1972), and rat liver (Inoue and Lowenstein, 1972; Nakanishi and Numa, 1970; Tanabe et al., 1975) has been characterized in the laboratories of Lane, Numa, and Lowenstein (Table 1). Acetyl-CoA carboxylase exists in at least two major forms: an active polymer and an inactive protomer. Dissociation to the protomeric form is favored by palmityl CoA as well as low protein concentration, Cl^-, pH greater than 7.5, and carboxylation of the enzyme to produce carboxybiotin. The equilibrium toward the aggregated polymeric form is favored by citrate as well as acetyl CoA, high protein concentration, or pH 6.5–7.0. The electron microscopic appearance of the enzyme varies markedly with the state of aggregation. The inactive protomeric form appears as particles with a maximum dimension of 100–300 Å. The active polymeric form appears as a network of filaments 70–100 Å in width and up to 4,000 Å in length. The filaments exhibit longitudinal periodicity of about 120–140 Å, perhaps representing the individual protomeric units (Lane et al., 1974). These observations have led to the speculation that the network of filaments might provide a basic structural matrix for organization of the other enzymes involved in lipid synthesis (Gregolin et al., 1966a; Kleinschmidt et al., 1969).

The most detailed studies of possible subunits of animal acetyl-CoA carboxylase have involved the avian and rat liver enzymes (Gregolin et al., 1968b; Guchhait et al., 1974b; Inoue and Lowenstein, 1972; Lane et al., 1970; Tanabe et al., 1975). Chicken liver acetyl-CoA carboxylase has been resolved by polyacrylamide gel electrophoresis in 6 M urea - 0.1% sodium dodecyl sulfate (SDS) into polypeptide chains with molecular weights of 139,000; 129,000; and 117,000. Consideration of the mass ratios, estimated by gel scanning, and the molecular weights of the three chains indicates a molar stoichiometry of 1.0:1.0:1.8 for the 139,000; 129,000; and 117,000 subunits, respectively, which is consistent with a tetrameric structure. Microbiological assay of biotin in each band revealed that covalently bound biotin is associated with the lightest polypeptide chain (117,000), and it was deter-

TABLE 1   Molecular Properties of Animal Acetyl
CoA Carboxylases

Source of enzyme	Molecular form	Molecular weight	Biotin content
Avian liver	Polymer	4–10 million	Many
	Protomer	410,000	0.93
Rat liver	Polymer	–	Many
	Protomer	215–230,000	1
Bovine adipose tissue	Polymer	Several million	Many
	Protomer	560,000	2

mined further that there is one biotin prosthetic group per 488,000 daltons. This indicated that only one of the two light chains possesses a biotin prosthetic group. Thus, the biotin content—that is, one biotinyl group per 488,000 daltons—as well as the subunit stoichiometry indicated that avian liver acetyl-CoA carboxylase was tetrameric. Lane and co-workers proposed that four apparently nonidentical subunits comprise the fundamental protomeric unit of avian liver acetyl-CoA carboxylase. One polypeptide chain of 117,000 carries the prosthetic group, and each protomeric unit possesses a single biotinyl moiety (Lane et al., 1970). The protomers *per se* appear to be identical. That the subunits are nonidentical is further supported by the fact that only one biotinyl prosthetic group, one acetyl CoA binding site, one bicarbonate loading site, and one tight citrate binding site are present per protomer (Gregolin et al., 1968b). Nevertheless, the possibility cannot be ruled out that these observations of four subunits from avian liver carboxylase were caused by proteolytic modification of the enzyme during the isolation procedures.

Inoue and Lowenstein (1972) purified to homogeneity the acetyl-CoA carboxylase of rat liver, and some apparent differences from the avian enzyme are evident. Thus, SDS gel electrophoresis resolved the rat liver enzyme into bands with estimated molecular weights of 215,000; 125,000; and 118,000. The latter two peptides appeared to be derived from the 215,000 species. Therefore, the enzyme apparently contains at least two types of unlike subunits. One mol (0.91) of biotin was found per 215,000 daltons, and thus the rat liver enzyme appears to have twice the biotin content of the chicken liver enzyme. The enzyme was also found to contain 2.1 mol of phosphate per 215,000 daltons, and Lowenstein raised the possibility that the activity of the enzyme is regulated by phosphorylation and dephosphorylation, as is the case with pyruvate dehydrogenase complex (Linn et al., 1969) and phosphorylase (Fischer et al., 1970). The recent studies of rat liver acetyl-CoA carboxylase by Numa and coworkers (Tanabe et al., 1975) may be of extreme significance for the interpretation of the various studies of subunits of animal carboxylases. Thus, these workers present data leading to the conclusions that the rat liver carboxylase contains a single subunit of molecular weight 230,000 and that this subunit can be converted to the smaller polypeptides by proteolytic modification. Thus, endogenous proteases or trypsin and chymotrypsin resulted in cleavage of the large polypeptide into the smaller fragments. Acetyl-CoA carboxylase isolated from crude rat liver extracts by means of immunoprecipitation with specific antibody invariably showed only the large polypeptide. The biotin content of the enzyme was found to be 1 mol per 237,000 g protein. These observations are of great interest because they suggest that the rat liver carboxylase contains the biotin carboxylase, the biotin carboxyl carrier protein, and the carboxyl transferase apparently bound covalently in a single subunit. Such a structure would represent a distinctive evolutionary modification of the organization of this multienzyme complex and would be closely analogous to the organization of the animal fatty acid synthetase multienzyme complex (see discussion below).

Subunit functions. All attempts to dissociate the acetyl-CoA carboxylase of animals and yeast have been unsuccessful. In contrast, the acetyl-CoA carboxylases of *E. coli* and plants are readily dissociated into active subunits, and the functions of the various subunits have been defined primarily by study of these systems.

Initial studies of the acetyl-CoA carboxylase of *E. coli* revealed that the enzyme is composed of three proteins, which are involved in the two half-reactions, as demonstrated in reactions 5 and 6 (Alberts et al., 1969, 1971; Alberts and Vagelos, 1968; Dimroth et al., 1970; Fall et al., 1971; Fall and Vagelos, 1972; Guchhait et al., 1971; Nervi et al., 1971).

$$ATP + HCO_3^- + BCCP \xrightarrow{\text{biotin carboxylase/Mg}^{2+}} CO_2^- -BCCP$$
$$+ ADP + P_i \quad (5)$$

$$CO_2^- -BCCP + \text{acetyl-CoA} \xrightarrow{\text{transcarboxylase}} BCCP + \text{malonyl-CoA} \quad (6)$$

The three proteins are biotin carboxylase, BCCP and transcarboxylase.

Biotin Carboxylase. Biotin carboxylase catalyzes the first half-reaction, the carboxylation of the biotinyl moiety of the biotin carboxyl carrier protein. This enzyme, purified to homogeneity and crystallized by Lane and co-workers (Dimroth et al., 1970; Guchhait and Mukherjee, 1972), has a molecular weight of 98,000 and contains two apparently identical subunits of molecular weight 51,000. The enzyme does not contain biotin but has a binding site for biotin. Model reactions have been utilized to study the mechanism of the reaction catalyzed by biotin carboxylase (Polakis et al., 1974). Biotin carboxylase catalyzes a biotin-dependent phosphoryl transfer from carbamyl phosphate (an analog of carbonic-phosphorous anhydride) to ADP to form ATP, and this fact suggests that the carboxylation of biotin may proceed via a carbonic-phosphorous anhydride intermediate. Biotin does not appear to participate directly in the phosphoryl transfer reaction, but instead occupies the biotin binding site on the biotin carboxylase to induce a conformational change in the enzyme which orients functional groups at the sites for HCO_3^- and ATP and thereby activates carbonic-phosphoric anhydride formation. Thus, these data suggest another role for biotin in the acetyl-CoA carboxylase reaction, in addition to the role of carboxyl acceptor.

Biotin Carboxyl Carrier Protein. Biotin carboxyl carrier protein plays a central role in the carboxylation of acetyl CoA. It is carboxylated to form $CO_2^- -BCCP$ in the biotin carboxylase reaction, and the carboxyl group of $CO_2^- -BCCP$ is transferred to acetyl CoA to form malonyl CoA in the reaction catalyzed by the transcarboxylase. The protein has been shown to contain 1.0 residue of biotin per 22,000 daltons (Fall et al., 1971; Fall and Vagelos, 1972, 1973; Nervi et al., 1971). The apparent native form of the protein is best represented by a dimeric structure. Biotin has been shown to be bound to the ε-amino group of a lysine residue of the protein (Knappe et al., 1963; Waite and Wakil, 1962). Lynen and co-workers (Himes et al., 1963; Knappe et al., 1961, 1963; Lynen, 1967; Lynen et al., 1961) determined the mode of binding of the carboxyl group to the biotin prosthetic group by carrying out the model reaction of carboxylation of free biotin with β-methylcrotonyl-CoA carboxylase, methylating the product and identifying the methylated product as 1′-*N*-carboxymethylbiotin methyl ester. Similar experiments, carried out with carboxylated enzyme, led to the conclusion that the site of carboxylation on biotin is the 1′-ureido-N (Knappe et al., 1963; Numa et al., 1964). The current concept of the function of BCCP is that the carboxyl moiety is attached to the 1′-N of the bicyclic ring of the prosthetic group, and the latter, which resides at the distal end of a flexible 14 Å side chain (Mildvan et al., 1966), acts as a "mobile carboxyl carrier" between the catalytic centers of the biotin carboxylase and the transcarboxylase (Lane et al., 1971).

Transcarboxylase. The transcarboxylase component of acetyl-CoA carboxylase catalyzes the reversible transfer of carboxyl groups from CO_2^- BCCP to acetyl CoA to form malonyl CoA (Alberts et al., 1971; Guchhait et al., 1971; Polakis et al., 1974). This component has a molecular weight of 130,000 and is composed of nonidentical polypeptide chains of 30,000 and 35,000 daltons (Guchhait et al., 1974a). The enzyme has a binding site for biotin, acetyl CoA, and malonyl CoA. That the two acyl CoA derivatives are bound at a common site was shown by the following (Alberts et al., 1971). The malonyl CoA binding site was demonstrated directly by isolating the [^{14}C]malonyl-transcarboxylase intermediate by Sephadex G-50 chromatography after reacting [2-^{14}C]malonyl CoA with the purified enzyme. That the site for acetyl CoA was common to that for malonyl CoA was shown when addition of unlabeled acetyl CoA decreased the amount of [^{14}C]malonyl CoA bound to the transcarboxylase.

Regulation. Allosteric Effects. Although acetyl-CoA carboxylase is frequently cited as the rate-limiting enzyme in fatty acid synthesis, evidence to support this contention is not decisive. Early observations indicated that hepatic carboxylase activity is very much lower than fatty acid synthetase activity under a variety of nutritional conditions (Ganguly, 1960; Numa et al., 1961). However, later observations (Chang et al., 1967; Liou and Donaldson, 1973; Majerus et al., 1968; Numa et al., 1970) of the carboxylase, fully activated and assayed under optimal conditions, revealed enzymatic activity that is similar to that for fatty acid synthetase. Thus, the degree to which the carboxylase is activated *in vivo* must play a decisive role in determining the extent to which this enzyme directs the rate of fatty acid synthesis. Perhaps most important, recent observations by Guynn et al. (1972) indicate that acetyl-CoA carboxylase may be the rate-limiting enzyme in the short-term control of fatty acid synthesis and that fatty acid synthetase may be the rate-limiting enzyme in long-term control. Thus, in short-term experiments—that is, animals refed for 3 hr after a 45 hr fast—there resulted in liver a sharp increase in the malonyl CoA concentration and in the rate of fatty acid synthesis, as measured by the ^3H_2O method. The rise in malonyl CoA concentration suggested that the site of this short-term control was before the fatty acid synthetase step. Detailed studies of substrate levels indicated that control was not related to limitation of substrates for acetyl-CoA carboxylase, and thus appeared to be at the level of acetyl-CoA carboxylase *per se*. Further support for acetyl-CoA carboxylase as the rate-limiting enzyme in short-term regulation is provided by the studies of the effects of glucagon and manno-heptulose *in vivo* and of exogenous fatty acids in cultured cells (see relevant sections below).

Citrate and long-chain fatty acyl CoA derivatives. Allosteric regulators considered to be of prime physiological importance are tricarboxylic acids and long-chain fatty acyl CoA derivatives. The initial observation that citrate stimulates fatty acid synthesis from acetate (Brady and Gurin, 1952) was explained by the discovery that citrate and other Krebs cycle intermediates cause polymerization and activation of rat adipose tissue acetyl-CoA carboxylase (Martin and Vagelos, 1962; Vagelos et al., 1962, 1963). This fundamental observation was confirmed by studies of acetyl-CoA carboxylase from rat liver (Matsuhashi et al., 1964b; Numa et al., 1965a, 1965b), avian liver (Goto et al., 1967; Gregolin et al., 1966a, 1966b; Lane et al., 1970; Numa et al., 1966), bovine adipose tissue (Kleinschmidt et al., 1969), and rat mammary gland (Miller and Levy, 1969). Activation by citrate is accompanied by polymerization of inactive protomers to active polymeric filaments and is clearly associated with a conformational change of the enzyme (Goto et al., 1967; Gregolin et al., 1966a, 1966b; Martin and Vagelos, 1962; Matsuhashi et al., 1964b; Numa et al., 1965a, 1965b, 1966; Vagelos et al., 1962). Kinetic analyses of acetyl-CoA carboxylase of rat liver (Numa et al., 1964), avian liver (Gregolin et al., 1968a; Ryder et al., 1967), and bovine adipose tissue have established that the major effect of the activators is on the maximal velocity of the enzyme rather than on the K_m values for substrates.

The locus of citrate activation has been studied particularly in the laboratories of Lynen (Matsuhashi et al., 1964a) and Lane (Gregolin et al., 1966b, 1968a; Lane et al., 1970, 1971; Moss and Lane, 1972a; Ryder et al., 1967). Both half-reactions of acetyl CoA carboxylation are activated by citrate. Lynen and co-workers utilized exchange reactions to study the two partial reactions and showed that both partial reactions of the rat liver enzyme are activated by citrate. This was confirmed for the avian liver carboxylase by Lane and co-workers (Gregolin et al., 1966b, 1968a; Moss et al., 1972). Using model compounds, Lane and co-workers were able to perform more detailed kinetic analyses than were possible with the very rapid exchange reactions. The first half-reaction was followed by the carboxylation of free (+)-biotin, a model of the prosthetic group, and the second by transcarboxylation of acetylpantetheine, a model of acetyl CoA. Again, both half-reactions were markedly stimulated by citrate. Several lines of evidence indicate that the biotin prosthetic group is intimately associated with the locus of the citrate-induced conformational changes (Landman and Dakshinamurti, 1975; Lane et al., 1971; Moss and Lane, 1972a, 1972b; Ryder et al., 1967). First, the biotinyl moiety is involved in both half-reactions that are stimulated by citrate. Second, kinetic analysis of the avian liver enzyme has revealed that the citrate-induced conversion to the polymeric state renders the biotinyl moiety inaccessible to avidin. Third, although citrate has been shown to activate all of the reactions of the carboxylase that are avidin-sensitive, the avidin-insensitive decarboxylation of malonyl CoA by acetyl-CoA carboxylase is unaffected by the activator. Fourth, apoenzyme of mammalian adipose tissue does not aggregate under conditions favoring the aggregation of the holoenzyme to the polymeric form.

Long-chain acyl CoA thioesters in micromolar concentrations inhibit acetyl-CoA carboxylase from rat liver (Bortz and Lynen, 1963b; Numa et al., 1965a, 1965b), avian liver (Goodridge, 1972), and rat mammary gland (Miller and Levy, 1969). This inhibition is competitive with respect to citrate but noncompetitive with respect to acetyl CoA, bicarbonate, or ATP (Numa, 1965a, 1965b). The most potent inhibitors, CoA thioesters of C_{16}–C_{18} fatty acids, occur abundantly in animal tissues. Because long-chain acyl CoA derivatives are potent detergents and, in fact, inhibit a variety of enzymes of diverse metabolic function on the basis of detergent properties (Taketa and Pogell, 1966), the physiological importance of these observations was questioned initially. The physiological significance of regulation of acetyl-CoA carboxylase activity by palmityl CoA in chicken liver was critically reexamined by Goodridge (1972). It was recognized that the concentration of palmityl CoA as well as the relative affinity of the carboxylase for this thioester are important determinants. In the presence of bovine serum albumin (25 mg/ml), palmityl CoA (100 μM) inhibited incorporation of [^{14}C]citrate into fatty acids by a 100,000 x g supernatant solution of chicken liver and inhibited the activity of acetyl-CoA carboxylase purified from chicken liver. Under similar conditions, palmityl CoA (200 μM) did not inhibit other lipogenic enzymes, such as fatty acid synthetase, ATP-citrate lyase, malic enzyme, and NADP-linked isocitrate dehydrogenase, or two other enzymes, pyruvate kinase and glutamate dehydrogenase, previously reported to be inhibited by long-chain fatty acyl CoA derivatives (Taketa and Pogell, 1966; Tsutsumi and Takenaka, 1969). This "specific" inhibition of acetyl-CoA carboxylase was reversed in one of three ways: (1) by increasing the concentration of albumin, (2) by increasing the concentration of citrate, or (3) by addition of (+)-palmitylcarnitine. Palmitylcarnitine may act as a structural analog that binds to the enzyme at the same site as palmityl CoA but does not inhibit enzymatic activity. That the inhibition by palmityl CoA was unlikely to be nonspecific detergent inactivation was supported by its relative specificity, failure to increase with time of incubation, and reversibility and competition with a potentially physiological activator, citrate.

Although it is apparent from the data reviewed that citrate activates and palmityl CoA inhibits acetyl-CoA carboxylase, considerable controversy exists over the occurrence of such phenomena *in vivo*. Over 70% of the citrate in mammalian liver is associated with mitochondria (Schneider et al., 1956); estimates of concentrations of citrate in the cytoplasmic fraction are 0.1–0.2 mM (Greenbaum et al., 1971). Since citrate activates acetyl-CoA carboxylase with an apparent K_m of 2–6 mM, the data suggest that the carboxylase may not be activated fully *in vivo*. However, the extent of compartmentalization of citrate within the cytoplasm is entirely unknown. The total concentration of long-chain fatty acyl CoA derivatives in mammalian and avian liver varies with the nutritional state of the animal, but values of 15–140 μM have been recorded (Bortz and Lynen, 1963a; Greenbaum et al., 1971; Tubbs and Garland, 1963, 1964; Yeh and Leveille, 1971). Since palmityl CoA inhibits acetyl-CoA carboxylase with an apparent K_i of 0.8–1.1 μM, the levels of such derivatives are well within the concentration range that inhibits the enzyme. However, in addition to the uncertainties of compartmentalization, factors such as the degree of binding of these derivatives to cellular proteins and the resulting concentration of acyl CoA derivatives available for inhibition of the carboxylase remain unknown.

Studies *in vivo* correlating rates of fatty acid synthesis with tissue levels of citrate or long-chain fatty acyl CoA derivatives have yielded conflicting results (Ballard and Hanson, 1969; Guchhait and Mukherjee, 1972; Guynn et al., 1972; Nishikori et al., 1973; Spencer and Lowenstein, 1967). Numa and co-workers recently correlated rates of fatty acid synthesis from acetate with levels of acetyl-CoA carboxylase and concentrations of citrate and long-chain acyl CoA derivatives in liver of rats during the first 48 hr of refeeding after starvation (Nishikori et al., 1973). In the first 8 hr of refeeding there was a severalfold increase in the rate of fatty acid synthesis and, during the same interval, an abrupt rise in citrate levels and fall in long-chain acyl CoA derivatives. No change occurred in the level of acetyl-CoA carboxylase. After 8 hr the increasing rate of fatty acid synthesis was accompanied by a rise in the level of acetyl-CoA carboxylase. The early increase in fatty acid synthesis was considered to be caused by an increase in acetyl-CoA carboxylase activation by citrate and a decrease in inhibition by long-chain acyl CoA derivatives without a change in the level of the enzyme (Nishikori et al., 1973). The later rise in both fatty acid synthesis and levels of acetyl-CoA carboxylase was considered to be caused by adaptive changes in content of the enzyme (see below). Similarly, in short-term experiments with isolated hepatocytes from neonatal chicks, Goodridge (1973d) observed a positive correlation of the citrate content of the isolated cells with fatty acid synthesis under all incubation conditions. The effect of citrate was considered to be at the level of acetyl-CoA carboxylase. Inhibition of fatty acid synthesis in the liver cells by free fatty acids was accompanied by an increase in the fatty acyl CoA level (Goodridge, 1973d). Goodridge suggested that inhibition of fatty acid synthesis by fatty acyl CoA might occur directly by inhibition of acetyl-CoA carboxylase or by inhibition of the mitochondrial citrate carrier (Halperin et al., 1972), thereby reducing the supply of citrate for activation of the carboxylase. An effect on the citrate carrier would also cause a reduction in the cytoplasmic production of acetyl CoA by the ATP-citrate lyase reaction and thus amplify the effect on fatty acid synthesis.

Phosphorylation-dephosphorylation. The possibility that acetyl-CoA carboxylase may be regulated by phosphorylation-dephosphorylation and thus exert short-term control of fatty acid synthesis is suggested by recent observations. Following the finding by Inoue and Lowenstein (1972) that pure rat liver acetyl-CoA carboxylase contains phosphate, Carlson and Kim (1973, 1974a, 1974b) presented data to indicate that the enzyme is inactivated by phosphorylation and activated by dephosphorylation. Partially but not highly purified acetyl-CoA carboxylase was inactivated by ATP in a reaction that was time- and temperature-dependent. A protein fraction that inactivated purified acetyl-CoA carboxylase in the presence of ATP was obtained in a 65–75% ammonium sulfate fraction that was devoid of carboxylase activity. Evidence that acetyl-CoA carboxylase was phosphorylated by added ATP was several-fold: (1) inactivation with $[\gamma\text{-}^{32}P]$ ATP but not $[U\text{-}^{14}C]$ ATP was accompanied by incorporation of acid-stable radioactivity into the enzyme; (2) when $[\gamma\text{-}^{32}P]$ ATP-inhibited enzyme was reactivated by Mg^{2+}, a time-dependent release of radioactivity occurred that paralleled the recovery of enzymatic activity; (3) on purification of acetyl-CoA carboxylase inactivated by $[\gamma\text{-}^{32}P]$ ATP, the ^{32}P label copurified with the enzyme; and (4) $[\gamma\text{-}^{32}P]$ ATP-inhibited enzyme was precipitated by anti-acetyl-CoA carboxylase antibody. The phosphorylating activity was called "acetyl-CoA carboxylase kinase" and the Mg^{2+}-dependent dephosphorylating activity "acetyl-CoA carboxylase phosphatase." An analogy with regulation of pyruvate dehydrogenase complex (Linn et al., 1969) was suggested (Carlson and Kim, 1973). The inactivated form of acetyl-CoA carboxylase was less sensitive to stimulation by citrate and more sensitive to inhibition by palmityl CoA than was the activated form (Carlson and Kim, 1974b). These interesting latter data indicate a means by which the effects of these important physiologic modulators could be amplified.

Rous (1974) attempted to demonstrate phosphorylation of acetyl-CoA carboxylase and/or fatty acid synthetase *in vivo* by injection of rats with $Na_2 H^{32}PO_4$ followed by purification of the hepatic enzymes 14 hr later. Specific radioactivity of acetyl-CoA carboxylase increased with purification of the enzyme, whereas radioactivity virtually disappeared from the protein fractions obtained during purification of fatty acid synthetase.

Despite these interesting findings, certain considerations prevent unequivocal acceptance of the concept of acetyl-CoA carboxylase regulation by phosphorylation-dephosphorylation. Thus, in the studies of Carlson and Kim (1973), the enzyme retained 35–50% of the original activity despite maximum incorporation of radioactivity from $[\gamma\text{-}^{32}P]$ ATP. This retention of activity is in marked contrast to findings with pyruvate dehydrogenase complex (Wieland and Siess, 1970), which included virtually no retained activity when the complex was maximally phosphorylated. In addition, confirmation of the results of Carlson and Kim has yet to be reported. In the study of Rous (1974) no attempt was made at characterization of the radioactivity bound to the enzyme, and thus it cannot be stated unequivocally that the carboxylase had been phosphorylated *in vivo*.

Hormones and cyclic AMP. A role for cyclic AMP and/or certain hormones in the short-term regulation of hepatic acetyl-CoA carboxylase has been suggested by recent observations. In short-term experiments, glucagon, a hormone known to increase hepatic levels of cyclic AMP (Robinson et al., 1971), markedly depressed hepatic fatty acid synthesis, measured by incorporation of radioactive acetate or glucose *in vitro* by liver slices, *in vivo* by perfused liver preparations, or in isolated hepatocytes (Exton et al., 1972; Goodridge, 1973a; Haugaard and Stadie, 1953; Klain and Weiser, 1973; Meikle et al., 1973; Regen and Terrell, 1968). Klain and Weiser (1973) demonstrated an approximately 60% reduction in fatty acid synthesis from glucose 15 min after infusion of glucagon and a 75% reduction after 30 min, and simultaneously acetyl-CoA carboxylase activity was reduced by 55 and 70%. No change occurred in activities of fatty acid synthetase, glucose-6-phosphate dehydrogenase, NADP-malic dehydrogenase, isocitric dehydrogenase, or citrate cleavage enzyme. These experiments strongly suggested that short-term regulation of fatty acid synthesis by glucagon was mediated by alterations of acetyl-CoA carboxylase. Similarly, a variety of *in vitro* and *in vivo* studies have indicated that cyclic AMP exerts short-term control over fatty acid synthesis (Akhtar and Bloxham, 1970; Allred and Roehrig, 1972; Bricker and Levy, 1972; Capuzzi et al., 1974; Goodridge, 1973a; Tepperman and Tepperman, 1972). A possible role for acetyl-CoA carboxylase in this regulation is suggested by the observations of Allred and Roehrig (1972) that lipogenesis, measured by incorporation of tritium from ^3H_2O by liver slices, was reduced by 75% after a 30 min preincubation with 1 mM dibutyryl cyclic AMP and that this depression was accompanied by an approximately 60% reduction in activity of acetyl-CoA carboxylase. Inhibition of acetyl-CoA carboxylase by approximately 50% could be attained by preincubation of tissue homogenates with 1 mM dibutyryl cyclic AMP. The mechanism of the short-term effect of cyclic AMP on acetyl-CoA carboxylase remains unknown, but a possibility worthy of consideration is that cyclic AMP activates a protein kinase that phosphorylates and inactivates the enzyme, as suggested by Carlson and Kim (1973). A second possibility is that cyclic AMP interacts with a regulatory protein through a mechanism similar to that described for this mononucleotide in bacterial systems (Emmer et al., 1970; Jost and Richenberg, 1971; Zubay et al., 1970). A third possibility is that both glucagon and cyclic AMP exert their short-term inhibitory effects by increasing hepatic concentrations of long-chain fatty acyl CoA derivatives. A glucagon- and cyclic AMP-sensitive lipase has been reported in liver (Claycomb and Kilsheimer, 1969; Menahan and Wieland, 1969).

Lee et al. (1973) have made related observations of adipose tissue acetyl-CoA carboxylase. Preincubation of acetyl-CoA carboxylase of epididymal adipose tissue for 60 min with epinephrine (10^{-7}–10^{-3} M) resulted in a 25–65% reduction in activity. Similarly, preincubation with dibutyryl cyclic AMP (10^{-3} M) resulted in a 60% reduction. Conversely, acetyl-CoA carboxylase of adipose tissue preincubated with insulin (3 units/ml) exhibited approximately a 50–85% increase in activity. The latter effect was seen only in tissue of fasted animals, and the authors suggested that acetyl-CoA carboxylase in adipose tissue of normally fed animals may occur "mostly in the activated state, whereas the inactivated state of the enzyme predominates in the starved animals." Thus, the possibility is raised that in starvation increased levels of epinephrine and glucagon maintain the enzyme in an active state, while during refeeding increased levels of insulin activate the enzyme. Perhaps related to these findings is the observation that 3 hr after parenteral administration to rats of mannoheptulose, a compound known to cause a rapid fall in plasma insulin and a rise in plasma glucagon, fatty acid synthesis from glucose and activity of acetyl-CoA carboxylase (but not fatty acid synthetase) are reduced approximately threefold (Klain and Meikle, 1974). Administration of insulin with the mannoheptulose prevented the decrease in carboxylase activity. Whether these factors produce their short-term effects on acetyl-CoA carboxylase through a phosphorylation-dephosphorylation mechanism remains to be established.

The potential short-term effectors of acetyl-CoA carboxylase activity are summarized in Table 2. Unlike the unequivocal evidence implicating adaptive changes in enzyme content in long-term regulation of acetyl-CoA carboxylase (see below), the data relative to short-term effectors of this enzyme are derived from studies with relatively crude systems. Further study in better characterized systems, particularly of the effects of hormones and cyclic AMP and the potential role of phosphorylation-dephosphorylation in the regulation of acetyl-CoA carboxylase, will be of great interest.

Prosthetic Group Metabolism. A role for biotin metabolism in regulation of acetyl-CoA carboxylase has been demonstrated in recent studies of biotin-deficient animals (Achuta Murthy and Mistry, 1974; Dakshinamurti and Desjardins, 1968; Desjardins and Dakshinamurti, 1971; Jacobs et al., 1970; Mason and Donaldson, 1972). Biotin deficiency results in a marked difference in response of the acetyl-CoA carboxylases of adipose tissue and liver (Dakshinamurti and Desjardins, 1968; Jacobs et al., 1970). Thus, after 1–2 wk

TABLE 2 Potential Short-Term Effectors of Animal
Acetyl-CoA Carboxylase[a]

Effector	Mechanism	Effect on acetyl-CoA carboxylase activity
Citrate	Enhance conversion to active polymeric form	Increase
Long-chain fatty acyl CoA derivatives	Enhance conversion to inactive protomeric form	Decrease
Unknown	Phosphorylation	Decrease
Unknown	Dephosphorylation	Increase
Glucagon	Unknown	Decrease
Insulin	Unknown	Increase
Epinephrine	Unknown	Decrease
Cyclic AMP	Unknown	Decrease

[a]See text for sources of enzyme and experimental details.

of biotin deprivation activity in liver is unchanged, after 3 wk it is depressed by 35%, and after 6-8 wk it is depressed by only 50%. In contrast, after 1-2 wk of biotin deprivation activity in adipose tissue is depressed threefold, and after 6-8 wk, by sixfold. When biotin was injected into the biotin-deficient animals, carboxylase activity in adipose tissue rose within 2 min to a level two- to threefold that observed in animals fed a biotin-supplemented diet (Jacobs et al., 1970). These data suggested that apoenzyme had accumulated in adipose tissue of the biotin-deficient rats. Quantitative precipitin analyses with anti-acetyl-CoA carboxylase antibody demonstrated that this was indeed the case. These analyses indicated that an enzymatically inactive but immunologically reactive enzyme species—that is, apoenzyme—was present in the deficient animals.

Synthesis of holoenzyme from apoenzyme was demonstrated *in vivo* by giving a pulse of [^{3}H]biotin followed by isolation of the labeled holoenzyme by immunoprecipitation. There was a 16-fold increase in incorporation of biotin into holoenzyme in adipose tissue of deficient rats as compared to nondeficient animals. The synthesis of holoenzyme was also demonstrated *in vitro* with crude extracts of adipose tissue. The synthesis was dependent on ATP and presumably proceeded via a biotinyl-AMP intermediate, as demonstrated for yeast acetyl-CoA carboxylase (Lynen and Rominger, 1963) and other acyl-CoA carboxylases (Siegel et al., 1965). These results have been confirmed by Desjardins and Dakshinamurti (1971). Recently, a similar ATP-dependent system for acetyl-CoA holocarboxylase synthesis was described in a 0-60% ammonium sulfate fraction of chicken liver (Achuta Murthy and Mistry, 1974). The important additional finding was that citrate (5 mM) stimulated holoenzyme synthesis by 100%. Whether citrate affects the substrate—that is, apocarboxylase—or the holocarboxylase synthetase is unknown. Nevertheless, the effect raises the possibility of an additional control point for citrate in regulation of fatty acid synthesis, increasing the relative amount of acetyl-CoA holocarboxylase. Most recently, Landman and Dakshinamurti (1975) have demonstrated that acetyl-CoA apocarboxylase in protomeric form, isolated by Sepharose-avidin chromatography (Landman and Dakshinamurti, 1973) of adipose tissue from biotin-deficient rats, is not converted to a polymeric form by citrate. Transition to polymeric carboxylase is possible only after the conversion of the apoenzyme to the holoenzyme *in vitro*. This observation indicates that conversion of apo- to holoenzyme could represent an additional site for regulation of acetyl-CoA carboxylase.

Adaptive Changes in Enzyme Content. Acetyl-CoA carboxylase activity of a variety of tissue undergoes relatively long-term regulatory changes secondary to nutritional, hormonal, developmental, genetic, neoplastic, and pharmacologic factors. The best-studied tissue has been liver, and the following discussion will emphasize the enzyme of this tissue (see Table 3). Changes in fatty acid synthetase and in fatty acid synthesis are usually coordinated with alterations in acetyl-CoA carboxylase, but many exceptions to this rule are known. For example, during the first 24 hr of fasting the rate of fatty acid synthesis in mammalian liver falls by 99%, whereas acetyl-CoA carboxylase activity falls by only 50% (Korchak and Masoro, 1962). Injection of glucose into unfed, neonatal chicks results, in 1½ hr, in a fivefold increase in the hepatic rate of fatty acid synthesis but no change in either acetyl-CoA carboxylase or fatty acid synthetase (Goodridge, 1973b). If neonatal chicks are not fed, hepatic acetyl-CoA carboxylase activity does not increase, whereas activity of fatty acid synthetase does. Similarly, when eggs are incubated in 100% oxygen for 24 hr hepatic fatty acid synthetase activity increases twofold whereas acetyl-CoA carboxylase activity is unchanged (Goodridge, 1973c). These and other data (relative to discoordinate changes in hepatic ATP-citrate lyase and malic enzyme) led Goodridge to suggest that there is no "fatty acid synthesis pathway operon." These data notwithstanding the observations of acetyl-CoA carboxylase to be outlined below are usually accompanied by qualitatively similar ones made for fatty acid synthetase and *de novo* fatty acid synthesis.

Nutritional factors. Acetyl-CoA carboxylase activity is markedly elevated in livers of animals fed a high-carbohydrate, fat-free diet and depressed in animals fasted or fed a high-fat diet (Allmann et al., 1965; Korchak and Masoro, 1962; Numa et al., 1970). The most striking alterations occur when fasted animals are refed a fat-free diet (Gibson et al., 1966). Similar effects have been described in adipose tissue (Saggerson and Greenbaum, 1970) and in intestinal mucosa (Hynie and Hahn, 1972). No change in the acetyl-CoA carboxylase of rat brain occurs with fasting or fat-free feeding (Kelley and Joel, 1973). When fasted animals are refed a fat-free diet supplemented with polyunsaturated fatty acids, the increase in hepatic carboxylase activity is strikingly diminished (Allmann and Gibson, 1965; Gibson et al., 1972; Muto and Gibson, 1970; Smith and Abraham, 1970a). Palmitate and oleate

TABLE 3 Long-Term Regulation of Hepatic Acetyl-CoA Carboxylase

Condition	Specific activity (units/mg protein)	Rate of enzyme Synthesis	Degradation
Nutritional[a]			
1. High-carbohydrate diet	↑[b]	↑	N
2. Fat-free diet	↑	↑	N
3. High-fat diet	↓	↓	—
4. Polyunsaturated fatty acids	↓	—	—
5. Fasted	↓	↓	↑
6. Choline deprivation	↑	—	—
7. Vitamin B_{12} deprivation	↑	—	—
8. Biotin deficiency (prolonged)	↓	—	—
Hormonal[c]			
1. Diabetes	↓	↓	N
2. Diabetes + insulin	N	N	—
3. Glucagon	↓	—	—
4. Hyperthyroid	↑	—	—
5. Hypophysectomized	↓	—	—
Development[d]			
1. Fetus	↓	—	—
2. Suckling	↓	—	—
3. Weaned	↑	—	—
Genetic (obese-hyperglycemic mouse)[e]			
1. Standard laboratory chow	↑	↑	±↓
2. Fasted	N	—	—
3. Fasted, refed fat-free diet	↓	—	—
4. Fasted, refed sesame oil	N	—	—
Neoplastic (Minimal Deviation Hepatoma)[f]			
1. Standard laboratory chow	±↑	—	—
2. Fasted	↑	—	—
3. Fasted, refed fat-free diet	↓	—	—
Pharmacologic[g]			
1. TPIA, CPIB	↓	—	—

[a]Comparisons are between animals administered standard laboratory chow or the indicated diets or factors.

[b]N, ↑, and ↓ indicate no difference from, greater than, less than control, respectively; — indicates no data available.

[c]Comparisons are between animals subjected to the indicated hormonal changes and normal controls.

[d]Comparisons are between adult animals and those of the indicated ages.

[e]Comparisons are between obese-hyperglycemic mice and normal mice subjected to the indicated dietary alterations.

[f]Comparisons are between neoplastic liver and normal liver from the same animal subjected to the indicated dietary alterations.

[g]Comparisons are between animals treated with the drug and normal controls.

are relatively ineffective and arachidonate is most effective in the production of this effect (Muto and Gibson, 1970). Administration of fat to fed animals also causes a decrease in acetyl-CoA carboxylase activity (Bortz et al., 1963). Deprivation of two important nutrients, choline and vitamin B_{12}, results in 50-100% elevations in hepatic acetyl-CoA carboxylase activity. The characteristics of these two effects have been studied in greatest detail in relation to accompanying changes of fatty acid synthetase and will be reviewed in the section on control of the synthetase.

Immunochemical techniques have been utilized to determine whether some of these nutritional effects are secondary to changes in content of acetyl-CoA carboxylase or to changes in catalytic efficiency of the enzyme (Majerus and Kilburn, 1969; Nakanishi and Numa, 1970). The data can be summarized by stating that every long-term regulatory effect studied in this regard has been shown to be associated with a change in enzyme content. For example, acetyl-CoA carboxylase antibody, which inactivated and precipitated both protomeric and polymeric forms of the enzyme, was used in quantitative precipitin analyses, which revealed identical equivalence points for extracts from fasted rats and rats fed fat-free, high-fat, and chow diets. Thus, there was a constant and equal amount of immunoprecipitable enzyme per unit of activity in each extract, and therefore differences in specific activity reflected differences in content of enzyme. To determine whether these differences in content of acetyl-CoA carboxylase reflected changes in enzyme synthesis, the Schimke technique (Schimke and Doyle, 1970) of pulse-labeling the enzyme and isolating the radioactive carboxylase by immunoprecipitation was used. Marked increases in the rate of hepatic enzyme synthesis were observed in the animals fed fat-free diets and marked decreases in those fasted and fed high-fat diets. Changes in enzyme synthesis quantitatively accounted for the changes in enzyme levels for all states except fasting. To determine whether changes in the rate of degradation of acetyl-CoA carboxylase contribute to the alterations in hepatic activity, the enzyme was labeled with [^{3}H]leucine, and decay of radioactivity in the carboxylase, isolated by immunoprecipitation, was determined over several days. The half-life ($t_{1/2}$) of acetyl-CoA carboxylase did not vary significantly during normal, fat-free, or high-fat feeding, the value obtained by Majerus and Kilburn (1969) being 48 hr and by Nakanishi and Numa (1970) 55-59 hr. However, a distinct acceleration of the rate of degradation was observed in liver of fasted animals; the former workers noting a $t_{1/2}$ of 18 hr, the latter 31 hr. Thus, during fasting both a decreased rate of enzyme synthesis and an increased rate of degradation contribute to the lowered level of acetyl-CoA carboxylase.

The mechanisms by which the nutritional alterations in acetyl-CoA carboxylase occur are essentially unknown, although they probably do not differ from those underlying similar changes in hepatic fatty acid synthetase (see below). A role for insulin is emphasized by the observation that the increases in hepatic activities of lipogenic enzymes with refeeding a fat-free diet are closely paralleled by increases in levels of plasma insulin (Gibson et al., 1972).

Hormonal factors. A role for insulin in the regulation of acetyl-CoA carboxylase is suggested by the observation of markedly decreased hepatic activity in rats made diabetic by injection of alloxan or streptozotocin (Nakanishi and Numa, 1970; Wieland et al., 1963). Similar observations have been made for adipose tissue (Saggerson and Greenbaum, 1970). Recovery of hepatic activity occurs with insulin replacement. Thus, in addition to its potential role as a short-term effector of acetyl-CoA carboxylase, insulin has a distinct role as a long-term effector. Another pancreatic hormone, glucagon, prevents the marked increase in hepatic activity of acetyl-CoA carboxylase that results when fasted animals are refed a fat-free diet (Volpe and Marasa, 1975a). No effect of glucagon was noted in adipose tissue. Thus, glucagon has both short-term and long-term regulatory effects on hepatic acetyl-CoA carboxylase. Animals made thyrotoxic by 7–9 days of injection of triiodothyronine exhibit approximately twofold higher carboxylase activities in liver and adipose tissue (Diamant et al., 1972). Similarly, hypophysectomized animals exhibit a marked reduction in hepatic carboxylase activity (Volpe and Marasa, 1975a), although animals made only hypothyroid have not been studied in this regard. The most significant alterations in acetyl-CoA carboxylase induced by adrenal steroids occur in adipose tissue (Volpe and Marasa, 1975a). Thus, adipose tissue carboxylase is reduced two- to fourfold by administration of glucocorticoids and is increased twofold by adrenalectomy. These enzymatic effects induced by hormonal factors have been approximately coordinated with measurements of fatty acid synthesis. The mechanisms of the effects are probably similar to those elucidated for fatty acid synthetase (see below).

Developmental factors. Striking changes in acetyl-CoA carboxylase activity in perinatal animals have been described in avian liver (Arinze and Mistry, 1970; Goodridge, 1973b; Ryder, 1970), mammalian liver (Lockwood et al., 1970; Smith and Abraham, 1970a), and mammary gland (Howanitz and Levy, 1965; Mellenberger and Bauman, 1974). Thus, acetyl-CoA carboxylase activity rises dramatically in avian liver after hatching, in mammalian liver at the time of weaning, and in maternal mammary gland during middle to late pregnancy and, again, early in lactation. Alterations in rates of fatty acid synthesis accompany the enzymatic changes, except that in mammalian liver near the time of birth hepatic lipogenesis (Ballard and Hanson, 1967; Taylor et al., 1967) is relatively high and acetyl-CoA carboxylase relatively low (but see development of hepatic fatty acid synthetase below). The regulatory factors of importance in liver under these circumstances are primarily nutritional. The increases in hepatic fatty acid synthesis and in lipogenic enzymatic activity after hatching and with weaning are related primarily to changes in diet from relatively high-fat to relatively low-fat compositions. This explanation is supported by the fact that injecting glucose into embryonic eggs or prematurely weaning mice to a fat-free diet elevates hepatic acetyl-CoA carboxylase (Donaldson et al., 1971; Smith and Abraham, 1970a).

Teraoka and Numa (1975) utilized immunochemical techniques to demonstrate that the rise in acetyl-CoA carboxylase activity in chicken liver between 1 and 9 days after hatching is associated with an increase in enzyme content and that this increase in enzyme content is caused by an increase in enzyme synthesis. Interestingly, no apparent degradation of enzyme was noted in the 1-day-old animals, whereas a degradative rate of 42 hr was present at 9 days. Similar data were obtained for another lipogenic enzyme, malic enzyme (Silpananta and Goodridge, 1971). Direct measurements of the mechanisms underlying the developmental changes in acetyl-CoA carboxylase of mammalian liver have not been carried out, but it might be predicted from the data cited above on the effects of fat-free feeding in mature animals that an increase in enzyme content secondary to an increase in enzyme synthesis is an important regulatory mechanism in the developing liver as well. Support for this prediction is provided by the finding that the increase in hepatic acetyl-CoA carboxylase activity at the time of weaning is blocked by actinomycin D or puromycin (Smith and Abraham, 1970a). Moreover, an increase in the synthesis of mammalian hepatic fatty acid synthetase at the time of weaning has been reported (see below).

Genetic factors. The most detailed studies of fatty acid synthesis in a genetic mutant have been carried out in the Bar Harbor *obese-hyperglycemic* mouse (Bray and York, 1971). These mice carry a single recessive mutant gene for obesity and hyperglycemia (Ingalls et al., 1950) and exhibit elevated hepatic activities of acetyl-CoA carboxylase (Chang et al., 1967), fatty acid synthetase (Chang et al., 1967), and ATP-citrate lyase (Kornacker and Lowenstein, 1964). Utilizing immunochemical techniques, Nakanishi and Numa (1971) demonstrated that the increased level of acetyl-CoA carboxylase activity reflects increased content of enzyme and that the latter is related to a 7.7-fold higher relative rate of synthesis in the obese animals and a 1.7-fold slower rate of degradation ($t_{1/2}$ in obese animals, 115 hr; $t_{1/2}$ in nonobese animals, 67 hr). Regulation of hepatic acetyl-CoA carboxylase by nutritional factors in these animals appears to be different from control in nonobese mice (Maragoudakis et el., 1974). Thus, when the obese animals were fasted for 48 hr and then refed a fat-free diet for 48 hr, hepatic acetyl-CoA carboxylase activity increased ninefold in nonobese animals but only twofold in the obese ones. The acetyl-CoA carboxylase activity observed under these dietary conditions thus became comparable in the nonobese and obese animals. Acetyl-CoA carboxylase from obese animals does not exhibit any significant differences from the enzyme of nonobese animals in terms of catalytic, kinetic, sedimentation, and immunochemical properties (Maragoudakis et al., 1974; Nakanishi and Numa, 1971). The mechanisms for the differences in regulation are probably similar to those elucidated for fatty acid synthetase in the mutants (see below).

Pharmacologic factors. Because of their use as agents in the therapy of *hyperlipidemia,* certain drugs have been studied in considerable detail in recent years (Maragoudakis, 1969, 1970a, 1970b, 1971b; Maragoudakis and Hankin, 1971a; Maragoudakis et al., 1972; Schacht and Granzer, 1970; Zakim et al., 1970). Prominent examples of such drugs with a major effect on fatty acid synthesis are 2-methyl-2-[*p*-(1,2,3,4-tetrahydro-1-napthyl)phenoxyl] propionic acid (TPIA) and 2(*p*-chlorophenoxy)-2-methyl propionic acid (CPIB-acid). Hepatic lipogenesis from acetate is depressed in rats treated with TPIA and in mammary gland cell cultures grown in the presence of TPIA and CPIB-acid (Maragoudakis, 1971b). TPIA was at least ten times more potent an inhibitor than CPIB-acid. At least one significant mechanism for the depression in fatty acid synthesis induced by these drugs is related to their effect on acetyl-CoA carboxylase. Maragoudakis (1969, 1970a, 1970b, 1971a) has shown that the drugs inhibit acetyl-CoA carboxylase of avian and rat liver and that the inhibition of the drugs is competitive with activation by citrate. The relevance of these findings to the *in vivo* data is suggested by the finding that *in vitro,* as in the whole animal and in cell culture, TPIA is at least ten times more potent an inhibitor of citrate acitvation than is CPIB-acid. Moreover, *in vivo* reduction of the specific activity of hepatic acetyl-CoA carboxylase accompanies the reduction in hepatic lipogenesis induced by TPIA or CPIB-acid.

The mechanism of the pharmacologic effect on acetyl-CoA carboxylase may be related to a direct interaction of the drug with the enzyme. Thus, when animals were treated with [^{14}C] TPIA and the carboxylase precipitated by ammonium sulfate, at least 50% of the labeled drug was also precipitated. The label could be removed by dialysis of the dissolved ammonium sulfate precipitate against a citrate-containing buffer, and under these conditions a direct relation was observed between restoration of acetyl-CoA carboxylase activity and removal of [^{14}C] TPIA by dialysis. Although these data suggested the possibility of an enzyme-drug complex, attempts to isolate such a complex by immunoprecipitation were unsuccessful. Nevertheless, the data do indicate that these lipid-lowering agents inhibit acetyl-CoA carboxylase *in vivo* and *in vitro.* However, the dramatic decreases in lipogenesis observed *in vivo* and in cell culture often are more extensive than the decreases in acetyl-CoA carboxylase activity, raising the possibility that the hypolipidemic effects are related in part to other effects of the agents. In support of this possibility are the findings that the drugs inhibit *in vivo* the activity of certain key enzymes of glycolysis (phosphofructokinase, pyruvate kinase) (Schacht and Granzer, 1970), gluconeogenesis (phosphoenolpyruvate carboxykinase (Schacht and Granzer, 1970), and lipogenesis (glucose-6-phosphate dehydrogenase) (Zakim et al., 1970), and *in vitro* (in relatively high concentrations) the activity of fatty acid synthetase (Zakim et al., 1970).

Fatty Acid Synthetase

Fatty acid synthetase is the multienzyme complex that catalyzes the synthesis of saturated fatty acids from malonyl CoA. Requirements of the reaction include acetyl CoA and NADPH, as indicated in the following equation:

$$CH_3CO\text{-}S\text{-}CoA + 7\ HOOCCH_2CO\text{-}S\text{-}CoA + 14\ NADPH + 14\ H^+ \rightarrow$$

$$CH_3CH_2(CH_2CH_2)_6CH_2COOH + 7\ CO_2 + 14\ NADP^+$$

$$+ 8\ CoA\text{-}SH + 6\ H_2O \qquad (7)$$

The stoichiometry of the reaction in animals was determined initially in pigeon liver (Wakil, 1961; Wakil and Ganguly, 1959), rat liver (Brady et al., 1960), and rat brain (Brady, 1960). The enzyme was discovered in yeast by Lynen (1961) as a multienzyme complex. Comparable complexes have been isolated and purified from pigeon liver (Hsu et al., 1965), chicken liver (Hsu and Yun, 1970), rat liver (Burton et al., 1968), human liver (Roncari, 1974b), rat (Smith and Abraham, 1970b), rabbit (Carey and Dils, 1970), guinea pig (Strong and Dils, 1972), and bovine mammary gland (Knudsen, 1972; Maitra and Kumar, 1974b), *Mycobacterium smegmatis* (Brindley et al., 1969), *Corynebacterium diphtheriae* (Knoche and Koths, 1973), and *Euglena gracilis* (Delo et al., 1971; Goldberg and Bloch, 1972).

Reaction sequence. Primarily on the basis of observations made with model compounds and the susceptibility of the enzyme complex to inactivation by sulfhydryl (SH) binding agents, Lynen (1961) originally proposed that the acyl intermediates in fatty acid biosynthesis are bound in thioester linkage to the component enzymes of the complex. Experiments in *E. coli* demonstrated that, indeed, a central component of the fatty acid synthetase is the acyl carrier protein (ACP) and that the intermediates are acyl groups bound in thioester linkage to the 4'-phosphopantetheine moiety of ACP (Majerus et al., 1965a). Study of *E. coli* synthetase, which is not a tightly associated complex, led to the delineation of the nature of the protein-bound intermediates as well as the details of the intermediate reactions of the fatty acid synthetase (Majerus et al., 1964; Majerus and Vagelos, 1967; Vagelos et al., 1966; Wakil et al., 1964). The following reaction sequence was elucidated:

$$CH_3CO\text{-}S\text{-}CoA + HS\text{-}ACP \rightarrow CH_3CO\text{-}S\text{-}ACP + CoA\text{-}SH \qquad (8)$$

$$CH_3CO\text{-}S\text{-}ACP + HS\text{-}E_{cond} \rightarrow CH_3CO\text{-}S\text{-}E_{cond} + ACP\text{-}SH \qquad (9)$$

$$HOOCCH_2CO\text{-}S\text{-}CoA + HS\text{-}ACP \rightarrow HOOCCH_2CO\text{-}S\text{-}ACP + CoA\text{-}SH \quad (10)$$

$$HOOCCH_2CO\text{-}S\text{-}ACP + CH_3CO\text{-}S\text{-}E_{cond} \rightarrow CO_2$$

$$+ HS\text{-}E_{cond} + CH_3COCH_2CO\text{-}S\text{-}ACP \qquad (11)$$

$$CH_3COCH_2CO\text{-}S\text{-}ACP + NADPH + H^+ \rightarrow NADP^+$$

$$+ CH_3CHOHCH_2CO\text{-}S\text{-}ACP \qquad (12)$$

$$CH_3CHOHCH_2CO\text{-}S\text{-}ACP \rightarrow H_2O + CH_2CH=CHCO\text{-}S\text{-}ACP \quad (13)$$

$$CH_3CH=CHCO\text{-}S\text{-}ACP + NADPH + H^+ \rightarrow$$

$$CH_3CH_2CH_2CO\text{-}S\text{-}ACP + NADP^+ \quad (14)$$

In reaction 8 the enzyme acetyl-CoA-ACP transacylase catalyzes the transfer of an acetyl group from the SH group of CoA to that of ACP to form acetyl-S-ACP. When the latter acetyl group is transferred in turn to an SH group (a cysteine residue) of the condensing enzyme (reaction 9), ACP is liberated and can accept a malonyl group (reaction 10), transferred by malonyl-CoA-ACP transacylase. The condensation reaction follows, and the β-ketoacyl derivative formed then undergoes the first (reaction 12) of the two reductions catalyzed by the fatty acid synthetase. A dehydration (reaction 13) and the second reduction (reaction 14) then result in the formation of a four-carbon saturated acyl-ACP thioester. This can then react with the condensing enzyme in reaction 9 to form the acyl-enzyme intermediate, liberating ACP to react with another malonyl group and thus initiate another sequence of condensation, reduction, dehydration, and reduction. The synthetase of *E. coli,* like that of the animal and plant systems, gives rise *in vitro* to free palmitate as the final product due to the action of a long-chain thioesterase. However, *in vivo* in *E. coli,* palmityl-S-ACP probably reacts directly with glycerol 3-phosphate and a specific membranous acyltransferase to form lysophosphatidic acid, the first intermediate in the pathway of phospholipid biosynthesis (Ailhaud and Vagelos, 1966; Goldfine et al., 1967; Van den Bosch and Vagelos, 1970). The additional observation that ACP in *E. coli* is localized on or very near the inner aspect of the cell membrane strongly suggests that the product of the synthetase reaction is well positioned for direct incorporation into the phospholipids of the cell membrane (Van Den Bosch et al., 1970).

Acyl carrier protein. The ACP of fatty acid synthetase plays a central role in fatty acid synthesis, as illustrated in the reactions of the enzyme system (equations 8-14). The discovery, isolation, and demonstration of the important structural and functional properties of *E. coli* ACP have been reviewed recently (Prescott and Vagelos, 1972) and will not be reiterated here. Nevertheless, it should be emphasized that the most significant feature of all ACPs is the 4'-phosphopantetheine prosthetic group, initially discovered in *E. coli* (Majerus et al., 1965a) and illustrated below:

```
serine
  |
  O        H₃C      O H              O H
  |         |       ‖ |              ‖ |
HO—P—O—CH₂—C—CH—C—N—CH₂—CH₂—C—N—CH₂—CH₂—SH
  ‖         |  |
  O        H₃C OH
```

The acetyl intermediates in fatty acid synthesis are bound in thioester linkage to the SH group of the 4'-phosphopantetheine, and the latter is bound to the protein as a phosphodiester with the hydroxyl of a serine residue (Majerus et al., 1965b; Pugh and Wakil, 1965).

Acyl Carrier Protein of Animals. The nature of the ACP of animal fatty acid synthetase has been an important topic for recent research, because elucidation of the structure and mode of interaction of this protein within the tightly associated multienzyme complex would provide considerable insight into the function and organization of such systems. Although unequivocal isolation of animal ACP in pure form has not yet been accomplished, the primary structure of rat liver ACP at the site of the 4'-phosphopantetheine moiety has been elucidated (Roncari et al., 1972). Rat fatty acid synthetase was labeled in its 4'-phosphopantetheine moiety by injecting animals with radioactive pantothenate. The radioactive synthetase was subjected to proteolytic digestion and radioactive peptides were characterized (Roncari et al., 1972). The sequence of 13 residues around the active serine residue was shown to be: Leu-Gly-*Ser*-Leu-Asx-Leu-Gly-Glx-*Gly*-Glu-*Asp-Ser**-*Leu*. The asterisk refers to the serine to which the 4'-phosphopantetheine was bound, and the italicized residues are homologous with those surrounding the active serine of *E. coli* ACP (Vanaman et al., 1968b).

Relatively small peptides considered to represent animal ACP have been isolated recently from pigeon liver (Qureshi et al., 1975b), dog liver (Roncari, 1974a), and chicken liver (Bratcher and Hsu, 1975). Porter and co-workers successfully separated the approximately half-molecular-weight subunits of pigeon liver by affinity chromatography (Lornitzo et al., 1974) (see below). One such subunit contained all of the radioactivity incorporated into the fatty acid synthetase on injection of [^{14}C]pantothenate into pigeons. When this subunit was allowed to stand overnight in 0.1 M Tris-phosphate buffer, pH 8.5, at 0°–4°C and then was concentrated by means of PM-10 ultrafiltration, 10% of the radioactivity was found in the filtrate (Qureshi et al., 1974). A radioactive peptide, isolated from the filtrate, migrated in a similar manner to *E. coli* ACP when subjected to high-voltage electrophoresis and cochromatographed with the bacterial protein on Sephadex G-50. The pigeon liver ACP peptide was an acceptor for an acetyl group from acetyl CoA and a malonyl group from malonyl CoA when incubated in the presence of the second subunit of pigeon liver fatty acid synthetase—that is, the transacylase subunit. Sulfhydryl analyses of the pigeon liver ACP peptide showed one SH equivalent per 9,000 daltons, and the peptide contained 82 amino acids and one β-alanine residue. No specific attempts to eliminate or assess proteolysis in the isolation procedures were carried out. Virtually simultaneously, Roncari (1974a) reported that SDS treatment of purified dog liver fatty acid synthetase, labeled in its 4'-phosphopantetheine group, led to release of a small radioactive peptide. The molecular weight determined by gel elctrophoresis and by gel filtration chromatography was in the range 9,000–13,500. The peptide could not be isolated when the purified synthetase was treated only with guanidine-HCl and urea, without SDS. When the proteolytic inhibitor, phenylmethylsulfonyl fluoride, was present throughout all procedures, similar results were obtained.

Most recently, Bratcher and Hsu (1975) have isolated a peptide of molecular weight 6,000 from the dissociated chicken liver synthetase. Details of the characterization of this peptide are yet to be reported. Although these findings, with the animal fatty acid synthetase complexes, of ACP-like peptides with molecular weights similar to that of *E. coli* ACP are intriguing, it is not yet clear that such peptides represent animal ACP. Thus, Wakil and co-workers (Stoops et al., 1975) have shown that the fatty acid synthetases of chicken and rat liver are composed of two polypeptide chains of molecular weight 220,000–250,000. Highly purified preparations have been shown to contain protease that becomes activated in SDS, guanidine-HCl, or urea. Inactivation of the protease made it possible to dissociate the complex in the presence of SDS, guanidine-HCl, urea, or a combination thereof, into polypeptides of ~220,000 daltons. Labeling fatty acid synthetase with [^{14}C]pantothenate, [^{14}C]acetyl, or [^{14}C]malonyl groups resulted in labeling only these two polypeptides. Similar findings have been obtained with purified fatty acid synthetases from rat and human liver and from Chang liver cells grown in culture (Alberts et al., 1976). These data lead decisively to the conclusion that the synthetase of animal liver is composed of two polypeptides, one (or both) of which contains the prosthetic group, 4'-phosphopantetheine (ACP). This conclusion is analogous to that reached earlier by Schweizer et al. (1973), based on studies of fatty acid synthetase mutants in yeast (see below). The yeast complex appears to be composed of two different polypeptide chains; ACP is not an individual protein component of the synthetase complex but rather a distinct region of one of the polypeptide chains.

Structure-Function Relationships. The role of ACP as acyl carrier for all of the intermediates in fatty acid synthesis indicates that protein-protein interactions are critical in its function. Elucidation of the structure-function relationships of ACP, therefore, could make a significant contribution to our understanding not only of ACP but of protein-protein interactions in general. Delineation of the complete amino acid sequence of *E. coli* ACP by Vanaman et al. (1968b) was an important step toward this goal. The most critical feature of the sequence is the serine residue to which the prosthetic group is attached at position 36, approximately the middle of the 77 amino acid peptide. Although considerable insight into structure-function relationships has been gained in recent years by analyses of peptide fragments produced by chemical modification and proteolytic digestion, the most decisive definition of the structure-function relationships of ACP was made possible by the synthesis of apo-ACP by solid-phase techniques (Merrifield, 1963). The data derived from these studies have been recently reviewed (Volpe and Vagelos, 1976).

Prosthetic Group Turnover. A pantothenate auxotroph of *E. coli* was utilized to establish that CoA is the immediate precursor of the 4′-phosphopantetheine prosthetic group of ACP (Alberts and Vagelos, 1966). The synthesis of holo-ACP from apo-ACP is catalyzed by the enzyme holo-ACP synthetase according to:

$$\text{CoA} + \text{apo-ACP} \xrightarrow{\text{Mg}^{2+}} \text{holo-ACP} + \text{adenosine-3}′,5′\text{-diphosphate} \qquad (15)$$

Another enzyme of *E. coli,* ACP hydrolase, catalyzes the hydrolysis of ACP to yield the prosthetic group and the apoprotein, according to:

$$\text{holo-ACP} \xrightarrow{\text{Mn}^{2+}} \text{apo-ACP} + 4′\text{-phosphopantetheine} \qquad (16)$$

The 4′-phosphopantetheine is converted to CoA through expenditure of two molecules of ATP:

$$4′\text{-Phosphopantetheine} \xrightarrow{\text{ATP} \rightarrow \text{PP}_i} \text{dephospho CoA} \xrightarrow{\text{ATP} \rightarrow \text{ADP}} \text{CoA} \qquad (17)$$

Holo-ACP synthetase and ACP-hydrolase have been purified and partially characterized from *E. coli* (Elovson and Vagelos, 1968; Prescott et al., 1969; Vagelos and Larrabee, 1967) but these enzymes have not yet been isolated from mammalian tissue.

These enzymes participate in a remarkably rapid turnover of the 4′-phosphopantetheine prosthetic group in *E. coli* (Powell et al., 1969). A similar rapid turnover of the prosthetic group occurs in mammalian cells and may be of regulatory significance (see discussion of regulation below).

Multienzyme complexes. Yeast. The fatty acid synthetase of yeast purifies as a homogenous protein with a molecular weight of 2,300,000 (Lynen, 1961, 1969; Lynen et al., 1964), and contains 3.5–6.0 mol of 4′-phosphopantetheine per mole of enzyme (Schweizer et al., 1970). Lynen's studies of this enzyme system provided the first major insight into the chemical details of fatty acid synthesis from acetyl CoA and malonyl CoA. The work also provided an understanding of the mode of action of the fatty acid synthetases that occur as tightly associated multienzyme complexes—those of animals and yeast. The overall reaction catalyzed by the yeast enzyme is

$$\text{CH}_3\text{CO-S-CoA} + n \text{ COOHCH}_2\text{CO-S-CoA} + 2n \text{ NADPH} + 2n \text{ H}^+ \rightarrow$$

$$\text{CH}_3(\text{CH}_2\text{CH}_2)_n\text{CO-S-CoA} + n \text{ CO}_2 + n \text{ CoA} + 2n \text{ NADP}^+ + n \text{ H}_2\text{O} \qquad (18)$$

The similarity to the reaction for *E. coli* (reaction 7) is obvious; the most important difference is the product obtained *in vitro*—that is, acyl CoA thioesters, rather than free long-chain fatty acids as in bacteria and animals.

Structural and functional organization. Important insight into the structural and functional organization of the yeast, and probably fatty acid synthetase multienzyme complexes of animals, has been provided by the studies of Schweizer and co-workers with various fatty acid synthetase mutants of *Saccharomyces cerevisiae* (Burkl et al., 1972; Kuhn et al., 1972; Schweizer and Golling, 1970; Schweizer et al., 1971, 1973). Because of its extreme importance and probable relevance for animal synthetases, this work will be considered in detail. Detailed genetic studies, based on complementation analyses and assay of all the component enzymes of the fatty acid synthetase by model reactions, indicate that in yeast the multienzyme complex is encoded by two polycistronic and genetically distinct gene loci, designated *fas* 1 and *fas* 2. The structural genes for four of the seven different fatty acid synthetase components have been allocated to distinct regions within these loci. One locus (*fas* 2) contains the cistrons for β-ketoacyl synthetase and β-ketoacyl reductase, and other (*fas* 1) for enoyl reductase and dehydrase. The protein structure encoded by these genetic loci has been demonstrated by dissociating the purified yeast synthetase in SDS with or without guanidine-HCl. SDS gel electrophoresis resolves two major components, designated A and B, with molecular weights of 185,000 and 180,000. Pantothenate is bound to the A component.

The genetic locus that contains the cistron for the prosthetic group of the yeast synthetase was defined recently by the study of pantetheine-deficient mutants (Schweizer et al., 1973). The mutants were shown to be unable to incorporate [^{14}C]pantothenate into the fatty acid synthetase multienzyme complex. The mutants apparently lacked only the pantetheine prosthetic group, rather than the entire ACP, because on SDS gel electrophoresis no differences in molecular weight could be observed between the protein components of the 4'-phosphopantetheine-free mutant fatty acid synthetase and those of the wild-type complex. It was not possible to determine whether the defect involved ACP or holo-ACP synthetase. When the purified 4'-phosphopantetheine-free fatty acid synthetase of the mutant was tested for the seven known components of the complex, only the β-ketoacyl synthetase activity was found to be impaired. This finding is in keeping with previous observations with model substrates that only the β-ketoacyl synthetase is strictly specific for ACP derivatives. It was further shown that the 4'-phosphopantetheine is bound to the same polypeptide chain as the β-ketoacyl synthetase—component A—which is encoded by the *fas* 2 genetic locus. It was thus concluded that ACP of the yeast fatty acid synthetase is represented by a specific region of a large, multifunctional polypeptide chain rather than by an individual protein component. This finding has direct relevance to the search for the ACP of the animal complexes and may explain the difficulty of dissociating a small ACP peptide from these complexes.

Taken together, the data of Schweizer and co-workers suggest that the yeast multienzyme complex is composed of two different polypeptide chains multiply combined in an undetermined ratio in the complex. This would account for the molecular weight (2,300,000) and pantothenate composition of the complex. The polypeptide chains are clearly multifunctional. The difficulty in isolating individual enzyme components from the complex is explained by their *covalent* association within multifunctional chains. This type of organization for a multienzyme complex represents an evolutionary advance when compared to a heteropolymeric aggregate of individual component enzymes. The problem of subunit assembly and stoichiometry are solved in a unique and efficient way (Schweizer et al., 1973).

Reaction mechanism. The details of the reaction mechanism of yeast fatty acid synthetase were elucidated primarily by kinetic and inhibition studies, isolation of acyl intermediates, and study of model reactions. These details have been reviewed recently (Volpe and Vagelos, 1976).

Liver. Fatty acid synthetase has been purified to homogeneity as a tightly associated multienzyme complex from liver of pigeon (Hsu et al., 1965), chicken (Hsu and Yun, 1970), rat (Burton et al., 1968), and human (Roncari, 1974b). The enzyme from pigeon liver has a molecular weight of 450,000 (Yang et al., 1967); chicken liver, 508,000 (Hsu and Yun, 1970; Yun and Hsu, 1972); rat liver, 540,000 (Hsu and Yun, 1970); and human liver, 410,000 (Roncari, 1974b). Each of the complexes is inhibited by SH binding agents. Products of both the avian (Bressler and Wakil, 1962) and mammalian (Brady et al., 1960) synthetases *in vitro* are free fatty acids, primarily palmitate, rather than thioesters of CoA as in yeast.

All attempts to dissociate the multienzyme complexes of animals or yeast into individual enzyme components have been unsuccessful. Attempts with detergents like palmityl CoA or SDS (Butterworth et al., 1967; Dorsey and Porter, 1968; Roncari, 1974b), maleate (Butterworth et al., 1967), or phenol-acetic acid-urea (Yang et al., 1967) have led to a variable number of bands when preparations were subjected to gel electrophoresis. Enzymatically active components were not isolated from these procedures. Moreover, these experiments were carried out under conditions that could easily be complicated by proteolysis. Less drastic procedures have led to the dissociation of the complexes of pigeon (Butterworth et al., 1967; Kumar et al., 1970; Muesing et al., 1975; Yang et al., 1965), rat (Burton et al., 1968), and chicken (Yun and Hsu, 1972) liver into approximately half-molecular-weight subcomplexes. This is accomplished most easily with the enzyme from pigeon liver, and the most detailed studies of this phenomenon have been carried out with this system by Porter and co-workers. This dissociation can be accomplished by storage in 2-mercaptoethanol (aging), reaction with carboxymethylsulfide, or exposure to low ionic strength, high pH, or low temperature.

Stability is enhanced by phosphate ions (Kumar et al., 1972), fructose 1,6-diphosphate (Jacobs et al., 1970), and NADPH (Kumar and Porter, 1971). The mechanism of the dissociative process is not understood. Dissociation can occur without oxidation of SH groups, and inactivation by oxidation of SH groups can occur without dissociation (Kumar et al., 1972; Yun and Hsu, 1972). The relative contributions of changes in hydrophobic and electrostatic interactions remain unclear. Comparison of the rates of reassociation, as determined by ultracentrifugation studies, and the kinetics of reactivation led to the conclusion that an intact complex inactive for fatty acid synthesis is formed before reactivation (Muesing et al., 1975). The nature of the change in the complex that leads to reactivation is unknown.

Structural and functional organization. Important insight into the structure and function of the fatty acid synthetase of animal liver was gained by study of the approximately half-molecular-weight subcomplexes formed by dissociation by low ionic strength of the pigeon liver enzyme. These two components catalyze all of the partial reactions of the intact complex, except for the condensation reaction (Kumar et al., 1970, 1972). Recently, the half-molecular-weight components of the pigeon liver enzyme have been separated by an affinity chromatography column containing ε-aminocaproyl-pantetheine bound to cyanogen bromide-activated Sepharose through the ε-amino group (Lornitzo et al., 1974). When dissociated 4'-phospho[^{14}C]-pantetheine-labeled pigeon liver fatty acid synthetase was passed over the column, the subunit containing 4'-phospho[^{14}C]pantetheine, and presumably the ACP of the complex, was only slightly retarded, whereas the subunit free of label was strongly adsorbed. The two subunits were then further purified by sucrose density gradient centrifugation. Recombination of the purified subunits under appropriate conditions yielded an enzymatically active fatty acid synthetase complex. The subunit containing the ACP also contained the β-ketoacyl reductase activity, and the other subunit contained the acetyl-CoA transacylase activity. These data are of particular interest in view of Schweizer's demonstration that the yeast complex is composed of two polypeptide chains and that the component that contains the ACP also contains the β-ketoacyl reductase. If, as now seems probable, the animal multienzyme complex is composed, like the yeast multienzyme complex, of two polypeptide chains with the component proteins covalently attached, a clear explanation will be apparent for the great difficulty encountered in dissociating the synthetase into individual, active enzymes, as well as ACP. Moreover, a new mode of structural organization for multienzyme complexes in animals will be defined. The recent data indicating a similar type of organization for the components of animal acetyl-CoA carboxylase is of particular interest in this regard.

Reaction mechanism. The mechanism of action proposed for the animal fatty synthetase is similar to that proposed earlier by Lynen for the yeast multienzyme complex. The partial reactions of the synthetase were demonstrated with model substrates (Kumar et al., 1970). These features have been reviewed recently (Volpe and Vagelos, 1976).

Other Multienzyme Complexes. Fatty acid synthetase has been purified to homogeneity as a multienzyme complex from mammary gland of the rat (Smith and Abraham, 1970b), rabbit (Carey and Dils, 1970), guinea pig (Strong and Dils, 1972), and cow (Knudsen, 1972; Maitra and Kumar, 1974b), certain advanced bacteria (e.g., *Mycobacterium smegmatis* Brindley et al., 1969; Vance et al., 1973), *Corynebacterium diphtheriae* (Knoche et al., 1973; Knoche and Koths, 1973)), and a unicellular phytoflagellate, *Euglena gracilis* (Delo et al., 1971; Goldberg and Bloch, 1972). The distinctive features of these synthetases have been reviewed recently (Volpe and Vagelos, 1976).

Primer specificity. Recent studies indicate that the primer for fatty acid synthetase of mammary gland and mammalian liver is butyryl CoA rather than acetyl CoA (Lin and Kumar, 1971, 1972; Maitra and Kumar, 1974a, 1974b; Nandedkar and Kumar, 1969; Smith and Abraham, 1971). We have drawn a similar conclusion on the basis of current work with synthetase purified from mammalian brain (Volpe, unpublished). Since the initial work on the fatty acid synthetases of pigeon liver, yeast, and bacteria, systems that do preferentially utilize acetyl CoA as primer, it has been assumed that the universal primer for the reaction is acetyl CoA. Kumar and co-workers have demonstrated in the soluble fraction of mammary tissues enzymes that catalyze the reversal of the β-oxidation steps from butyryl CoA to acetyl CoA (thus, the term β-reductive enzymes). The steps involved are:

$$\text{2 Acetyl CoA} \xleftrightarrow[\text{thiolase}]{\beta\text{-ketoacyl-CoA}} \text{acetoacetyl CoA + CoASH} \qquad (19)$$

$$\text{Acetoacetyl CoA + NADH + H}^+ \xleftrightarrow[\text{reductase}]{\beta\text{-ketoacyl}} \beta\text{-hydroxybutyryl CoA + NAD}^+ \qquad (20)$$

$$\beta\text{-Hydroxybutyryl CoA} \xrightleftharpoons[\text{hydratase}]{\text{enoyl-CoA}} \text{crotonyl CoA + H}_2\text{O} \qquad (21)$$

$$\text{Crotonyl CoA + NADPH + H}^+ \xrightarrow[\text{(fatty acid synthetase)}]{\text{enoyl-CoA reductase}} \text{butyryl CoA + NADP}^+ \qquad (22)$$

The first three reactions are catalyzed by enzymes that precipitate between 30 and 60% ammonium sulfate saturation, and the last reaction is catalyzed by an enzyme that precipitates between 0 and 30% ammonium sulfate saturation. This enoyl-CoA reductase step is, in fact, an inherent property of FAS. [This was proved conclusively by the demonstration that the crotonyl-CoA reductase and the synthetase activities of lactating bovine mammary gland copurified with a constant ratio of the two activities, cochromatographed on Sephadex, had comparable K_m values for crotonyl CoA, and exhibited similar loss and recovery of activity when the complex was dissociated and reassociated (Maitra and Kumar, 1974a, 1974b).]

Lin and Kumar (1972) showed that the synthetases of rat and rabbit liver, as well as of mammary gland, were more active with butyryl CoA than with acetyl CoA as primer. We have obtained preliminary data concerning the primer specificity of fatty acid synthetase of mammalian brain and have observed a higher V_{max} and lower K_m when butyryl CoA rather than acetyl CoA is used as primer (Volpe, unpublished). In addition, by (1) incubating particle-free supernatant solution in a reaction mixture suitable for fatty acid synthesis and the β-reductive steps, containing [1-^{14}C] acetyl CoA and unlabeled malonyl-CoA, and (2) subjecting the fatty acids formed to Kuhn-Roth oxidation, it was demonstrated that 90% of the acetyl CoA was converted to butyryl CoA prior to condensation with malonyl CoA (Lin and Kumar, 1972).

The first reaction of the β-reductive pathway is catalyzed by acetoacetyl-CoA thiolase. A cytosolic form of this enzyme has been described in mammalian liver (Williamson et al., 1968; Middleton, 1973). The enzyme was isolated from avian liver and characterized by Lane and co-workers (Clinkenbeard et al., 1973). That this cytosolic thiolase is distinct from the mitochondrial thiolase was shown by isoelectric focusing. The cytosolic thiolase is involved in regulation of cholesterol synthesis, as discussed below. The formation of acetoacetyl CoA by this reaction—that is, the reaction in the condensation rather than in the thiolytic direction—is thermodynamically unfavorable. However, the reaction can be driven in the condensation direction in fatty acid synthesis when coupled with the thermodynamically favorable β-ketoacyl reductase reaction. (As will be discussed below, the thiolase reaction may also be driven in the condensation direction in cholesterolgenesis when coupled with the HMG-CoA synthase reaction). It is noteworthy that this cytoplasmic acetoacetyl-CoA reductase differs from the mitochondrial enzyme of β-oxidation in its ability to oxidize D(−)-β-hydroxybutyryl CoA at a faster rate than the CoA derivative of the L(+) isomer (Nandedkar and Kumar, 1969). The conversion of β-hydroxybutyryl CoA to crotonyl CoA can proceed relatively freely, and the final fatty acid synthetase-catalyzed enoyl-CoA reductase reaction proceeds readily to butyryl CoA. Butyryl CoA is then utilized as the preferred primer in the synthetase reaction for palmitate synthesis.

Since acetoacetyl CoA lies at a branch point in cholesterol as well as fatty acid synthesis, regulation at this level may be of considerable importance in lipogenesis. Thus, consideration of this β-reductive pathway in the overall scheme of lipid biosynthesis from acetyl CoA (Fig. 1) leads to the conclusion that an important first committed step in fatty acid synthesis is the

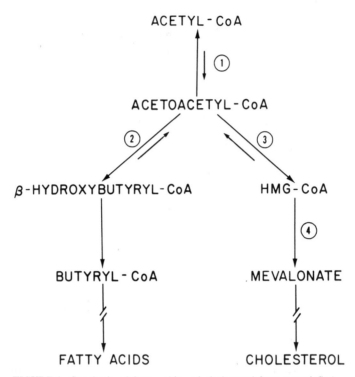

FIGURE 1 Synthesis of fatty acids and cholesterol from acetyl CoA, with emphasis on acetoacetyl CoA as an important intermediate. Reactions 1–4 are catalyzed by acetoacetyl-CoA thiolase, β-ketoacyl-CoA reductase, HMG-CoA synthase, and HMG-CoA reductase. Butyryl CoA is utilized as primer to be elongated by malonyl CoA in the synthesis of fatty acids by fatty acid synthetase.

conversion of acetoacetyl CoA to β-hydroxybutyryl CoA by the β-ketoacyl-CoA reductase. Since this reaction is probably best considered as coupled to the thiolase, the thiolase and reductase are good candidates for regulation of fatty acid synthesis. As will be discussed in more detail below, the aceto-acetyl-CoA thiolase is also coupled to the first committed step in cholesterol synthesis, that is, the HMG-CoA synthase reaction.

    Regulation. Allosteric Effects. Fatty acid synthetase undergoes rapid catalytic changes under certain circumstances *in vitro*. The physiological significance of these changes is obscure, and at the present time no study has established unequivocally a physiological role for synthetase in short-term regulation. The most important potential mechanisms for such regulation are discussed next.

    Hexose phosphates. Wakil and co-workers (Plate et al., 1968; Wakil et al., 1966) first made the intriguing observation that the fatty acid synthetases of pigeon liver and *E. coli* are stimulated by phosphorylated sugars, especially fructose 1,6-diphosphate. At comparable concentrations (20 m*M*) lesser degrees of stimulation were observed with glucose 1-phosphate, glucose 6-phosphate, α-glycerol phosphate, pyrophosphate, and orthophosphate (Wakil et al., 1966). These observations were of particular interest because they suggested a means whereby fatty acid synthesis could be attuned to glucose metabolism, and certaintly the stimulatory effect of carbohydrate consumption on lipogenesis in animals is the best established of all regulatory responses studied. Hepatic levels of fructose 1,6-diphosphate and fatty acid synthesis are enhanced when carbohydrate is readily available (Brunengraber et al., 1973). Kinetic studies with the avian liver synthetase suggested that the effect of phosphorylated sugars was related to inhibition of the synthetase by malonyl CoA, and this inhibition was competitive with respect to NADPH (Plate et al., 1968). The K_m for NADPH was decreased by fructose 1,6-diphosphate, and the sugar reversed inhibition by malonyl CoA. It was suggested that hexose diphosphate acted either by competing for a regulatory site or by binding at a specific site to promote a conformational change of the enzyme, rendering it insensitive to malonyl CoA inhibition. The effect of the hexose diphosphate on the K_m for NADPH may be more important than reversal of malonyl CoA inhibition. Thus, purified synthetase of human liver is not inhibited by malonyl CoA (Roncari, 1975). However, the human synthetase is stimulated two- to threefold by 10 m*M* fructose 1,6-diphosphate and five- to sixfold by 100 m*M* concentrations. Less striking stimulation is seen with fructose 6-phosphate and glucose 6-phosphate and none with phosphoenolpyruvate or glycero-3-phosphate. Nevertheless, the significance of these findings is difficult to interpret for several reasons. First, Porter and co-workers were unable to show any effect of hexose diphosphates on the enzyme activities of purified pigeon or rat liver fatty acid synthetases (Porter et al., 1971), and no effect was observed with the synthetase of rat mammary gland (Smith and Abraham, 1970b). Similarly, we have been unable to demonstrate any effect with the synthetase of rat brain (Volpe, unpublished). Second, the concentration of phosphorylated sugars tested *in vitro* are well above physiological concentrations (Porter et al., 1971). (The possibility of compartmentalization of relatively high concentrations of the sugars has not been ruled out.) Third, concentrations of malonyl CoA as high as 100 μ*M* had no effect on binding of NADPH to the pigeon liver fatty acid synthetase, as determined by fluorescence emission spectroscopy (Dugan and Porter, 1970). Thus, although a physiological role for this apparent allosteric effect of hexose phosphates on hepatic fatty acid synthetase remains unproved, further studies will be of interest.

Long-chain fatty acyl CoA derivatives. Palmityl CoA and other long-chain acyl CoA derivatives inhibit *in vitro* the fatty acid synthetase of pigeon liver (Dorsey and Porter, 1968), rat liver (Tubbs and Garland, 1963), human liver (Roncari, 1975), and rat brain (Robinson et al., 1963). The idea of feedback inhibition as an important regulatory mechanism received support from findings that liver concentrations of long-chain acyl CoA derivatives are elevated in starvation and high-fat feeding when hepatic synthetase activity is low (Bortz and Lynen, 1963b; Tubbs and Garland, 1963). However, the effect of palmityl CoA on the pigeon liver enzyme was questioned by Dorsey and Porter (1968). Inhibition by the thioester depended on the molar ratio of palmityl CoA to protein, and this suggested that palmityl CoA acts as a detergent and is not a site-specific inhibitor. The inhibition was irreversible and similar to that produced by SDS, another detergent. Similar findings were recorded by Roncari (1975) with purified human liver synthetase. Moreover, palmityl CoA has been shown to inhibit nonspecifically a wide variety of enzymes via its detergent properties (Taketa and Pogell, 1966). Perhaps most important, as discussed above in relation to the regulation of acetyl-CoA carboxylase, fatty acid synthetase of animal liver does not exhibit the competitive, reversible inhibition by long-chain acyl CoA that is seen with acetyl-CoA carboxylase. Thus, the sum of current information does not support a role for long-chain acyl CoA derivatives in short-term regulation of fatty acid synthetase. A possible role for these compounds in long-term regulation is suggested by data to be reviewed below.

Phosphorylation-dephosphorylation. Porter and co-workers (Qureshi et al., 1975a) have recently separated, by affinity chromatography on Sepharose ε-aminocaproylpantetheine, purified avian liver holo-FAS into a high specific activity form (holo-a) and a low specific activity form (holo-b). When animals were injected with $^{32}PO_4^{2-}$ prior to enzyme isolation, ^{32}P was found to be incorporated into the purified synthetase. After isolation by affinity chromatography, holo-b was found to contain a much greater amount of radioactivity than holo-a. The low-activity holo-b synthetase (^{32}P-labeled) could be converted to high-activity holo-a synthetase after incubation with Mg^{2+} and a phosphatase fraction isolated from 0–40% ammonium sulfate precipitation of the 105,000 x g supernatant solution. A marked decrease in the amount of ^{32}P associated with the enzyme accompanied the 20-fold activation. The high-activity holo-a synthetase could be converted to low-activity holo-b synthetase after incubation with $[\gamma\text{-}^{32}P]$ ATP and a kinase fraction isolated from 55–75% ammonium sulfate precipitation of the 105,000 x g supernatant solution. A marked increase in the amount of ^{32}P associated with the enzyme accompanied the 15-fold decrease in activity. (The phosphatase fraction was obtained from 48 hr fasted and 12 hr refed birds, while the kinase fraction was obtained from 48 hr refed and 12 hr fasted birds.) These data suggest the possibility that fatty acid synthetase of animal liver can be regulated by phosphorylation-dephosphorylation. When considered with the evidence suggesting that acetyl-CoA carboxylase may also be regulated by phosphorylation-dephosphorylation, the possibility of coordinate control of these two important lipogenic enzymes by phosphorylation-dephosphorylation is raised. The inability of Rous (1974) to isolate ^{32}P-fatty acid synthetase from livers of rats fed *ad libitum* and injected with $^{32}PO_4^{2-}$ supports the possibility that the nutritional state of the animal plays a role in this regulation.

Prosthetic Group Metabolism. A potential mechanism for regulation of fatty acid synthetase involves the critical 4'-phosphopantetheine prosthetic group. If the synthetase is in the apo form, clearly it will be inactive. The occurrence of aposynthetase in animal liver has been demonstrated recently by Porter and co-workers (Qureshi et al., 1975b). Utilizing affinity gel chromatography, these workers separated apo and holo fatty acid synthetase from pigeon liver. When [^{14}C] pantetheine-labeled synthetase complex was separated, the enzymatically active holo form contained all of the ^{14}C label. Preliminary data indicated that the apoenzyme is present in largest amounts after a 48 hr fast and that this form is an intermediate in the synthesis of holosynthetase on refeeding a starved animal. These data suggest the possibility of an apo-holo enzyme system for control of fatty acid synthetase activity.

The possibility that an apo-holo system exists for *short-term* regulation of fatty acid synthetase is suggested by the demonstration of rapid turnover of the prosthetic group in several mammalian tissues by a process that is apparently analogous to that occurring in *E. coli.* Thus, Larrabee and co-workers (Tweto et al., 1971) studied prosthetic group turnover in rat liver by pulse-labeling with [^{3}H] pantothenate and determining the specific radioactivity of the 4'-phosphopantetheine of purified fatty acid synthetase and CoA. Maximum specific radioactivity of CoA was reached before that of the synthetase, supporting a precursor role of CoA for the 4'-phosphopantetheine group of ACP. Specific radioactivity of the 4'-phosphopantetheine of fatty acid synthetase remained low until about 6 hr after injection, when it rose rapidly to reach a maximum 8 hr later. The turnover rate of the prosthetic group was at least an order of magnitude faster than that of the whole complex, which has a $t_{1/2}$ of about 70 hr (see below). The likelihood that only the prosthetic group participates in the rapid turnover, as described in *E. coli,* was supported by the failure to detect any extremely rapidly turning over peptide isolated from the fatty acid synthetase of rat liver after tryptic digestion or treatment with SDS (Tweto et al., 1972). Rapid prosthetic group turnover is probably a general phenomenon in mammalian tissues. Thus, it was demonstrated also in the fatty acid synthetase of mammalian brain and adipose tissue (Volpe and Vagelos, 1973a). In brain the prosthetic group is replaced completely in 10–11 hr and, as in liver, this is an order of magnitude faster than the turnover of the enzyme complex, previously shown to occur with a $t_{1/2}$ of 6.4 days (Volpe et al., 1973).

Because of the possibility that this turnover is involved in short-term regulation of the synthetase, studies of the process in starved animals and those fed a fat-free diet have been carried out (Tweto and Larrabee, 1972; Volpe and Vagelos, 1973a). During the 24–48 hr after the onset of starvation or refeeding of a fat-free diet, marked changes in prosthetic group exchange were observed. During starvation the process in liver was markedly diminished, and during fat-free feeding, moderately accelerated. In brain no changes in prosthetic group exchange occurred either during starvation or refeeding a fat-free diet (Volpe and Vagelos, 1973a). It is noteworthy in this regard that the turnover of the brain multienzyme complex is also not altered by these nutritional alterations, although the hepatic synthetase undergoes marked changes (Volpe et al., 1973). The physiological significance of the alterations in prosthetic group exchange in liver is unknown. Attempts with immuno-chemical techniques to demonstrate apoenzyme in the liver of the starved animal have not been successful (Volpe and Vagelos, 1973a; Yu and Burton, 1974a). Moreover, the mechanisms of the changes in prosthetic group turnover in liver are unknown. This is related in part to the inability to isolate from mammalian tissues the enzymes responsible for prosthetic group turnover—holo-ACP synthetase (reaction 15) and ACP hydrolase (reaction 16). In addition, the possibility that effects occur at the level of CoA metabolism has not been ruled out entirely.

Yu and Burton (1974a, 1974b) recently presented evidence suggesting the presence of enzymatically inactive, immunologically reactive fatty acid synthetase in rat liver during the first 3 hr of refeeding after a 48 hr fast. Thus, crude liver extracts from animals refed for 1, 2, and 3 hr were shown to contain increasing amounts of material that competed with pure synthetase for binding sites on antisynthetase antibody. After 3–5 hr of refeeding, it was not possible to demonstrate the competition because of the marked increase in active synthetase relative to the inactive species. Extracts from starved animals had little or no ability to compete in the assay devised by Yu and Burton (1974a). Purification of the cross-reacting material was not carried out. However, the possibility that the immunologically reactive material was indeed inactive fatty acid synthetase was supported by pulse-labeling the enzyme in the refed rats with [^{3}H] amino acids and measuring the radioactivity incorpo-rated into the protein precipitated by antisynthetase antibody. A marked increase in specific radioactivity during the first 3 hr of refeeding was observed, while synthetase specific activity remained unchanged. Nearly maxi-mal rates of synthesis occurred by 5 hr of refeeding. When [^{14}C] pantothenate was injected into refed rats, no incorporation of radioactivity into immuno-precipitable enzyme was observed until 4 hr of refeeding, and thereafter the rate of increase of enzyme-bound pantothenate paralleled the rate of increase of synthetase specific activity. These findings suggested that apoenzyme is synthesized rapidly in the first several hours of refeeding and then converted to active holoenzyme in the following hours. Porter and co-workers reached a similar conclusion on the basis of observations of isolated liver cells studied both by immunochemical and direct purification techniques (Lakshamanan et al., 1975b).

Recent attempts to demonstrate the activities of holo-ACP synthetase and ACP hydrolase in liver of starved and refed rats have produced provoca-tive data. Pursuing their observations suggesting conversion of apoenzyme to holoenzyme in refed rats, Yu and Burton (1974b) demonstrated generation of fatty acid synthetase activity in liver extracts of animals refed for 3 hr by incubating the extract with CoA, ATP, and a 20–40% ammonium sulfate fraction of liver from animals refed for 12 hr (the synthetase had been removed from the latter extract by immuno-precipitation). CoA could be replaced by *E. coli* ACP. It was assumed that the liver extract from the animal refed for 12 hr imparted the capacity to synthesize holoenzyme from apoenzyme and that this capacity was lacking in the liver of the animal refed for 3 hr. However, whether or in what manner this capacity was related to an enzymatic activity was not established. When [^{14}C]CoA was utilized in the reaction mixture, radioactivity was found associated with TCA-precipitable protein. Upon mild alkaline hydrolysis, a procedure that cleaves the phosphodiester linkage of the 4'-phosphopantetheine of ACP, 62% of the radioactivity was released. However, the radioactive product was not characterized in more detail. A more decisive demonstration of the capacity to synthesize holoenzyme was provided by Qureshi et al. (1975b). The enzymatically inactive aposynthetase, isolated by affinity gel chromatography as described above, was converted to active holosynthetase after incubation with CoA, ATP, and a 20-50% ammonium sulfate fraction of pigeon liver.

ACP hydrolase was sought in liver extracts of rats starved for 72 hr (Roncari, 1975). Substrate quantities of [^{14}C]fatty acid synthetase, labeled in its 4'-phosphopantetheine moiety, were incubated in the presence of Mg^{2+} and crude extract (700 x *g* supernatant solution) of liver from the fasted animals. When the products of the reaction were chromatographed on Sephadex G-50, the major portion of the radioactivity was discovered in the inclusion volume of the column. This radioactivity was identified as 4'-phosphopantetheine by DEAE-cellulose and paper chromatography. No significant release of radioactivity from the labeled synthetase occurred when crude extract of liver from animals fed *ad libitum* was used in lieu of that from fasted animals. Roncari concluded that cleavage of the prosthetic group of the synthetase by crude extracts from fasted rats had occurred and was the result of an enzymatic activity that might mediate rapid control of synthetase activity (Roncari, 1975). The enzymatic activity was not characterized further. Again, although these data may represent the first demonstration of ACP hydrolase activity in mammalian liver, more detailed studies will be of great importance.

All of the above data suggest that an apo-holo enzyme system for control of fatty acid synthetase activity may be operative in mammalian liver and that such a system may provide a means for rapid regulation. Demonstration of the operation and control of such a system may be accomplished more readily by the use of isolated liver cells or cultured cell lines than by studies performed *in vivo*.

Adaptive Changes in Enzyme Content. Like acetyl-CoA carboxylase, fatty acid synthetase activity of a variety of tissues undergoes relatively long-term regulatory changes secondary to nutritional, hormonal, developmental, genetic, and neoplastic factors. Liver has been studied in greatest detail, and the following discussion will emphasize the enzyme of this tissue (see Table 4). Although evidence for a physiological role for fatty acid

TABLE 4 Long-Term Regulation of Hepatic Fatty Acid Synthetase

Condition	Specific activity (units/mg protein)	Rate of enzyme	
		Synthesis	Degradation
Nutritional[a]			
1. High-carbohydrate diet	↑[b]	↑	N
2. Fat-free diet	↑	↑	N
3. High-fat diet	↓	—	—
4. Polyunsaturated fatty acids	↓	—	—
5. Fasted	↓	↓	↑
6. Choline deprivation	↑	—	—
7. Vitamin B_{12}	↑	↑	±↑
Hormonal[c]			
1. Diabetes	↓	↓	—
2. Diabetes + Insulin	N	N	—
3. Diabetes + fructose feeding	N	N	—
4. Glucagon	↓	↓	—
5. Theophylline	↓	↓	—
6. Dibutyryl cyclic AMP	↓	↓	—
7. Hyperthyroid	↑	—	—
8. Hypothyroid	↓	—	—
9, Hypophysectomized	↓	—	—
Development[d]			
1. Fetus	↓	—	—
2. Newborn	↓-N	—	—
3. Suckling	↓	↓	N
4. Weaned	↑	↑	N
Genetic (obese-hyperglycemic mouse)[e]			
1. Standard laboratory chow	↑	↑	N
2. Fasted	↑	↑	
3. Fasted, refed fat-free diet	↑	—	—
4. Triiodothyronne for 7 days	N	—	—
Neoplastic (minimal deviation hepatoma)[f]			
1. Standard laboratory chow	↓	—	—
2. Fasted	↑	—	—
3. Fasted, refed fat-free diet	↓	—	—

[a]Comparisons are between animals administered standard laboratory chow or the indicated diets or factors.

[b]N, ↑, and ↓ indicate no difference from, greater than, less than control, respectively; — indicates no data available.

[c]Comparisons are between animals subjected to the indicated hormonal changes and normal controls.

[d]Comparisons are between adult animals and those of the indicated ages.

[e]Comparisons are between obese-hyperglycemic mice and normal mice subjected to the indicated dietary alterations.

[f]Comparisons are between neoplastic liver and normal liver from the same animal subjected to the indicated dietary alterations.

synthetase in rapid regulation of fatty acid synthesis is scant, considerable information indicates that the synthetase is a critical enzyme in relatively long-term regulation, that is, over hours to days. This conclusion will become apparent in the discussion that follows.

Nutritional factors. The most profound alterations of hepatic fatty acid synthetase activity induced by nutritional alterations occur in animals refed a high-carbohydrate, fat-free diet after a 48 hr fast (Gibson et al., 1966). Thus, specific activity in fasted animals is very low and with refeeding rises 10- to 50-fold (for examples see Allmann and Gibson, 1965; Allmann et al., 1965; Burton et al., 1969; Butterworth et al., 1966; Craig et al., 1972a, 1972b; Hicks et al., 1965; Muto and Gibson, 1970; Volpe and Kishimoto, 1972; Zakim and Ho, 1970). The importance of fatty acid synthetase and not acetyl-CoA carboxylase as the rate-limiting step in fatty acid synthesis during long-term, high-carbohydrate feeding is demonstrated by simultaneous measurements of malonyl CoA, which indicate that the utilization of malonyl CoA by the synthetase is limiting under such circumstances (Guynn et al., 1972). Changes similar to those described for hepatic synthetase with fasting and refeeding are observed with the synthetase of adipose tissue (Saggerson and Greenbaum, 1970) and, to a lesser extent, intestinal mucosa (Zakim and Ho, 1970). No change in fatty acid synthetase of brain occurs with fasting or refeeding (Volpe and Kishimoto, 1972; Volpe et al., 1973).

The effects of carbohydrate on fatty acid synthetase differ according to the nature of the sugar utilized, and these differences may have important implications for the mechanism of regulation by other compounds as well. Thus, fructose feeding results in two- to threefold higher hepatic synthetase activities than does glucose feeding (Bruckdorfer et al., 1972; Volpe and Vagelos, 1974). The converse effect is seen in adipose tissue. The mechanism whereby fructose leads to increased hepatic synthetase is probably related to the metabolism of this carbohydrate. Fructose is phosphorylated in liver by fructokinase to fructose 1-phosphate (Leuthardt and Testa, 1951). This intermediate is converted by an aldolase to glyceraldehyde, and the latter is converted to glyceraldehyde 3-phosphate by a triokinase (Hers and Kusaka, 1953). This pathway is very active in liver (Sillero et al., 1969) and, in fact, fructose can be phosphorylated in liver at a much faster rate than glucose (Spiro and Hastings, 1958; Zakim et al., 1967). By this active pathway, fructose bypasses the first two slow steps in glycolysis, catalyzed by glucokinase and phosphofructokinase; in fact, fructose feeding results in 40–70% higher levels of pyruvate, acetyl CoA, and malate in liver than does glucose feeding (Zakim et al., 1967). It may be possible that an intermediate(s) at the triose phosphate step or beyond (e.g., acetyl CoA, citrate) leads to the induction of fatty acid synthetase. [This hypothesis may also account for the stimulation of other hepatic lipogenic enzymes by *glycerol* administration (Takeda et al., 1967).] The rapid rise in hepatic synthetase activity on refeeding after a fast is paralleled by a similar rise in levels of plasma insulin

(Gibson et al., 1972), which would also result in an increase in such potentially stimulatory intermediates. The difference in response to fructose feeding of fatty acid synthetase of adipose tissue is also consistent with this hypothesis. Thus, in adipose tissue fructokinase is not present (Adelman et al., 1967) and fructose must be phosphorylated to fructose 6-phosphate by hexokinase (type II isoenzyme) (Katzen and Schimke, 1965). The latter enzyme has a 20-fold higher affinity for glucose than fructose, and therefore any potentially stimulatory intermediates would be lower in concentration in adipose tissue on feeding of fructose rather than glucose. On the basis of studies correlating rates of fatty acid synthesis and activities of acetyl-CoA carboxylase and fatty acid synthetase with levels of a variety of intermediates of carbohydrate and fatty acid metabolism, Goodridge (1973a, 1973b) has proposed an analogous hypothesis—that is, that the concentrations of the lipogenic enzymes are regulated by concentrations of intermediates in the lipogenic pathway.

The effects of fat on fatty acid synthetase in liver vary with the nature of the lipid administered (for examples see Allmann and Gibson, 1965; Bartley and Abraham, 1972; Gibson et al., 1972; Liou and Donaldson, 1973; Muto and Gibson, 1970; Wiegand et al., 1973). Differences in results are related not only to the type of fat administered but to the species of animal studied, the mode of fat administration, prior nutritional alterations such as fasting, and so on. Nevertheless, two major conclusions concerning hepatic regulation seem warranted: (1) high-fat feeding leads to a diminution in fatty acid synthesis and activities of fatty acid synthetase as well as acetyl-CoA carboxylase, and (2) polyunsaturated fatty acids (arachidonate $>$ linoleate) are most effective in the production of such a response, and completely saturated fatty acids are generally ineffective.

An important role for fatty acid synthetase in the biochemical pathology of B_{12} deprivation is indicated by the occurrence of odd-numbered and/or branched-chain fatty acids in tissues of humans (Frenkel, 1971; Kishimoto et al., 1973) and animals (Cardinale et al., 1970; Frenkel, 1972) and in cultured glial cells (Barley et al., 1972) subjected to deprivation of this vitamin. The basis for the fatty acid abnormalities is related to the accumulation of propionyl CoA and methylmalonyl CoA as a result of a block in the mutase-catalyzed conversion of methylmalonyl CoA to succinyl CoA, a reaction that requires deoxyadenosyl B_{12}. Odd-numbered fatty acids result when propionyl CoA replaces acetyl CoA as primer for the synthetase, and branched-chain fatty acids when methylmalonyl CoA replaces malonyl CoA during chain elongation. Recently, another effect of B_{12} deprivation on fatty acid synthesis has been recorded (Frenkel et al., 1973, 1974). When animals were made B_{12}-deficient, hepatic activity of fatty acid synthetase was two- to threefold that in B_{12}-supplemented animals. Hepatic acetyl-CoA carboxylase was increased approximately twofold. Physiological significance for these effects was suggested because rates of fatty acid synthesis, measured by the tritiated water method, were also higher in the B_{12}-deprived animals (Frenkel et al., 1973).

A role for fatty acid synthetase in the production of the fatty liver of choline deficiency has been suggested by recent observations of rats fed a choline-deficient diet (Rosenfeld, 1973). Thus, animals on the diet for only 2 days exhibited a 60% increase in hepatic synthetase activity; no further increase was seen after 4 days. Increases in the relative and absolute amounts of palmitic acid in hepatic triglycerides were considered to be caused by the elevated activity of fatty acid synthetase (Rosenfeld, 1973). An approximately similar stimulation of hepatic acetyl-CoA carboxylase has also been observed (Chalvardjian, 1969). Impairment of lipoprotein synthesis and secretion has been suggested as a mechanism for the accumulation of triglycerides in the liver of the choline-deficient rat (Lombardi et al., 1968; Mookerjea, 1971). However, the impairment of lipoprotein synthesis and secretion in choline deficiency is much less striking than in orotic acid-fed rats (Windmueller, 1964), which exhibit a similar increase in hepatic triglycerides. Thus, the possibility might be considered that increased hepatic fatty acid synthetase activity is at least an additional factor causing the fatty infiltration in choline-deficient animals (Rosenfeld, 1973).

Every study directed toward elucidation of the mechanisms causing the dramatic adaptive changes in hepatic synthetase activity has led to the conclusion that these changes are associated with concomitant alterations in enzyme *content*. Thus, Porter and co-workers demonstrated that the content of the synthetase, determined by direct purification, was considerably lower in liver of fasted than of fat-free fed pigeons (Butterworth et al., 1966) and rats (Burton et al., 1969). Accelerated synthesis of enzyme on refeeding starved animals a fat-free diet was demonstrated by pulse-labeling *in vivo* with [^{14}C]leucine and purifying the synthetase; a striking increase of incorporation of radioactivity into the enzyme was noted 6 hr after refeeding (Burton et al., 1969). By pulse-labeling with [U-^{14}C]amino acids and isolating the synthetase by purification, Tweto and Larrabee (1972) showed that the rate of synthesis of the complex in liver of starved rats fell to its lowest values after approximately 16 hr of fasting. Isotopic-immunochemical experiments, similar to those described above for acetyl-CoA carboxylase, were utilized to define rate constants of synthesis and degradation (Craig et al., 1972b; Volpe et al., 1973). An approximately 20-fold difference in synthetase activity and content per gram of liver was noted between starved rats and those fed fat-free diets (Volpe et al., 1973). The rate of *synthesis* of hepatic fatty acid synthetase per gram of liver in the fat-free fed rats was sixfold greater than that in liver of starved rats. The rate of degradation of the enzyme was nearly fourfold greater in the livers of starved rats ($t_{1/2}$ in starved animals = 18 hr). Thus, the observed 20-fold difference in activity per gram of liver is close to the difference predicted on the basis of the changes in rates of enzyme synthesis and degradation (Volpe et al., 1973). The remarkable acceleration of degradation plays a major role in determining the lower hepatic synthetase activity in starved animals. This mechanism of enzyme regulation is operative for two other lipogenic enzymes: acetyl-CoA carboxylase (Majerus and Kilburn, 1969; Nakanishi and Numa, 1970) and malic enzyme (Silpananta and Goodridge, 1971). The rate of degradation of hepatic synthetase in animals fed a fat-free diet ($t_{1/2}$ = 2.7 days) was essentially identical to that for normally fed animals ($t_{1/2}$ = 2.8 days) (Volpe et al., 1973). Thus, the increase in hepatic fatty acid synthetase activity and content in fat-free fed animals was entirely related to an acceleration of enzyme synthesis. Similarly, fructose feeding was shown to increase hepatic fatty acid synthetase at the level of enzyme synthesis (Volpe and Vagelos, 1974). None of these nutritional states was accompanied by a change in content, synthesis, or degradation of brain synthetase. Utilizing a similar experimental approach, Frenkel et al. (1974) demonstrated that the elevated hepatic synthetase activity in B_{12}-deprived rats was caused primarily by an increase in synthetase synthesis.

To obtain insight into the factors controlling synthesis of fatty acid synthetase, Vagelos and co-workers studied the components for the synthesis of this protein according to methods developed in Schimke's laboratory (Shapiro et al., 1974; Taylor and Schimke, 1973, 1974). To identify the polyribosomes synthesizing fatty acid synthetase, a purified, monospecific antisynthetase antibody was prepared by affinity chromatography and iodinated with [125]I (Alberts et al., 1976). Antibody was incubated with polysomes and the mixture then subjected to sucrose density gradient configuration. Fatty acid synthetase nascent peptides were identified in association with the heavier polysomes. Correlative evidence that [125I]anti-synthetase antibody binds to the nascent chains of fatty acid synthetase on the polysomes was obtained by using an *in vitro* translation system with the polysomes (Strauss et al., 1976). In these studies the nascent chains bound to the polysomes that had been initiated *in vivo* were completed and the products immunoprecipitated and identified by SDS gel electrophoresis. When [3H]leucine was used as a label, the synthetase peptide(s) of molecular weight 240,000 contained most of the counts. This suggested that fatty acid synthetase is indeed synthesized as two large peptides of this size, and an analogy is immediately apparent between the synthesis of the mammalian and yeast fatty acid synthetases. When polysomes of fasted and refed animals were studied, a slight increase in rate of synthesis of synthetase peptides occurred after 2½ hours of refeeding, but by 5 hr the rate of synthesis in refed animals was approximately 19-fold higher than in fasted animals, and by 16 hr it was approximately 95-fold higher. The sharp increases in synthesis after 5 hr of refeeding correlated with increases in activity of fatty acid synthetase, suggesting that any apoenzyme synthesized was rapidly converted to active enzyme. These data show that control of the rate of translation of synthetase peptides is critical in the "adaptive synthesis" of fatty acid synthetase seen with refeeding after a fast. Further studies of this system will define whether the translational effects observed are related to changes in initiation rates, amounts of messenger RNA for fatty acid synthetase, and so on. Thus, it is clear that the stage is set for investigations designed to elucidate the mode of regulation of synthetase synthesis in mammals, whether it be at the transcriptional, translational, or posttranslational level.

Hormonal factors. The best studied of the hormone-dependent changes of fatty acid synthetase are the effects of the diabetic state on the enzyme of rat liver. Thus, in diabetic animals the hepatic synthetase is markedly decreased (Gibson and Hubbard, 1960), and this decrease is caused by a diminution in synthesis of enzyme (Lakshmanan et al., 1972; Volpe and Vagelos, 1974). Insulin administration corrects these deficits (Gibson and Hubbard, 1960; Lakshmanan et al., 1972; Nepokroeff et al., 1974; Volpe and Vagelos, 1974). Similar observations have been made for synthetase of adipose tissue (Saggerson and Greenbaum, 1970; Volpe and Vagelos, 1974). Studies in diabetic animals of the effects of feeding of fructose, a carbohydrate that is metabolized by liver in the absence of insulin, revealed that regulation of hepatic synthetase is not absolutely dependent on insulin (Volpe and Vagelos, 1974). Thus, fructose feeding to diabetic animals resulted in a complete correction of the deficit in synthesis of hepatic fatty acid synthetase. This result further supports the importance in the regulation of synthetase synthesis of stimulatory intermediates at the triose phosphate steps or beyond. Fructose feeding did not correct the deficit in synthetase of diabetic adipose tissue. This observation also supports the importance of such intermediates because in adipose tissue fructose must be phosphorylated by hexokinase (Katzen and Schimke, 1965), the activity of which is depressed in diabetic animals (McLean et al., 1966). Therefore, no significant increase in potentially stimulatory intermediates could be expected to occur in this tissue in diabetic animals.

Glucagon plays an important role in the long-term regulation of fatty acid synthetase (Lakshmanan et al., 1972; Volpe and Marasa, 1975a), acetyl-CoA carboxylase (Volpe and Marasa, 1975a), and, as a consequence, fatty acid synthesis in liver (Volpe and Marasa, 1975a). A marked decrease in the induction of these three parameters on refeeding a fat-free diet to a starved animal occurs when glucagon is administered concurrently with the refeeding. The administration of the methylxanthine, theophylline, causes an intermediate decrease. Immunochemical experiments determined that the decreases in hepatic synthetase induced by glucagon and/or theophylline were caused by decreases in enzyme synthesis (Volpe and Marasa, 1975a).

The mechanism by which glucagon and theophylline decrease synthetase synthesis may involve cyclic AMP. Hepatic levels of cyclic AMP can be increased by glucagon (Robinson et al., 1971), an effect presumably secondary to stimulation of adenyl cyclase by the hormone (Birnbaumer and Rodbell, 1969). A possible role for cyclic AMP in the inhibition of fatty acid synthesis in short-term experiments *in vivo* or *in vitro* was discussed above (see control of acetyl-CoA carboxylase). Administration of dibutyryl cyclic AMP to rats in long-term experiments—that is, during refeeding for 2 days after starvation—results in reductions of hepatic glucose-6-phosphate dehydrogenase (Rudack et al., 1971) and fatty acid synthetase (Lakshmanan et al., 1972) that are comparable to those observed when glucagon is administered. The observation that theophylline, a drug whose major metabolic effects is inhibition of phosphodiesterase (Jost and Richenberg, 1971), causes an intermediate reduction in fatty acid synthesis and synthesis of fatty acid synthetase, and glucagon a marked reduction of these processes, further supports the likelihood that the effects of glucagon are mediated by cyclic AMP. The mechanism whereby cyclic AMP causes a decrease in synthesis of fatty acid synthetase remains unknown. One possibility is that the mononucleotide produces the response indirectly as a consequence of one or more of its other well-recognized metabolic effects. For example, cyclic AMP prevents the induction of hepatic glucokinase (Ureta et al., 1970) and causes a drastic reduction in the conversion of glucose to CO_2 by liver slices. Such an effect might be expected to include also a decrease in hepatic concentration of intermediates of the glycolytic pathway or beyond, and thus lead to decreased synthesis of fatty acid synthetase by a mechanism essentially similar to that discussed above.

The role of thyroid hormone in the regulation of fatty acid synthetase has been demonstrated by several observations. Animals injected with thyroid hormone for 7-9 days exhibited two- to three-fold higher activities of synthetase in liver and adipose tissue than did saline-injected controls (Diamant et al., 1972; Volpe and Kishimoto, 1972; Volpe and Marasa, 1975a, 1975c). Similarly, hepatic activity is reduced by production of hypothyroidism (Volpe and Kishimoto, 1972) or by hypophysectomy (Volpe and Marasa, 1975a). These changes in synthetase activity are coordinate with similar changes in acetyl-CoA carboxylase and in fatty acid synthesis.

The most significant alterations in fatty acid synthetase induced by adrenal steroids occur in adipose tissue (Volpe and Marasa, 1975a). Thus, animals treated with glucocorticoids for 7-10 days showed a four- to five-fold reduction in synthetase specific activity, whereas adrenalectomized animals exhibited a two-fold increase in enzymatic activity (Volpe and Marasa, 1975a). The effect was shown to be caused by a decrease in synthetase synthesis. The mechanism by which synthetase synthesis is decreased may be related to the diminution of glucose uptake by adipose tissue that is induced by glucocorticoids (Fain, 1964; Munck, 1971). Since uptake is the rate-limiting step in glucose metabolism in adipose tissue (Munck, 1971), the generation of potentially stimulatory intermediates of the glycolytic pathway or beyond would be expected to decrease.

Developmental factors. Striking changes in fatty acid synthetase during the perinatal period have been described in avian liver (Goodridge, 1973b), mammalian liver (Smith and Abraham, 1970a; Volpe and Kishimoto,

1972; Volpe et al., 1973), mammalian brain (Volpe and Kishimoto, 1972; Volpe et al., 1973), and mammary gland (Mellenberger and Bauman, 1974). The major alterations are similar to those described for acetyl-CoA carboxylase. Thus, synthetase activity rises dramatically in avian liver after hatching, in mammalian liver transiently around the time of birth and then permanently after weaning, and in maternal mammary gland during middle to late pregnancy and, again, early in lactation. In contrast, synthetase activity in brain is highest in late fetal and young suckling animals and decreases with maturation (Volpe and Kishimoto, 1972). Nutritional factors are important in the control of the developmental changes in mammalian liver. Thus, prematurely weaning suckling mammals to a high-carbohydrate, low-fat diet induces a dramatic increase in synthetase activity (Smith and Abraham, 1970a; Volpe and Kishimoto, 1972). Similarly, glucose injection into embryonic eggs is followed after 4 days by a distinct elevation of hepatic synthetase (Donaldson et al., 1971). Moreover, although hepatic synthetase activity rises slowly after hatching in the absence of feeding, high-carbohydrate feeding results in a markedly accelerated rate of increase (Goodridge, 1973b). Hormonal influences may be more important than nutritional ones in regulation of the development of brain synthetase. Thus, suckling animals made hypothyroid exhibited a marked reduction in brain synthetase activity (Volpe and Kishimoto, 1972).

The mechanisms underlying the changes in fatty acid synthetase activity of developing liver and brain have been elucidated by immunochemical techniques (Volpe et al., 1973). All changes in both tissues were shown to reflect changes in enzyme content. The 15-fold rise in hepatic activity at the time of weaning was accompanied by a 12-fold increase in rate of synthetase synthesis. Degradation of fatty acid synthetase was similar in liver of suckling and weaned animals.

Genetic factors. Regulation of fatty acid synthetase has been studied in the genetic mutant, the Bar Harbor obese-hyperglycemic mouse. The mechanisms underlying the regulatory changes were defined by immunochemical techniques (Volpe and Marasa, 1975c). The major conclusions were as follows: (1) Although the hepatic specific activity of fatty acid synthetase is higher in obese than in nonobese animals fed chow (Chang et al., 1967; Volpe and Marasa, 1975c), no difference in hepatic activities is apparent in animals fed a fat-free diet. (2) The higher enzymatic activity in obese animals fed chow is related to a higher content of enzyme, and this higher content is associated with a higher rate of enzyme synthesis. (3) The decrease in hepatic synthetase activity with starvation is distinctly more striking in nonobese than in obese animals, and the changes in activity reflect changes in content of enzyme. (4) With starvation, there is a decrease in synthesis of enzyme in obese and nonobese animals, but *only in nonobese animals* is there also a marked increase in the rate of synthetase *degradation* ($t_{1/2} = 24$ hr during starvation, $t_{1/2} = 76$ hr during normal feeding). (5) Refeeding starved mice a fat-free diet results in a more striking increase in hepatic synthetase activity in nonobese than in obese animals. (6) Administration of triiodothyronine causes a more marked increase in hepatic synthetase activity in nonobese than in obese animals. Thus, a variety of clear differences in regulation of hepatic synthetase is apparent between the mutant and normal animals.

The mechanism that underlies the accelerated synthesis of fatty acid synthetase in the mutant animal appears to be qualitatively similar to at least one of the mechanisms that underlie this process in normal animals. The important difference between the mutant and normal animal is a quantitative one. Regulation of synthetase synthesis by carbohydrate is perhaps the most well established of the mechanisms operative in normal mammalian liver (Volpe and Marasa, 1975a; Volpe and Vagelos, 1973b, 1974), and there is good evidence to suggest that this is the important mechanism operative in liver of the obese animal. As pointed out above, the stimulatory effect of insulin on hepatic synthetase synthesis in the normal animal is probably mediated by the effects of this hormone on glucose metabolism, and in this regard it is noteworthy that a particularly well documented metabolic feature of the obese-hyperglycemic mouse is hyperinsulinemia (Bray and York, 1971; Christophe et al., 1959). Despite evidence indicating a degree of insulin "resistance" in these mutants (Freychet et al., 1972; Kahn et al., 1973; Stauffacher et al., 1971; Stauffacher and Renold, 1969; Yen and Steinmetz, 1972), important glycolytic enzymes, including the insulin-responsive gluco-kinase, phosphofructokinase, and pyruvate kinase, exhibit distinctly elevated hepatic activities in the obese mouse (Seidman et al., 1967, 1970). Thus, an abundance of the potentially stimulatory intermediates acting on synthetase synthesis might be expected in the mutant animal.

The failure of the rate of hepatic synthetase degradation to increase in the obese animal during starvation may provide important insight into the mechanism by which such degradation is regulated in the normal animal. The failure of synthetase synthesis in the obese mouse to fall abruptly in the first 24 hr after the onset of starvation may be significant in this regard. Thus, it is possible that the marked acceleration of synthetase degradation observed in the normal starved mouse is "triggered" by the abrupt fall in enzyme synthesis. The failure of enzyme synthesis to decrease markedly in the obese animal may be related to the failure of insulin levels to decrease markedly in the mutant as they do in the normal mouse (Christophe et al., 1959).

Neoplastic factors (minimal deviation hepatoma). The failure of fatty acid synthetase of minimal deviation hepatoma to respond to fasting or refeeding is similar to the failure of acetyl-CoA carboxylase of the tumor to respond (Majerus et al., 1968). This interesting phenomenon has been discussed in the section on control of acetyl-CoA carboxylase.

Regulation of *de Novo* Fatty Acid Synthesis in Cell Culture

The preceding discussions make clear the insight into regulation of fatty acid synthesis in animals gained by studies performed *in vivo* and *in vitro*.

Nevertheless, it is also clear that the most complicated questions remain unanswered, and the search for systems that are less complicated and better defined has led to a growing use of cells in culture. Cultured cells are particularly valuable for studies of lipid regulation for two major reasons. First, nutritional and hormonal conditions can be defined clearly, and effects of specific regulators can be isolated. *In vivo,* the complicated interplay of various effectors frequently makes precise interpretation of observations impossible. Second, certain tissues, such as brain, exhibit marked cellular heterogeneity, and the contributions of different cell types can be defined only rarely from studies carried out *in vivo.* By the use of cells in culture, these specific cell types can be studied in pure form. For example, neuronal and glial cells that exhibit many biochemical properties of cells *in situ* have been grown in culture (Nelson, 1975).

For the purpose of the following discussion, we will consider studies that are relevant to either short-term or long-term regulation. Particular emphasis will be given to work concerned with regulation at the enzyme level.

Short-term regulation. A role for lipid in short-term regulation of fatty acid synthesis in cultured human fibroblasts was suggested initially by the observation that addition of serum to the medium of cells previously maintained in lipid-deficient serum cause a twofold reduction in acetate incorporation into fatty acids within 20 min (Jacobs et al., 1973). Moreover, when cells previously maintained in a serum-containing medium were exposed to a medium with lipid-deficient serum, a twofold increase in incorporation of acetate into fatty acids was observed within approximately 1 hr (Jacobs et al., 1973). More detailed study of this phenomenon indicated that the regulatory lipid in the serum was probably fatty acid. Thus, when cells maintained in medium containing lipid-deficient serum or no serum at all were exposed to the same medium plus albumin-bound palmitic acid, a twofold reduction in acetate incorporation into fatty acids was observed within 10 min (Jacobs and Majerus, 1973). Of various albumin-bound fatty acids tested, stearic acid was the most effective, producing 67% inhibition. Palmitic acid, oleic acid, arachidonic acid, and linoleic acid produced 48, 45, 30, and 26% inhibition, respectively. Stearate was more effective than palmitate in similar studies performed with isolated chick hepatocytes and Ehrlich ascites tumor cells (Goodridge, 1973d; McGee and Spector, 1974). In contrast, palmitate was most effective in studies with C-6 glial cells, and no definite differences among various fatty acids were observed in studies with neuroblastoma cells (Volpe and Marasa, 1977).

The inhibitory effects in all of the studies appeared before adaptive changes in the level of acetyl-CoA carboxylase were observed. Cellular concentrations of possible positive and negative regulators of acetyl-CoA carboxylase activity, such as citrate and long-chain acyl CoA compounds, were found not to correlate with the observed changes in fatty acid synthesis in the human fibroblasts. Such negative correlative data, however, do not exclude the possibilities that uptake of free fatty acid results in a change in the concentration of citrate or long-chain acyl CoA derivatives in the specific cellular compartment occupied by acetyl-CoA carboxylase and/or fatty acid synthetase. Moreover, in short-term experiments with isolated chick hepatocytes, an inverse correlation *was* observed between concentrations of long-chain acyl CoA derivatives and rates of fatty acid synthesis (Goodridge, 1973d). Similarly, glucagon led to an increase in concentration of fatty acyl CoA derivatives and a decrease in fatty acid synthesis in these cells (Goodridge, 1973d). Lipid synthesis in isolated chick hepatocytes was also markedly inhibited by dibutyryl cyclic AMP (Capuzzi et al., 1974), but long-chain acyl CoA derivatives were not measured.

The possibility that the short-term regulation of fatty acid synthesis by exogenous lipid occurs at the level of 2-carbon metabolism is suggested by the coordinate changes in synthesis of both fatty acids and cholesterol induced by exogenous lipid in the media of various cultured cell types (Capuzzi et al., 1974; Howard et al., 1974). Since the pathways for synthesis of fatty acids and sterols diverge after formation of acetyl CoA (Barth et al., 1973), a reaction that could affect both syntheses involves the generation of acetyl CoA from acetate, CoA, and ATP and is catalyzed by acetyl-CoA synthetase. This enzyme undergoes regulatory changes in adipose tissue and liver of animals subjected to nutritional alterations that affect lipid synthesis (Barth et al., 1972; Murthy and Steiner, 1972; Steiner and Cahill, 1966). Bailey and co-workers (Howard et al., 1974) demonstrated that in the first 3 hr after removal or addition of serum to cultured L-cells, two to threefold changes in acetyl-CoA synthetase activity accompanied appropriate changes in fatty acid synthesis from acetate. The effect appeared to be on catalytic efficiency rather than quantity of enzyme, because the changes in enzymatic activity occurred in the presence of cycloheximide, actinomycin D, or mitomycin C. These inhibitors of protein, RNA, and DNA synthesis also did not prevent the changes in fatty acid synthesis induced by changes in medium lipid. The mechanism of the effect on catalytic efficiency of acetyl-CoA synthetase was not elucidated. Alteration of this enzymatic activity is not likely to be the exclusive mediator of short-term regulation of L-cells. Thus, the relative magnitudes of the stimulation and inhibition of enzymatic activity were somewhat less than the changes in acetate incorporation into lipid. Moreover, an important role for this enzyme in short-term regulation of fatty acid synthesis has not been shown in any other cell line. Indeed, the dramatic short-term regulatory effects observed in C-6 glial cells are not accompanied by any alteration in acetyl-CoA synthetase activity (Volpe and Marasa, 1977).

Long-term regulation. The most well-studied effector in the long-term regulation of fatty acid synthesis is lipid, specifically fatty acid. When cells are grown in medium that has high levels of fatty acids bound to albumin (Spector et al., 1969), such as serum, the fatty acid composition of cellular lipids reflects that of serum (Bailey et al., 1972; Geyer et al., 1961) and the synthesis of fatty acids is very low (Bailey, 1966; Howard and Kritschevsky, 1969). Growth in medium free of fatty acids results in increased incorporation of acetate or glucose into fatty acids (Alberts et al., 1974; Bailey, 1966; Jacobs and Majerus, 1973; Jacobs et al., 1973; Raff, 1970; Volpe and Marasa, 1975b) and in increased activity of acetyl-CoA carboxylase and/or fatty acid synthetase in certain liver, fibroblast, and glial cell lines (Alberts et al., 1974; Jacobs et al., 1973; Volpe and Marasa, 1975b). However, culture of cells in serum-free media does not invariably result in such effects. Thus, in certain other liver and fibroblast cell lines, no increase was observed in the activities of fatty acid synthetase and/or acetyl-CoA carboxylase after 48 hr in serum-free media (Alberts et al., 1974; Watson, 1972).

The precise nature of the intracellular regulatory lipid or lipid product remains unknown, but it is well established that fatty acids in the medium are taken up by mammalian cells in culture and are incorporated into various cellular lipids (Geyer, 1967; Spector, 1972). The inhibitory effect of serum on activities of acetyl-CoA carboxylase and/or fatty acid synthetase, as well as on fatty acid synthesis, was mimicked by addition of various albumin-bound fatty acids to cultured fibroblast (Jacobs and Majerus, 1973), glial cells (Volpe and Marasa, 1975b), and chick hepatocytes (Goodridge et al., 1974). Palmitate was a more effective inhibitor than stearate in the mammalian cells, although differences were small, whereas stearate was a distinctly more effective inhibitor in the avian cells. These effects of long-chain fatty acids on acetyl-CoA carboxylase and fatty acid synthetase are accompanied by alterations in content rather than catalytic efficiency of enzyme (Jacobs et al., 1973; Volpe and Marasa, 1975b), and isotopic-immunochemical studies in glial cells have shown that the changes in fatty acid synthetase content are caused by changes in synthesis of enzyme (Volpe and Marasa, 1975b).

Studies of long-term regulation of lipid synthesis by hormones have indicated a role for insulin and dibutyryl cyclic AMP in liver cells and fibroblasts (Alberts et al., 1974), for glucagon, cyclic AMP, and thyroid hormone in chick hepatocytes (Goodridge et al., 1974), and for glucocorticoid (Volpe and Marasa, 1976a) and theophylline (Volpe and Marasa, 1976b) in C-6 glial cells. Thus, in Chang liver cells, fatty acid synthetase activity increased approximately twofold when in serum-free medium for 48 hr, but the increase was more than fivefold when insulin was added after 24 hr. The induction of fatty acid synthetase was prevented by inhibitors of protein or RNA synthesis, suggesting that enzyme synthesis is involved. A combination of dibutyryl cyclic AMP and theophylline also markedly decreased the induction caused by insulin. Similarly, the marked induction of fatty acid synthesis and fatty acid synthetase activity after 3–4 days in culture observed in embryonic chick hepatocytes was markedly inhibited by glucagon or cyclic AMP in the growth medium. This induction required undialyzed serum, and this suggested that a low-molecular-weight factor was critical. Insulin was not the responsible factor since chicken insulin failed to stimulate fatty acid synthesis. However, thyroid hormone was clearly involved because the induction of fatty acid synthesis was inhibited by addition of thyroxine-binding prealbumin and this inhibition was reversed by addition of triiodothyronine.

Indeed, the increase in fatty acid synthesis observed in cells grown in undialyzed serum was mimicked in cells grown in dialyzed serum plus triiodothyronine. Hydrocortisone in the growth medium of C-6 glial cells caused an approximately twofold reduction in activity of fatty acid synthetase after approximately 1 wk (Volpe and Marasa, 1976a). Immunochemical techniques were utilized to show that the glucocorticoid-induced decrease in synthetase activity reflected a decrease in synthetase content, and that this decrease in synthetase content was caused by a decrease in enzyme synthesis. Since hydrocortisone causes a decrease in glucose uptake into C-6 glial cells, this would be expected to lead to a decrease in concentration of those intermediates at the triose phosphate step or beyond that we postulate as important modulators of synthetase synthesis. Thus, the mechanism of the inhibitory effect of hydrocortisone on synthesis of fatty acid synthetase in C-6 glial cells may be similar to that postulated for the hormone's effect in adipose tissue. Theophylline causes an approximately twofold reduction in synthetase activity in C-6 glial cells within 48 hr after addition to the growth medium (Volpe and Marasa, 1976b). Immunochemical techniques demonstrated that the effect was also mediated by a decrease in synthetase synthesis.

CHOLESTEROL BIOSYNTHESIS

Introduction

The enzymatic synthesis of cholesterol from acetyl CoA was defined primarily by the pioneering studies from the laboratories of Bloch, Lynen, and Popjak. Several recent reviews describe various aspects of the biosynthetic pathway (Bortz, 1973; Dempsey, 1974; Dietschy and Wilson, 1970; Rodwell et al., 1973; Scallen et al., 1975). In animal cells the biosynthesis of cholesterol occurs via proteins in the cytoplasm and microsomes and is conveniently considered in four major phases:

1. Acetyl CoA → mevalonate
2. Mevalonate → squalene
3. Squalene → lanosterol
4. Lanosterol → cholesterol

The generation of mevalonate from acetyl CoA requires enzymes, which are described in more detail below. The primary regulation of cholesterol biosynthesis in animal tissues occurs in this sequence of the synthesis. Mevalonate is converted to squalene through several phosphorylated intermediates. Squalene undergoes attack by molecular oxygen in the presence of a mixed-function oxidase to form squalene-2(3)-epoxide, and a cyclase then catalyzes formation of lanosterol, the first 3-β-OH sterol in the pathway. Lanosterol is converted to cholesterol through several steps that include the removal of three methyl groups, saturation of the double bond of the side chain, and a shift of a double bond from one ring to another. The conversion of squalene to cholesterol requires the interaction of a number of microsomal enzymes and cytoplasmic protein(s), and the latter may function both as carriers for the water-insoluble substrates and as enzyme constituent(s) that facilitate catalysis (Scallen et al., 1975). Regulation of cholesterol synthesis probably occurs at one or more sites in the biosynthetic pathway after synthesis of mevalonate, but these are more likely to represent secondary regulatory sites than primary ones (see discussion below).

Synthesis of mevalonate. The synthesis of mevalonate proceeds via the following reactions:

$$2 \text{ Acetyl CoA} \rightleftharpoons \text{acetoacetyl CoA} \tag{23}$$

$$\text{Acetoacetyl CoA} + \text{acetyl CoA} \rightleftharpoons \text{HMG CoA} \tag{24}$$

$$\text{HMG CoA} \rightarrow \text{mevalonate} \tag{25}$$

Reactions 23–25 are catalyzed by acetoacetyl-CoA thiolase, HMG-CoA synthase, and HMG-CoA reductase, respectively.

The immediate precursor of mevalonate, β-hydroxy-β-methylglutaryl CoA (HMG CoA), until recently was considered to be of mitochondrial origin and produced as part of the cycle of enzymes involved in ketogenesis (in ketogenesis, HMG CoA in the mitochondrion is converted to acetoacetate and acetyl CoA by HMG-CoA lyase). If this were the case, HMG-CoA reductase, a microsomal enzyme, would be the first committed step in cholesterol biosynthesis and a likely target for regulation. Indeed, this enzyme is a target for regulation of cholesterol biosynthesis (see discussion below), but in view of recent data, this is probably not the first committed step in cholesterol biosynthesis.

A considerable body of recent data indicates that there are dual locations in the cell for HMG CoA synthesis, in the mitochondria for ketogenesis, and in the cytosol for cholesterolgenesis. First, acetoacetyl-CoA thiolase and HMG-CoA synthase have been isolated from the cytosol of animal tissues, and the cytosolic enzymes have been shown to exhibit distinct differences from the mitochondrial enzymes (Clinkenbeard et al., 1973, 1975a, 1975b; Middleton, 1973; Sugiyama et al., 1972). Second, cholesterol as well as fatty acid synthesis is blocked by (−)-hydroxycitrate, which inhibits ATP:citrate lyase, the major source for *cytosolic* acetyl CoA (Barth et al., 1972; Sullivan et al., 1972). This indicates that cytosolic acetyl CoA is the precursor of both cholesterol and fatty acids. Third, studies with perfused liver have demonstrated that different pools of acetyl CoA are involved in ketogenesis and cholesterolgenesis (Dietschy and McGarry, 1974).

Recent work by Lane and co-workers (Clinkenbeard et al., 1973, 1975a, 1975b; Sugiyama et al., 1972) has characterized the coupled system responsible for cytosolic HMG CoA synthesis—that is, acetoacetyl-CoA thiolase and HMG-CoA synthase. *Cytosolic acetoacetyl-CoA thiolase* constituted 70% of the total thiolase in avian liver and approximately 50% of the total in rat liver (Clinkenbeard et al., 1973). Isoelectric focusing revealed distinct differences between the mitochondrial and cytosolic enzymes. For cholesterol synthesis this cytosolic thiolase must catalyze reaction 23 in the condensation direction (generation of acetoacetyl CoA), which is thermodynamically unfavorable. However, the unfavorable equilibrium of the thiolase-catalyzed condensation reaction can be overcome by coupling acetoacetyl CoA formation to the thermodynamically favorable HMG-CoA synthase reaction (reaction 24). The availability of homogeneous preparations of both thiolase and synthase from avian liver enabled Lane and co-workers to demonstrate that the coupled reaction proceeds rapidly to an equilibrium at which 68% of the available acetyl CoA is converted to HMG CoA (Clinkenbeard et al., 1973). *Cytosolic HMG-CoA synthase* was isolated from avian and rat liver. The cytosolic synthase of avian liver was shown to differ from the mitochondrial enzyme by isoelectric focusing, elution behavior on ion exchange chromatography, and mobility on disc gel electrophoresis (Clinkenbeard et al., 1975b). Cytosolic synthase was demonstrated in many tissues of the chicken, including brain, whereas the mitochondrial synthase was confined to tissues capable of ketogenesis—that is, liver and kidney (Clinkenbeard et al., 1975a, 1975b). The potential importance of thiolase and synthase in regulation of cholesterol synthesis is indicated by alterations of these enzymes under conditions of cholesterol feeding, fasting, and cholestyramine administration (see discussion below).

Link between cholesterol and fatty acid biosynthesis. An important link between cholesterol and fatty acid synthesis is indicated by these data and those recorded above concerning the β-reductive enzymes and fatty acid synthesis. Such a link can be depicted according to the scheme shown in Fig. 1. Central importance is clear for acetoacetyl CoA synthesis from acetyl CoA and the coupling of this reaction (1) to the β-ketoacyl reductase reaction that generates crotonyl-CoA, precursor of butyryl-CoA, the preferred primer for fatty acid synthesis, or (2) to the HMG-CoA synthase reaction for cholesterol synthesis.

Regulation

In large part because of the great importance of cholesterol in cardiovascular disease, biosynthesis of this material and regulation thereof have been the subject of an enormous literature. Approximately 80–95% of the cholesterol in mammals is synthesized in liver and intestine (Bortz, 1973; Dietschy and Siperstein, 1967; Rodwell et al., 1973). The major fates of the synthesized cholesterol in mammals include secretion and carriage by lipoproteins, synthesis of bile acids, synthesis of cholesterol esters, synthesis of glucocorticoids and sex hormones, and incorporation into cellular membranes. The first of these predominates in liver, whereas synthesis of hormones occurs particularly in endocrine glands, especially the adrenal. Synthesis of cholesterol for incorporation into cellular membranes is an important process in proliferating or differentiating tissues.

The regulation of cholesterol biosynthesis has been studied in by far the greatest detail in liver. The major factors involved in the regulation of cholesterol synthesis and the critical rate-limiting enzyme, HMG-CoA reductase, are summarized in Table 5. Conspicuously absent from Table 5 are indications of whether changes in HMG-CoA reductase activity are caused by changes in enzyme synthesis and/or degradation. With few exceptions (see discussion below), this information is unavailable. Unlike the enzymes of *de novo* fatty acid biosynthesis, acetyl-CoA carboxylase and fatty acid synthetase, which are found in the cytosolic fraction, are readily purified, and thus can be studied by immunochemical techniques, HMG-CoA reductase is microsomal-bound, resistant to purification, and thus difficult to study by immunochemical techniques. However, very recently Scallen and co-workers succeeded in purifying hepatic HMG-CoA reductase 975-fold by the use of Blue Dextran-Sepharose 4B affinity chromatography (Tormanen et al., 1976). The purified enzyme had a specific activity many times higher than that of any preparation previously reported and by SDS polyacrylamide gel electrophoresis contained only "trace" impurities. It appears that a homogeneous preparation is attainable, and thus production of antibodies should be possible. Since the enzyme can be solubilized from crude extracts of microsomes simply by freeze-thawing (Heller and Gould, 1973, 1974), immunochemical methods for studying enzyme content, synthesis and degradation in the presence of critical regulatory effectors appear quite feasible for use in the near future.

Cholesterol feeding and the importance of HMG-CoA reductase. The importance of HMG-CoA reductase in regulation of cholesterol synthesis in liver is widely accepted. This was shown first in relation to the inhibition of cholesterol synthesis by cholesterol feeding. This end-product regulation was first shown by Gould and Taylor (1950), and localization to a step prior to mevalonic acid and after HMG-CoA was shown several years later (Bucher et al., 1960; Gould and Popjak, 1957; Siperstein and Guest, 1960; Siperstein and Fagan, 1966). An unequivocal demonstration that HMG-CoA reductase is the step involved was made by Linn (1967). The mechanism of the effect of cholesterol will be considered in more detail in the discussion of cholesterol synthesis in cultured cells.

A variety of *in vivo* studies suggest that cholesterol leads to a decrease in *content* of HMG-CoA reductase and that this decrease is caused by a

TABLE 5 Regulation of Hepatic HMG-CoA Reductase

Condition	Specific activity (units/mg protein)
Enterohepatic[a]	
1. Fasting	↓[b]
2. Cholesterol feeding	↓
3. Bile acid feeding	↓
4. Removal of bile acids	↑
Bile duct obstruction	
Bile duct fistula	
Cholestyramine feeding	
Ileal bypass	
Hormonal[c]	
1. Diabetes	↓
2. Diabetes + Insulin	N
3. Insulin	↑
4. Glucagon	↓
5. Hyperthyroid	↑
6. Hypothyroid	↓
7. Hypophysectomized	↓
8. Glucocorticoid	↓
9. Cyclic AMP	↓
Development[d]	
1. Perinatal	↑
2. Suckling	↓
3. Weaned	↑
Neoplastic (hepatomas)[e]	
1. Cholesterol feeding	↑
2. Choloestyramine feeding	↓
3. Triton injection	↓
Pharmacologic[f]	
1. Clofibrate	↓
2. Triton	↑

[a]Comparisons are between animals administered standard laboratory chow or the indicated diets or factors.

[b]N, ↑, and ↓ indicate no difference from, greater than, less than control, respectively; — indicates no data available.

[c]Comparisons are between animals subjected to the indicated hormonal changes and normal controls.

[d]Comparisons are between adult animals and those of the indicated ages.

[e]Comparisons are between obese-hyperglycemic mice and normal mice subjected to the indicated dietary alterations.

[f]Comparisons are between neoplastic liver and normal liver from the same animal subjected to the indicated dietary alterations.

decrease in enzyme *synthesis* (Rodwell et al., 1973). Direct measurements of enzyme content and synthesis by immunochemical techniques indicated that during the early phase of cholesterol feeding inactivation of reductase may also occur, since enzyme activity declined more rapidly than did either the rate of enzyme synthesis or the amount of protein precipitated by anti-HMG-CoA reductase antibody (Higgins and Rudney, 1973). After 24 hr of cholesterol feeding, neither enzyme protein nor activity was detectable, indicating that enzyme synthesis was repressed.

Diurnal variation. Cholesterol synthesis and the activity of HMG-CoA reductase undergo a remarkable diurnal variation (Bach et al., 1969; Edwards et al., 1972; Kandutsch and Saucier, 1969a; Shapiro and Rodwell, 1969). Lowest levels of synthesis and activity occur at midmorning, and five-to tenfold higher levels at a double peak about midnight to 2 p.m. (Shapiro and Rodwell, 1972). Reverse lighting and forced-feeding experiments suggest a relation to feeding (Dugan et al., 1972; Edwards and Gould, 1972; Huber and Hamprecht, 1972), although the rhythm persists to some extent in the fasted rat (Shapiro and Rodwell, 1972). The cyclic rise was shown to be related to an increase in enzyme synthesis by experiments utilizing inhibitors of messenger RNA and protein synthesis (Edwards and Gould, 1972; Kandutsch and Saucier, 1969a; Shapiro and Rodwell, 1969), by comparisons of the kinetic properties of the enzyme at the peak and nadir of the rhythm (Shapiro and Rodwell, 1971), and by measuring the rate of incorporation of [^{3}H] leucine into enzyme purified from rats killed at various times during the cycle (Higgins et al., 1971). Related experiments indicated that the cyclic decline in reductase levels was caused by complete cessation of enzyme synthesis, and this was utilized to estimate a $t_{1/2}$ of HMG-CoA reductase of 4.2 hr (Edwards and Gould, 1972). In similar experiments a $t_{1/2}$ of approximately 2 hr has been estimated (Edwards and Gould, 1974; Dugan et al., 1972). Thus, this enzyme is capable of very rapid turnover, and relatively rapid regulation by alterations in enzyme synthesis and degradation rather than by allosteric effects is possible.

Bile factors. Cholesterol synthesis and the activity of HMG-CoA reductase can be regulated by factors present in bile. Thus, bile feeding or removal of bile (by creation of a bile duct fistula or ileal bypass, or by feeding cholestyramine) leads to a decrease or increase, respectively, in cholesterol synthesis and in HMG-CoA reductase activity (for reviews see Bortz, 1973; Rodwell et al., 1973). Moreover, the low reductase activity in the liver of the suckling rat can be raised nearly to the activity of the adult by severing the bile duct (Harris et al., 1967; McNamara et al., 1972). In addition, the possibility of an inhibitor in the cytosol of the suckling liver was suggested by mixing experiments (McNamara et al., 1972). It is thus of considerable interest that McNamara and Rodwell (1975) purified from bovine bile a high-molecular-weight lipoprotein, similar in density and lipid composition to serum β-lipoprotein, that inhibits the activity of HMG-CoA reductase. The inactivation occurred in the presence of microgram quantities of the protein, was irreversible, and could not be reproduced by physiologic concentrations of cholesterol or bile acid. Consideration of bile flow to the liver under physiological conditions leads to the hypothesis that this protein could regulate cholesterol synthesis *in vivo*. An interesting and still broader conclusion from this work is that the regulation of cholesterol synthesis and primarily HMG-CoA reductase need not be attributed solely to alterations in the rates of enzyme synthesis and degradation, but might also be secondary to changes in concentration of inhibitory proteins.

   Developmental aspects. The developmental aspect of hepatic cholesterol synthesis and reductase activity are of considerable interest. There are two major developmental changes (McNamara et al., 1972); the first rise in reductase activity occurs during late fetal life, and this is followed by a precipitous postnatal decline. Regulation of this rise and fall is not understood, although by analogy with other enzymes with similar perinatal changes, we would suggest that the prenatal rise is related to thyroid hormone and the postnatal fall to glucagon (Greengard, 1971). A second rise occurs at the time of weaning and is related to the change in diet. This latter conclusion is supported by the ability to induce the rise earlier than the usual age by premature weaning and to delay the rise by late weaning. The increase of activity from suckling to normal adult daytime levels does not appear to involve protein synthesis and may reflect relief of inhibition of reductase activity consequent to the change in diet (McNamara et al., 1972). The findings of inhibitors in cytosol of suckling rat liver, in rat milk, and in bile may be relevant in this regard, although precise delineation of the physiological significance of these inhibitors remains to be accomplished (see the discussion above of protein inhibitor in bile). At the time of weaning, marked increases in incorporation of mevalonate to total nonsaponifiable lipids as well as to digitonin-precipitable sterols also occur (Shah, 1973). These latter secondary regulatory steps occur at the levels of conversion of mevalonate to squalene and squalene to cholesterol. Similar postmevalonate regulation was delineated by the enzymatic studies of Porter and co-workers with adult animals (see discussion below).

   Hormones and cyclic AMP. Interplay of Hormones and the Diurnal Variation. The effects of various hormones on cholesterol synthesis and HMG-CoA reductase activity have been studied in several laboratories over the past 20 yr. Some particularly important recent data, obtained by Porter and co-workers (Dugan et al., 1974; Lakshmanan et al., 1973, 1975a; Ness et al., 1973), indicate that the levels of hepatic HMG-CoA reductase and of cholesterol synthesis can be regulated by the relative amounts of stimulatory hormones, such as insulin and thyroid hormone, and of inhibitory hormones, such as glucagon and glucocorticoids. Thus, hepatic HMG-CoA reductase activity increased two- to sevenfold after subcutaneous administration of insulin into normal or diabetic animals. The maximum effect occurred in 2-3 hr and could be elicited in animals that did not have access to food. Animals made diabetic exhibited after 7 days a marked decrease in hepatic HMG-CoA reductase activity (values were approximately 5% of those of normal animals) (Dugan et al., 1974). Moreover, the marked diurnal variation in enzyme activity was abolished in the diabetic animal and was restored by insulin administration. These data suggested that insulin is necessary for the diurnal rise in HMG-CoA reductase activity.

The fact that plasma insulin exhibits a diurnal variation (Kaul and Berdanier, 1972), associated with feeding and similar to that of reductase activity, supports the notion that insulin is intimately involved in the diurnal change of reductase activity. Other hormones may also be involved. Thus, the restorative effect of insulin on hepatic HMG-CoA reductase in diabetic animals is partially or completely suppressed by simultaneous administration of glucagon or glucocorticoid (Dugan et al., 1974). The diurnal rise in reductase activity in liver of normal animals can also be suppressed markedly by administration of glucagon, cyclic AMP, or glucocorticoid.

Since glucagon exhibits a diurnal variation opposite to that of insulin (Harris et al., 1967), the data lead to the conclusion that the relative concentrations of insulin and glucagon play important roles in the regulation of the diurnal variation of hepatic HMG-CoA reductase activity. The data on glucocorticoid are also of interest in this regard. Plasma glucocorticoids exhibit a diurnal variation (David-Nelson and Brodish, 1969) but the temporal aspects are not compatible with a fast-acting inhibitory role. Moreover, there are conflicting data concerning the effect of adrenalectomy on the diurnal variation of the reductase (Edwards, 1973; Hickman et al., 1972; Huber et al., 1972). Nevertheless, in view of these observations of Porter and co-workers, glucocorticoids, as well as glucagon and insulin, clearly have the capacity to regulate hepatic HMG-CoA reductase.

Cyclic AMP. The data discussed above suggest a role for cyclic AMP in the relatively long-term regulation of HMG-CoA reductase and cholesterol biosynthesis. Recent experiments suggest a role for the cyclic mononucleotide in *short-term* regulation as well. Utilizing rat liver slices, Bricker and Levey (1972) demonstrated that incubation with 5×10^{-3} M cyclic AMP led to a more than 80% decrease in conversion of acetate to cholesterol. Only a minimal effect was noted at a concentration of 5×10^{-4} M. Similar effects have been observed with comparable concentrations of dibutyryl cyclic AMP with liver slices (Allred and Roehrig, 1972; Edwards, 1975) and isolated hepatocytes (Capuzzi et al., 1974). Utilizing cell-free preparations (10,000 $\times$ g supernatant solution), Bloxham and Akhtar (1973) demonstrated a tenfold reduction in cholesterol biosynthesis with 5 mM cyclic AMP in the incubation medium. The inhibition was noted when acetate, mevalonate, squalene, or lanosterol was used as precursor. No effect was seen with cholest-7-en-β-ol as precursor. Thus, inhibition of the conversion of lanosterol to this sterol was suggested as the site of the cyclic AMP effect.

Somewhat different data were obtained by Gibson and co-workers (Beg et al., 1973), who also utilized cell-free preparations (5,000 × g supernatant solutions) of rat liver. Thus, these workers observed a five- to sixfold reduction in cholesterol biosynthesis from acetate when 2.5 mM cyclic AMP was added to the incubation. No effect on conversion of mevalonate to cholesterol was noted, and this suggested that HMG-CoA reductase was the enzyme affected. Indeed preincubation of liver slices, isolated cells, or the 5,000 × g supernatant solution for 60 min in the presence of 5 × 10^{-3} M cyclic AMP resulted in decreased activities of HMG-CoA reductase, although the maximal effect on the enzyme was only an approximately twofold reduction. Moreover, utilizing isolated hepatocytes prepared by improved techniques, Edwards (1975) demonstrated that the increase in HMG-CoA reductase activity noted in these cells on addition of 10% rat serum was inhibited by at least 90% when cells were incubated for 3 hr in 3 × 10^{-4} M dibutyryl cyclic AMP. Gibson and co-workers suggested the possibility that reductase activity is regulated by a cyclic AMP-dependent phosphorylation-dephosphorylation mechanism because (1) washed microsomes preincubated with ATP, Mg^{2+}, and a cytosolic fraction exhibited a tenfold reduction in HMG-CoA reductase activity, (2) addition of 10^{-6} M cyclic AMP to the ATP and Mg^{2+} accentuated the inhibition, and (3) a second preincubation with a separate cytosolic fraction (precipitating between 65 and 75% ammonium sulfate saturation) resulted in some reversal of the inactivation.

The *physiological* significance of these observations with cyclic AMP was questioned by recent studies (Chow et al., 1975; Raskin et al., 1974). Although Raskin et al. (1974) confirmed the effects of high concentrations of cyclic AMP on cholesterol synthesis by liver slices, in perfusion experiments the addition of glucagon sufficient to cause a 50-fold increase in hepatic cyclic AMP levels resulted, in 30 min, in no significant change in cholesterol synthesis from acetate or octanoate or in HMG-CoA reductase activity. Moreover, Rudney and co-workers (Chow et al., 1975) reexamined the inhibitory effect of ATP and Mg^{2+} in more detail and found that inhibition of HMG-CoA reductase by these factors varied from zero to complete. They could not demonstrate a requirement for a cytosolic fraction. Most important, utilizing specific antibody to precipitate the enzyme after incubation with ATP labeled uniformly with ^{14}C in the adenine portion and ^{32}P in the terminal phosphate, these workers were unable to demonstrate labeling of the protein. These data led to the conclusion that the mechanism of inhibition in the presence of ATP does not involve phosphorylation or adenylization of the enzyme protein and to the suggestion that competition between enzyme substrate and ATP might be responsible for the inhibition. Thus, at present, a physiologic role for cyclic AMP in the short-term regulation of cholesterol synthesis is unproved.

Thyroid Hormone. A role for thyroid hormone in the regulation of hepatic HMG-CoA reductase appears well established. Thyroidectomy leads to a more than 50% decrease in reductase activity and administration of thyroid hormone restores the activity to normal after approximately 30 hr (Guder et al., 1968). Normal animals given thyroid hormone approximately 2 days before exhibit reductase activities at 1,400 hr that are as high as those occurring at 2,200 hours in the treated or untreated animals (Ness et al., 1973). However, if the *hypophysectomized* animal is given thyroid hormone under · similar circumstances, activities are very high at both times of day and are, in fact, fourfold higher than the highest attained in the normal animals injected with thyroid hormone. This suggests that one of the pituitary hormones acts to oppose the stimulatory effect of thyroid hormone, either by itself or through its target endocrine hormone. The data reviewed above on the inhibitory effects of glucocorticoid raise the distinct possibility that the stimulation of HMG-CoA reductase by thyroid hormone in the normal animal is inhibited by glucocorticoid, which is absent in the hypophysectomized animal. The fact that hypophysectomized animals do not exhibit a detectable diurnal variation in HMG-CoA reductase activity (Edwards, 1973; Guder et al., 1968) suggests that pituitary hormones and/or the secretion of their target glands may be involved in the diurnal changes.

Interplay of Hormones and Dietary Factors. A recent study of the effects of hormones and dietary factors on hepatic HMG-CoA reductase and on serum and hepatic cholesterol levels provides insight into the interaction of these various regulatory effectors (Lakshmanan et al., 1975a). Normal animals, those that had been hypophysectomized with or without subsequent treatment with thyroid hormone, and those that had been made diabetic with or without subsequent treatment with insulin were studied under the following dietary conditions: normal feeding, cholestyramine administration, cholesterol feeding, or fasting. The results demonstrated that cholestyramine administration stimulated HMG-CoA reductase activity in animals depleted of insulin or thyroid hormone. Thus, these hormones are not absolute requirements for the synthesis of cholesterol and HMG-CoA reductase. Under certain conditions the results were consistent with a model in which cholesterol functions as a feedback repressor of HMG-CoA reductase. However, a number of dietary and hormonal manipulations produced little or no change in the level of serum or hepatic cholesterol, while producing widely different reductase activities. Thus, regulation is clearly more complex than simple cholesterol feedback, and regulatory mechanisms clearly differ in various states of dietary or hormonal function.

Catecholamines. Another category of hormones involved in the regulation of cholesterol synthesis is composed of the catecholamines. Bortz (1968) observed a twofold stimulation of cholesterol synthesis from acetate 12 hr after intraperitoneal administration of norepinephrine, 0.1 mg/100 g body weight. No effect on conversion of mevalonate to cholesterol was observed, and the effect on acetate → cholesterol was prevented when puromycin was administered with the norepinephrine. These data suggested that norepinephrine administration led to an increase in cholesterol synthesis by an increase in synthesis of HMG-CoA reductase. This suggestion received support by the demonstration of an 80% increase in hepatic HMG-CoA reductase activity 3 hr after injection of epinephrine, 0.05 mg/100 g body weight (Edwards and Gould, 1974). Actinomycin D injected at the same time as (but not 1 hr after) the epinephrine prevented the stimulation, suggesting that the effect is dependent on mRNA synthesis. Edwards (1975) recently reproduced the effect in isolated hepatocytes, indicating that the catecholamines act directly on the liver cell.

    Genetic factors. Three recessive mutations in the mouse result in severely defective myelination of the central nervous system: the "jimpy," myelin synthesis deficiency, and "quaking" animals. Kandutsch and Saucier (1969b, 1972) have demonstrated diminished rates of cholesterol synthesis from acetate and mevalonic acid and diminished levels of HMG-CoA reductase activity in brain of these animals. In general, the defects became more prominent with maturation, although quantitative differences among the three mutants were apparent. It is not likely that the defect in sterol synthesis is the primary defect in these mutants. Indeed, in the quaking mouse a defect in the microsomal system for chain elongation of behenyl CoA is the probable primary defect (Goldberg et al., 1973). Nevertheless, the fact that sterol synthesis is altered under conditions in which myelination is severely deranged suggests a link between regulation of these two processes.

    Pharmacologic factors. Although a number of drugs affect cholesterol synthesis, a well-studied example in clinical use is clofibrate, the ethyl ester of *p*-chlorophenoxyisobutyric acid (CPIB). The drugs have a variety of metabolic effects (see discussion of acetyl-CoA carboxylase), one of which involves HMG-CoA reductase. Thus, when rats were fed clofibrate (0.3% in the diet), an 86% decrease in conversion of acetate to cholesterol by liver slices was observed after only 1 day (White, 1971). There was no disturbance of conversion of acetate to CO_2 or fatty acids nor of mevalonate to cholesterol. HMG-CoA reductase activity was diminished by 72% after 1 day of the drug and by 90% after 3 days. The mechanism of the effect of clofibrate on HMG-CoA reductase has not been elucidated.

    Regulatory sites other than HMG-CoA reductase. Although the dominance of HMG-CoA reductase in the regulation of hepatic cholesterol biosynthesis is without question, the possibility of other sites of regulation has been suggested by several studies. Earlier reports indicated involvement prior to the reductase step—that is, the synthesis of HMG-CoA (White and Rudney, 1970)—as well as after—the synthesis of cholesterol from mevalonic acid (Gould and Swyryd, 1966; Siperstein and Guest, 1960). A role for the coupled enzyme system that synthesizes HMG-CoA—acetoacetyl-CoA thiolase and HMG-CoA synthase—is strongly suggested by recent work of Lane and co-workers (Clinkenbeard et al., 1973, 1975a, 1975b; Sugiyama et al., 1972). Thus, cholesterol feeding to rats for 7 days resulted in reductions of hepatic acetoacetyl-CoA thiolase and HMG-CoA synthase activities to 29 and 15%, respectively, of control values. That the effect was specific for the cytoplasmic HMG-CoA generating system was shown by the demonstration that mitochondrial thiolase was unaffected by the cholesterol feeding. Cholestyramine feeding to rats for 3 days caused 1.8- and 2.6-fold increases in the cytoplasmic activities of hepatic thiolase and synthase, respectively, results again compatible with the involvement of these enzymes in cholesterol synthesis. Moreover, with fasting for 48 hr the total hepatic activities of thiolase and synthase were reduced to 46 and 24%, respectively, of those in rats fed *ad libitum.*

Thus, the adaptive responses of these enzymes under conditions known to be accompanied by changes in cholesterol synthesis suggest a regulatory role. Nevertheless, it should be pointed out that the adaptive responses of thiolase and synthase are somewhat slower and smaller than those for cholesterol synthesis overall and for HMG-CoA reductase activity. For example, cholesterol synthesis from acetate is reduced more than 95% and HMG-CoA reductase approximately 90% after only 24 hr of fasting; activities of thiolase and synthase do not reach such levels even after 48 hr of fasting (Clinkenbeard et al., 1975b; Slakey et al., 1972). Similar conclusions apply to the responses to cholesterol feeding, although the maximal responses of thiolase and synthase are quite marked by 7 days of feeding. These data thus suggest that while primary control may reside with HMG-CoA reductase, secondary regulation occurs at the level of HMG-CoA synthesis. Changes at this level might serve to amplify regulation at the HMG-CoA reductase step. Moreover, the possibility is raised that primary regulation at the level of HMG-CoA synthesis could occur under circumstances still to be defined.

Porter and co-workers have compared in rat liver the effects of fasting, refeeding, and time of day on the levels of enzymes catalyzing the conversion of HMG CoA to squalene and on the synthesis of nonsaponifiable and digitonin-precipitable lipids from acetate or mevalonate (Slakey et al., 1972). Their work suggests that there are at least two secondary regulatory processes active in controlling the flux of intermediates from mevalonate to cholesterol. The data support the proposal that the overall rate of cholesterol synthesis is controlled by the level of HMG-CoA reductase activity during most of the period of fasting and refeeding a fat-free diet. However, regulation of the flux through the entire pathway of cholesterol synthesis was not sufficiently described by the model of HMG-CoA reductase as a rate-limiting step. The incorporation of mevalonate into nonsaponifiable compounds was reduced 20-fold by 48 hr of fasting, and the recovery of synthesis of digitonin-precipitable material was slower than the recovery of synthesis of nonsaponifiable compounds. Thus, Porter and co-workers concluded that secondary regulatory sites exist between mevalonic acid and squalene and between squalene and digitonin-precipitable sterols.

Regulation in Cultured Cells

As discussed above in connection with *de novo* fatty acid synthesis, the use of cultured cells affords distinct advantages in the study of the regulation of lipid synthesis. As the following review will indicate, remarkable insight into the mechanisms of regulation of cholesterol synthesis has been attained by study of various cultured cell lines. Moreover, the use of readily sampled cells, such as fibroblasts and white blood cells, has provided the opportunity to study regulation in the normal and diseased human. This approach may shed considerable light on the role of deranged cholesterol synthesis and the regulation thereof in the genesis of atherosclerotic cardiovascular disease.

Lipid. Importance of Low-Density Lipoproteins. Cultured fibroblastic cell lines actively synthesize cholesterol from glucose or acetate, and the rate of synthesis can be controlled by the lipid content of the medium, as first shown by Bailey (1967). Inhibition was not observed when mevalonate was used as precursor, and this suggested that the enzymatic site of regulation is the HMG-CoA reductase step. Similar regulatory data have been obtained with other fibroblastic lines (Avigan et al., 1975; Brown et al., 1973a; Rothblat et al., 1971), hepatoma (Watson, 1972), swine aortic smooth muscle cells (Assman et al., 1975), and leukocytes (Fogelman et al., 1975). Particularly interesting recent studies of the regulation of HMG-CoA reductase have been concerned particularly with cultured human fibroblasts, hepatoma cells, mouse liver cells, and, leukocytes, described below.

The activity of HMG-CoA reductase in cultured human fibroblasts is regulated by the content of serum in the medium. Thus, activity is suppressed when cells are grown in 10% fetal calf serum and rises 12-fold over 12 hr when serum is removed (Goldstein and Brown, 1973). That the factor in serum is associated with the lipid fraction was shown by reproducing the effect of serum removal by delipidation of the serum. That the suppressing factor in serum was associated with cholesterol was shown by the observation that the suppressing effect of various sera correlated roughly with cholesterol concentration. However, at comparable cholesterol concentrations egg yolk had no effect, indicating that the mode of delivery of cholesterol to the cell is critical. The responsible factor in human serum was found in low density and very low density lipoprotein (LDL and VLDL). When added at equal cholesterol concentrations, high density lipoprotein (HDL) was much less effective than LDL in reducing reductase activity. This suggested that the apoprotein to which cholesterol is bound is critical. LDL and VLDL but not HDL contain apolipoprotein B. That this protein is intimately involved in the suppressing effect was shown by the finding that serum from a patient with abetalipoproteinemia did not suppress HMG-CoA reductase activity of cultured human fibroblasts (Brown et al., 1974). That the physiological suppressor of reductase activity is probably cholesterol was suggested by the observation that nonlipoprotein cholesterol was nearly as effective as LDL-cholesterol in producing the effect. That these effects on reductase activity are not caused by alterations in catalytic function is suggested by the inability to demonstrate inhibitory effects by various mixing experiments. That the stimulation of reductase activity by removal of LDL, in fact, is secondary to increased enzyme synthesis was shown by prevention of the effect by cycloheximide or actinomycin D (Brown et al., 1973b). A similar observation was made with hepatoma cells (Kirsten and Watson, 1974).

By the use of cycloheximide to prevent enzyme synthesis, Brown et al. (1974) measured the first-order decline in reductase activity and obtained a $t_{1/2}$ of 2.7 hr. A similar value (2.9 hr) was obtained in cells grown in lipoprotein-poor serum (LPPS). By similar techniques with hepatoma cells a $t_{1/2}$ of 4-5 hr was obtained. Analysis of the rate of decline in reductase activity of cells grown first in LPPS and then in serum lipoproteins resulted in a $t_{1/2}$ of 1.8-2.0 hr. These values are similar to those obtained with the liver enzyme and indicate a capacity for rapid regulation of HMG-CoA reductase by alterations in enzyme synthesis and degradation.

Analysis of the disturbance in regulation of cholesterol synthesis in cultured fibroblasts of patients with homozygous *familial hypercholesterolemia* has furthered understanding of regulation in normal cells (Brown et al., 1974; Goldstein and Brown, 1973). Cultured cells from the mutants showed a very high level of HMG-CoA reductase activity under all culture conditions, and there was a nearly complete failure of suppression of enzyme activity by LDL. [Subnormal though detectable suppression was noted in the cells of patients studied by Avigan et al. (1975).] When cholesterol was administered to the mutant cells in a nonlipoprotein form, a marked suppression of HMG-CoA reductase resulted, suggesting that the defect in these cells resided in the transfer of cholesterol from extracellular LDL to its presumed site of action on or within the cell (Brown et al., 1974; Goldstein and Brown, 1973).

These data indicating that LDL binding to the cell is related to suppression of HMG-CoA reductase and that such binding might be deficient in the familial hypercholesterolemic cells led to a study of the binding of LDL to fibroblasts and the effects of such binding (Brown and Goldstein, 1974a; Goldstein and Brown, 1974; Goldstein et al., 1974). Preparation of ^{125}I-labeled LDL allowed definition of high-affinity binding to fibroblasts, presumably representing binding to specific receptor sites on the cell surface. The high-affinity binding process exhibited saturation kinetics, competition by related molecules (e.g., VLDL), and destruction by limited treatment of the cells with pronase. Binding to the cells was followed by degradation of the [125I] LDL by proteolysis. After limited treatment of the cells with pronase binding was disturbed, and suppression of HMG-CoA reductase and degradation of LDL reduced. Cultured cells from patients with homozygous familial hypercholesterolemia, which were shown to lack the high-affinity binding process, were also resistant to suppression of HMG-CoA reductase by LDL and were deficient in the high-affinity degradation of LDL. These data suggested that a prerequisite to suppression of HMG-CoA reductase by LDL was binding of LDL to the high-affinity surface receptor sites.

   Role of Cholesterol Ester Formation. A third role of LDL binding to fibroblasts, in addition to suppression of reductase and stimulation of LDL degradation, may involve another process necessary for regulation of the enzyme. Thus, incubation of fibroblasts with LDL led to a 30- to 40-fold increase in the rate of cholesterol ester formation (Goldstein et al., 1974). The stimulation of cholesterol ester formation occurred despite nearly complete suppression of endogenous cholesterol synthesis. This stimulation did not occur in the hypercholesterolemic cells, which is consistent with the view that LDL binding is necessary for the effect and is defective in the mutant cells. Also consistent with this formulation is the finding that nonlipoprotein cholesterol can both stimulate cholesterol esterification and suppress cholesterol synthesis in these cells. The reciprocal decrease in free cholesterol synthesis and increase in cholesterol ester formation induced by LDL suggests that the increase in cholesterol esters is an intermediate event necessary for suppression of HMG-CoA reductase activity. This view is further supported by the recent observation that incubation of fibroblasts with certain oxygenated sterols (see discussion below), which leads to suppression of HMG-CoA reductase activity, also leads to an increase in the cellular content of cholesterol esters (Brown et al., 1975b). The enhanced capacity for esterification was associated with a marked increase in the activity of a membrane-bound fatty acyl-CoA:cholesteryl acyltransferase.

   Role of Sterol Flux into and out of the Cell. An additional view of the mechanism of regulation of HMG-CoA reductase has been suggested on the basis of recent studies of cholesterol synthesis in leukocytes (Fogelman et al., 1975). Thus, when these cells were transferred to lipid-free medium cholesterol synthesis from acetate, but not mevalonate, rose, and this was accompanied by induction of HMG-CoA reductase. These increases were more pronounced in cells of patients with heterozygous familial hypercholesterolemia. Moreover, when intracellular sterols were labeled by incubation of cells with [^{3}H]mevalonate and then cells were transferred to lipid-free medium, the heterozygous cells released significantly more [^{3}H]sterol into the medium than did the normal cells. This led to the suggestion that the abnormally high induction of HMG-CoA reductase in the heterozygous cells resulted from a more rapid dissociation within the cell of a sterol repressor of the system coding for the enzyme. The mutation would represent defective binding for a sterol repressor synthesized within the cell, with a major consequence being greater loss of sterol from the cell. The greater loss of sterol from the cell appears to trigger a mechanism for the maintenance of intracellular cholesterol at a constant level—that is, increase in HMG-CoA reductase activity and cholesterol synthesis.

   Further support for the importance of sterol influx and efflux in the regulation of cholesterol synthesis is derived from recent studies with isolated rat hepatocytes (Edwards, 1975; Edwards et al., 1976). Thus, incubation of the isolated hepatocytes in a sterol-free medium containing 1.5% albumin resulted in a loss of cholesterol from the cells and increased activity of HMG-CoA reductase. Addition of lecithin dispersions resulted in still greater rates of sterol efflux and increased levels of reductase. The enzyme levels observed after 3 hr of incubation with lecithin dispersions in the medium were directly proportional to the amount of cholesterol lost by the cells to the medium during the first 45 min of incubation. This was shown by incubating the hepatocytes for 45 min with various concentrations of the lecithin dispersions, removing the lecithin and determining the amount of cholesterol lost into the medium, and assaying HMG-CoA reductase after an additional 2.25 hr incubation in lecithin-free medium. Sterol loss preceded the change in reductase activity; essentially no increase in reductase activity occurred during the initial 45 min incubation. The data demonstrate that the activity of HMG-CoA reductase depends on the amount of cholesterol leaving the cell. Presumably, the rapid response of the cells to small losses of cholesterol by induction of HMG-CoA reductase is a mechanism for the maintenance of intracellular cholesterol content at a constant level. *In vivo* intracellular cholesterol could be altered in liver by changes in the rate of lipoprotein or bile acid secretion, or in proliferating or differentiating tissues by deposition of the sterol in cellular membranes. Indeed, catabolism of hepatic cholesterol to bile acids undergoes a diurnal rhythm with a peak at 9 p.m. while cholesterol synthesis exhibits a peak several hours later. An intriguing possibility that remains to be established firmly is that the diurnal "loss" of hepatic cholesterol to bile acids predetermines the activity of HMG-CoA reductase in that tissue (Edwards et al., 1976).

Cholesterol derivatives and analogs. A marked inhibiton of cholesterol synthesis and/or HMG-CoA reductase by oxygenated sterols has been demonstrated in primary liver cell cultures and in various cultured fibroblasts (Avigan et al., 1970; Brown and Goldstein, 1974b; Brown et al., 1975b; Kandutsch and Chen, 1973, 1974, 1975; Rothblat and Buchko, 1971; Rothblat et al., 1971). Utilizing liver cell cultures and L-cells, Kandutsch and Chen (1973) demonstrated that several steroids with 7-ketone and 7-hydroxyl functions led to nearly complete suppression of sterol synthesis and reductase activity after 6 hr of incubation. Sterol synthesis was more sensitive to inhibition in L-cells than in primary cultures of liver cells. In a more detailed study (Kandutsch and Chen, 1974), the same workers demonstrated that the time course of the decline in HMG-CoA reductase activity of L-cells incubated with 25-hydroxycholesterol and 20α-hydroxycholesterol was such that half of the enzyme activity was lost in 1–1.3 hr. If these derivatives act by repressing the synthesis of HMG-CoA reductase, the half-life of the enzyme must have been no greater than 1–1.3 hr, which is at the lower limit of the range of values reported for hepatic reductase *in vivo* and for cultured human fibroblasts and hepatoma cells (see discussions above). It is of particular interest that, of the inhibitory sterols studied, 7α-hydroxycholesterol and 20α-hydrocholesterol are of physiologic importance, since they are the first intermediates in production from cholesterol of bile acids and steroid hormones, respectively.

Brown and Goldstein (1974b) amplified these data still further, testing 47 steroid compounds for their ability to suppress HMG-CoA reductase activity in cultured human fibroblasts. The compounds included intermediates in cholesterol synthesis, cholesterol esters, various steroid hormones, and bile acids. The only consistent structural requirement for suppression of enzyme activity was the presence of an unesterified oxygen function at position 3 of the sterol nucleus. Compounds such as cholesterol, lanosterol, and desmosterol were effective inhibitors at concentrations of 5 and 32 μg/ml (24 hr incubations). [The possibility that cholesterol is not inhibitory in pure form and is converted by autoxidation to inhibitory derivatives during prolonged incubation has been raised by Kandutsch and Chen (1973, 1974), who studied mouse cells. However, marked decreases in activity of HMG-CoA reductase of isolated hepatocytes occur after incubations of only 3 hr with purified cholesterol-lecithin dispersions (Edwards, 1975).] The most potent C-27 derivative was 7-ketocholesterol, which suppressed reductase activity by more than 90% in 2 hr. When cells were cultured in the presence of 7-ketocholesterol and in the absence of LDL, the suppression of endogenous cholesterol synthesis by the steroid resulted in a marked inhibition of cell growth. This inhibition of growth could be prevented by the addition to the culture medium of either cholesterol or mevalonate, but not acetate. Thus, the activity of HMG-CoA reductase became the rate-limiting factor for both cholesterolgenesis and cell growth under conditions where exogenous cholesterol was not available. This interesting finding established culture conditions that may allow an analysis of the role of cholesterol in membrane function.

A role for cholesterol ester formation in the regulation of HMG-CoA reductase and cholesterol synthesis by oxygenated sterols (as by LDL) is suggested by recent observations of Brown et al. (1975b). Thus, under conditions whereby incubation with 7-ketocholesterol or 25-hydroxycholesterol produced marked inhibition of HMG-CoA reductase, there was a marked increase in cholesterol ester formation. This increased esterification was associated with a marked increase in the activity of membrane-bound fatty acyl-CoA:cholesteryl transferase.

The extremely rapid suppression of reductase activity by 7-ketocholesterol suggests the possibility that the effect is mediated by an alteration in catalytic function rather than enzyme synthesis or degradation. Direct effects of the steroids have been ruled out by appropriate *in vitro* experiments. The data of Beg et al. (1973) reviewed above in relation to hepatic reductase—that is, inactivation by a possible cyclic AMP-augmented phosphorylation—are of interest in this regard. Brown et al. (1975a) have recently shown that HMG-CoA reductase of cultured human fibroblasts could be inactivated *in vitro* by a factor in the soluble fraction of fibroblast extracts in a reaction requiring either ATP or ADP and Mg^{2+} or Mn^{2+}. The inactivation factor was heat-labile, nondialyzable, and precipitable with ammonium sulfate. Addition of cyclic AMP had no effect. Kinetic studies suggested that the inactivation factor catalyzes the conversion of the microsomal enzyme from an inactive to an active form. Since solubilized preparations of HMG-CoA reductase were resistant to inactivation, the possibility was raised that some unidentified microsomal component may participate in the inactivation reaction. Preliminary attempts to demonstrate alterations in the activity of the inactivating system by various manipulations known to alter reductase activity in culture were not successful.

Hormones and cyclic AMP. In contrast to the relatively abundant information on regulation of cholesterol synthesis in cultured cells by lipoprotein fractions and oxygenated sterols, little data has been accumulated on regulation by hormones and/or cyclic AMP. When human fibroblasts were grown in the absence of serum and in the presence of 10^{-6}-10^{-8} M insulin for 24 hr, activities of HMG-CoA reductase were increased by approximately 60% (Brown et al., 1974). The effect is smaller than, although in the same direction as, that observed with insulin *in vivo*.

L-cells incubated in the presence of 3 mM cyclic AMP ± 1 mM theophylline or 1 mM dibutyryl cyclic AMP for 5 hr did not exhibit the reduced activity of HMG-CoA reductase that might have been predicted from studies of liver *in vivo* (Kandutsch and Chen, 1975).

Clearly, study of the regulation of cholesterol synthesis in cultured cells by hormonal and other factors has just begun. The striking effects described above in the section on regulation *in vivo* remain to be defined more precisely by such study. Here indeed is a fertile area for future work.

REFERENCES

Achuta Murthy, P. N. and Mistry, S. P. 1974. Synthesis of acetyl coenzyme A holocarboxylase *in vitro* by a cytosolic preparation from chicken liver. *Proc. Soc. Exp. Biol. Med.* 147:114–117.

Adelman, R. C., Ballard, F. J. and Weinhouse, S. 1967. Purification and properties of rat liver fructokinase. *J. Biol. Chem.* 242:3360–3365.

Ailhaud, G. P. and Vagelos, P. R. 1966. Palmityl-acyl carrier protein as acyl donor for complex lipid biosynthesis in *Escherichia coli. J. Biol. Chem.* 241:3866–3869.

Ailhaud, G. P., Vagelos, P. R. and Goldfine, H. 1967. Involvement of acyl carrier protein in acylation of glycerol 3-phosphate in *Clostridium butyricum*. I. Purification of *Clostridium butyricum* acyl carrier protein and synthesis of long chain acyl derivatives of acyl carrier protein. *J. Biol. Chem.* 242:4459–4465.

Akhtar, M. and Bloxham, D. P. 1970. The co-ordinated inhibition of protein and lipid biosynthesis by adenosine 3':5'-cyclic monophosphate. *Biochem. J.* 20:11P.

Alberts, A. W. and Vagelos, P. R. 1966. Acyl carrier protein. VIII. Studies of acyl carrier protein and coenzyme A in *Escherichia coli* pantothenate or β-alanine aurotrophs. *J. Biol. Chem.* 241:5201–5204.

Alberts, A. W. and Vagelos, P. R. 1968. Acetyl-CoA carboxylase. I. Requirement for two protein fractions. *Proc. Natl. Acad. Sci. U.S.A.* 59:561–568.

Alberts, A. W. and Vagelos, P. R. 1972. Acyl-CoA carboxylases. *Enzymes* 6:37–82.

Alberts, A. W., Nervi, A. M. and Vagelos, P. R. 1969. Acetyl-CoA carboxylase. II. Demonstration of biotin-protein and biotin carboxylase subunits. *Proc. Natl. Acad. Sci. U.S.A.* 63:1319–1326.

Alberts, A. W., Gordon, S. G. and Vagelos, P. R. 1971. Acetyl-CoA carboxylase: The purified transcarboxylase component. *Proc. Natl. Acad. Sci. U.S.A.* 68:1259–1263.

Alberts, A. W., Ferguson, K., Hennessy, S. and Vagelos, P. R. 1974. Regulation of lipid synthesis in cultured animal cells. *J. Biol. Chem.* 249:5241–5249.

Alberts, A. W., Strauss, A., Hennessy, S. and Vagelos, P. R. 1976. Regulation of the synthesis of hepatic fatty acid synthetase: Binding of fatty acid synthetase antibodies to polysomes. *Proc. Natl. Acad. Sci. U.S.A.* 72:3956–3960.

Allmann, D. W. and Gibson, D. M. 1965. Fatty acid synthesis during early linoleic acid deficiency in the mouse. *J. Lipid Res.* 6:51–62.

Allmann, D. W., Hubbard, D. D. and Gibson, D. M. 1965. Fatty acid synthesis during fat-free refeeding of starved rats. *J. Lipid Res.* 6:63–74.

Allred, J. B. and Roehrig, K. L. 1972. Inhibition of hepatic lipogenesis by cyclic-3',5'-nucleotide monophosphates. *Biochem. Biophys. Res. Commun.* 46:1135–1139.

Allred, J. B. and Roehrig, K. L. 1973. Inhibition of rat liver acetyl coenzyme A carboxylase by N^6, O^2-dibutyryl cyclic adenosine 3':5'-monophosphate *in vitro*. *J. Biol. Chem.* 248:4131–4133.

Arinze, J. C. and Mistry, S. P. 1970. Hepatic acetyl-CoA carboxylase, propionyl-CoA carboxylase and pyruvate carboxylase activities during embryonic development and growth in chickens. *Proc. Soc. Exp. Biol. Med.* 135:533–556.

Arslanian, M. J. and Wakil, S. J. 1975. Fatty acid synthetase from chicken liver. *Methods Enzymol.* 35:59–64.

Assman, G., Brown, B. G. and Mahley, R. W. 1975. Regulation of 3-hydroxy-3-methylglutaryl coenzyme A reductase activity in cultured swine aortic smooth muscle cells by plasma lipoproteins. *Biochemistry* 14:3996–4002.

Avigan, J., Williams, C. D. and Blass, J. P. 1970. Regulation of sterol synthesis in human skin fibroblast cultures. *Biochim. Biophys. Acta* 218:381–384.

Avigan, J. Bhathena, S. J. and Schreiner, M. D. 1975. Control of sterol synthesis and of hydroxymethylglutaryl CoA reductase in skin fibroblasts grown from patients with homozygous type II hyperlipoproteinemia. *J. Lipid Res.* 16:151–154.

Bach, P. Hamprecht, B. and Lynen, F. 1969. Regulation of cholesterol biosynthesis in rat liver: Diurnal changes of activity and influence of bile acids. *Arch. Biochem. Biophys.* 133:11–21.

Bailey, J. M. 1966. Lipid metabolism in cultured cells. VI. Lipid biosynthesis in serum and synthetic growth media. *Biochim. Biophys. Acta* 125:226–236.

Bailey, J. M. 1967. Cellular lipid nutrition and lipid transport. In *Lipid metabolism in tissue culture cells*, pp. 85–109. Philadelphia: Wistar Institute Press.

Bailey, J. M., Howard, B. V., Dunbar, L. M. and Tillman, S. F. 1972. Control of lipid metabolism in cultured cells. *Lipids* 7:125–134.

Lipid Metabolism   103

Ballard, F. J. and Hanson, R. W. 1967. Changes in lipid synthesis in rat liver during development. *Biochem. J.* 102:952–958.

Ballard, F. J. and Hanson, R. W. 1969. Measurement of adipose-tissue metabolites *in vivo*. *Biochem. J.* 112:195–202.

Barley, F. W., Sato, G. H. and Abeles, R. H. 1972. An effect of vitamin B$_{12}$ deficiency in tissue culture. *J. Biol. Chem.* 247:4270–4276.

Barth, C., Slader, M. and Decker, K. 1972. Dietary changes of cytoplasmic acetyl-CoA synthetase in different rat tissues. *Biochim. Biophys. Acta* 260:1–9.

Barth, C. A., Hackenschmidt, H. J., Weiss, E. E. and Decker, K. F. A. 1973. Influence of kynurenate on cholesterol and fatty acid synthesis in isolated perfused rat liver. *J. Biol. Chem.* 248:738–739.

Bartley, J. C. and Abraham, S. 1972. Dietary regulation of fatty acid synthesis in rat liver and hepatic autotransplants. *Biochim. Biophys. Acta* 260:169–177.

Beg, Z. H., Allman, D. W. and Gibson, D. M. 1973. Modulation of 3-hydroxy-3-methylglutaryl coenzyme A reductase activity with cAMP and with protein fractions of rat liver cytosol. *Biochem. Biophys. Res. Commun.* 54:1362–1369.

Birnbaum, J. 1969. Coenzyme repression of acetyl-CoA carboxylase by (+)-biotin. *Arch. Biochem. Biophys.* 132:436–441.

Birnbaumer, L. and Rodbell, M. 1969. Adenyl cyclase in fat cells. II. Hormone receptors. *J. Biol. Chem.* 244:3477–3482.

Bloxham, D. P. and Akhtar, M. 1971. Studies on the control of cholesterol biosynthesis: The adenosine 3':5'-cyclic monophosphate-dependent accumulation of a steroid carboxylic acid. *Biochem. J.* 123:275–278.

Bortz, W. 1968. Noradrenalin-induced increase in hepatic cholesterol synthesis and its blockade by puromycin. *Biochim. Biophys. Acta* 152:619–626.

Bortz, W. M. 1973. On the control of cholesterol synthesis. *Metabolism* 22:1507–1524.

Bortz, W. M. and Lynen, F. 1963a. The inhibition of acetyl CoA carboxylase by long chain acyl CoA derivatives. *Biochem. Z.* 337:505–509.

Bortz, W. M. and Lynen, 1963b. Elevation of long chain acyl CoA derivatives in livers of fasted rats. *Biochem. Z.* 339:77–82.

Bortz, W., Abraham, S. and Chaikoff, I. L. 1963. Localization of the block in lipogenesis resulting from feeding fat. *J. Biol. Chem.* 238:1266–1272.

Brady, R. O. 1960. Biosynthesis of fatty acids. II. Studies with enzymes obtained from brain. *J. Biol. Chem.* 235:3099–3103.

Brady, R. O. and Gurin, S. 1952. Biosynthesis of fatty acids by cell-free or water-soluble enzyme systems. *J. Biol. Chem.* 199:421–431.

Brady, R. O., Bradley, R. M. and Trams, E. G. 1960. Biosynthesis of fatty acids. I. Studies with enzymes obtained from liver. *J. Biol. Chem.* 235:3093–3098.

Bratcher, S. C. and Hsu, R. Y. 1975. Separation of active enzyme components from the fatty acid synthetase of chicken liver. *Fed. Proc.* 34:673.

Bray, G. A. and York, D. A. 1971. Genetically transmitted obesity in rodents. *Physiol. Rev.* 51:598–646.

Bressler, R. and Wakil, S. J. 1962. Studies on the mechanism of fatty acid synthesis. XI. The product of the reaction and the role of sulfhydryl groups in the synthesis of fatty acids. *J. Biol. Chem.* 237:1441–1448.

Bricker, L. A. and Levey, G. S. 1972. Evidence for regulation of cholesterol and fatty acid synthesis in liver by cyclic adenosine 3',5'-monophosphate. *J. Biol. Chem.* 247:4914–4915.

Brindley, D. N., Matsumara, S. and Bloch, K. 1969. *Mycobacterium phlei* fatty acid synthetase—A bacterial multienzyme complex. *Nature (Lond.)* 224:666–669.

Brooks, J. L. and Stumpf, P. K. 1966. Fat metabolism in higher plants. XXXIX. Properties of a soluble fatty acid synthesizing system from lettuce chloroplasts. *Arch. Biochem. Biophys.* 116:108–116.

Brown, M. S. and Goldstein, J. L. 1974a. Familial hypercholesterolemia: Defective binding of lipoproteins to cultured fibroblasts associated with impaired regulation of 3-hydroxy-3-methylglutaryl coenzyme A reductase activity. *Proc. Natl. Acd. Sci. U.S.A.* 71:788–792.

Brown, M. S. and Goldstein, J. L. 1974b. Suppression of 3-hydroxy-3-methylglutaryl coenzyme A reductase activity and inhibition of growth of human fibroblasts by 7-ketocholesterol. *J. Biol. Chem.* 249:7306–7314.

Brown, M. S., Dana, S. E. and Goldstein, J. L. 1973a. Regulation of 3-hydroxy-3-methylglutaryl coenzyme A reductase activity in human fibroblasts by lipoproteins. *Proc. Natl. Acad. Sci. U.S.A.* 70:2162–2166.

Brown, M. S., Goldstein, J. L. and Siperstein, M. D. 1973b. Regulation of cholesterol synthesis in normal and malignant tissue. *Fed. Proc.* 32:2168–2173.

Brown, M. S., Dana, S. E. and Goldstein, J. L. 1974. Regulation of 3-hydroxy-3-methylglutaryl coenzyme A reductase activity in cultured human fibroblasts. *J. Biol. Chem.* 249:789–796.

Brown, M. S., Brunschede, G. Y. and Goldstein, J. L. 1975a. Inactivation of 3-hydroxy-3-methylglutaryl coenzyme A reductase *in vitro*. *J. Biol. Chem.* 250:2502–2509.

Brown, M. S., Dana, S. E. and Goldstein, J. L. 1975b. Cholesterol ester formation in cultured human fibroblasts: Stimulation by oxygenated sterols. *J. Biol. Chem.* 250:4025–4027.

Bruckdorfer, K. R., Khan, I. H. and Yudkin, J. 1972. Fatty acid synthetase activity in the liver and adipose tissue of rats fed with various carbohydrates. *Biochem. J.* 129:439–446.

Brunengraber, H., Boutry, M. and Lowenstein, J. M. 1973. Fatty acid and 3-β-hydroxysterol synthesis in the perfused rat liver. *J. Biol. Chem.* 248:2656–2669.

Bucher, H. L. R., Overath, P. and Lynen, F. 1960. β-Hydroxy-β methylglutaryl coenzyme A reductase, cleavage and condensing enzymes in relation to cholesterol formation in rat liver. *Biochim. Biophys. Acta* 40:491–501.

Burkl, G., Castorph, H. and Schweizer, E. 1972. Mapping of a complex gene locus coding for part of the Saccharomyces cerevisiae fatty acid synthetase multienzyme complex. *Mol. Gen. Genet.* 119:315–322.

Burton, D. N., Haavik, A. G. and Porter, J. W. 1968. Comparative studies of the rat and pigeon liver fatty acid synthetases. *Arch. Biochem. Biophys.* 126:141–154.

Burton, D. N., Collins, J. M., Kennan, A. L. and Porter, J. W. 1969. The effects of nutritional and hormonal factors on the fatty acid synthetase level of rat liver. *J. Biol. Chem.* 244:4510–4516.

Butterworth, P. H. W., Guchhait, R. B., Baum, H., Olson, E. B., Margolis, S. A. and Porter, J. W. 1966. Relationship between nutritional status and fatty acid synthesis by microsomal and soluble enzymes of pigeon liver. *Arch. Biochem. Biophys.* 116:453–457.

Butterworth, P. H. W., Yang, P. C., Bock, R. M. and Porter, J. W. 1967. The partial dissociation and the reassociation of the pigeon liver fatty acid synthetase complex. *J. Biol. Chem.* 242:3508–3516.

Capuzzi, D. M., Rothman, V. and Margolis, S. 1974. The regulation of lipogenesis by cyclic nucleotides in intact hepatocytes prepared by a simplified technique. *J. Biol. Chem.* 249:1286–1294.

Cardinale, G. J., Carty, T. J. and Abeles, R. H. 1970. Effect of methylmalonyl coenzyme A, a metabolite which accumulates in vitamin B_{12} deficiency, on fatty acid synthesis. *J. Biol. Chem.* 245:3771–3775.

Carey, E. M. and Dils, R. 1970. Fatty acid biosynthesis. V. Purification and characterization of fatty acid synthetase from lactating-rabbit mammary gland. *Biochim. Biophys. Acta* 210:371–387.

Carlson, C. A. and Kim, K.-H. 1973. Regulation of hepatic acetyl coenzyme A carboxylase by phosphorylation and dephosphorylation. *J. Biol. Chem.* 248:378–380.

Carlson, C. A. and Kim, K.-H. 1974a. Regulation of hepatic acetyl coenzyme A carboxylase by phosphorylation and dephosphorylation. *Arch. Biochem. Biophys.* 164:478–489.

Carlson, C. A. and Kim, K.-H. 1974b. Differential effects of metabolites on the active and inactive forms of hepatic acetyl CoA carboxylase. *Arch. Biochem. Biophys.* 164:490–501.

Chalvardjian, A. 1969. Mode of action of choline. IV. Activity of the enzymes related to fatty acid synthesis and the levels of metabolic intermediates in choline-deficient rats. *Can. J. Biochem.* 47:917–926.

Chang, H.-C., Seidman, I., Teebor, G. and Lane, M. D. 1967. Liver acetyl CoA carboxylase and fatty acid synthetase: Relative activities in the normal state and in hereditary obesity. *Biochem. Biophys. Res. Commun.* 28:682–686.

Chow, J. C., Higgins, M. J. P. and Rudney, H. 1975. The inhibitory effect of ATP on HMG-CoA reductase. *Biochem. Biophys. Res. Commun.* 63:1077–1084.

Christophe, J., Dagenais, Y. and Mayer, J. 1959. Increased circulating insulin-like activity in obese-hyperglycaemic mice. *Nature (Lond.)* 184:61–62.

Claycomb, W. C. and Kilsheimer, G. S. 1969. Effect of glucagon adenosine-3′,5′-monophosphate and theophylline on free fatty acid release by rat liver slices and on tissue levels of coenzyme A esters. *Endocrinology* 84:1179–1183.

Clinkenbeard, K. D., Sugiyama, T., Moss, J., Reed, W. D. and Lane, M. D. 1973. Molecular and catalytic properties of cytosolic acetoacetyl coenzyme A thiolase from avian liver. *J. Biol. Chem.* 248:2275–2284.

Clinkenbeard, K. D., Reed, W. D., Mooney, R. A. and Lane, M. D. 1975a. Intracellular localization of the 3-hydroxy-3-methylglutaryl coenzyme A cycle enzymes in liver. *J. Biol. Chem.* 250:3108–3116.

Clinkenbeard, K. D., Sugiyama, T., Reed, W. D. and Lane, M. D. 1975b. Cytoplasmic 3-hydroxy-3-methylglutaryl coenzyme A synthase from liver. *J. Biol. Chem.* 250:3124–3135.

Craig, M. D., Dugan, R. E., Muesing, R. A., Slakey, R. A. and Porter, J. W. 1972a. Comparative effects of dietary regimens on the levels of enzymes regulating the synthesis of fatty acids and cholesterol in rat liver. *Arch. Biochem. Biophys.* 151:128–136.

Craig, M. D., Nepokroeff, C. M., Lakshmanan, M. R. and Porter, J. W. 1972b. Effect of dietary change on the rates of synthesis and degradation of rat liver fatty acid synthetase. *Arch. Biochem. Biophys.* 152:619–630.

Dakshinamurti, K. and Desjardins, P. R. 1968. Lipogenesis in biotin deficiency. *Can. J. Biochem.* 46:1261–1267.

David-Nelson, M. A. and Brodish, A. 1969. Evidence for a diurnal rhythm of corticotrophin-releasing factor (CRF) in the hypothalamus. *Endocrinology* 85:861–866.

Delo, J., Ernst-Fonberg, M. L. and Bloch, K. 1971. Fatty acid synthetases from *Euglena gracilis*. *Arch. Biochem. Biophys.* 143:384–391.

Deloach, J. R. and Aguanno, J. J. 1975. Prosthetic group exchange of acyl carrier protein in division synchronized cultures of *Escherichia coli*. *Fed. Proc.* 34:644.

Dempsey, M. E. 1974. Regulation of steroid biosynthesis. *Annu. Rev. Biochem.* 43:967–990.

Desjardins, P. R. and Dakshinamurti, K. 1971. Acetyl-CoA holocarboxylase synthesis in biotin-deficient rat adipose tissue. *Arch. Biochem. Biophys.* 142:292–298.

Diamant, S., Gorin, E. and Shafrir, E. 1972. Enzyme activities related to fatty-acid synthesis in liver and adipose tissue of rats treated with triiodothyronine. *Eur. J. Biochem.* 26:553–559.

Dietschy, J. M. and McGarry, J. D. 1974. Limitations of acetate as a substrate for measuring cholesterol synthesis in liver. *J. Biol. Chem.* 249:52–58.

Dietschy, J. M. and Siperstein, M. D. 1967. Effects of cholesterol feeding and fasting on sterol synthesis in seventeen tissues of the rat. *J. Lipid Res.* 8:97–104.

Dietschy, J. M. and Wilson, J. O. 1970. Regulation of cholesterol metabolism. *N. Engl. J. Med.* 282:1128–1138, 1179–1183, 1241–1249.

Dimroth, P., Guchhait, R. B., Stoll, E. and Lane, M. D. 1970. Enzymatic carboxylation of biotin: Molecular and catalytic properties of a component enzyme of acetyl CoA carboxylase. *Proc. Natl. Acad. Sci. U.S.A.* 67:1353–1360.

Dinello, R. K. and Ernst-Fonberg, M. L. 1973. Purification and partial characterization of an acyl carrier protein from *Euglena gracilis*. *J. Biol. Chem.* 248:1707–1711.

Donaldson, W. E., Mueller, N. S. and Mason, J. V. 1971. Intracellular localization of fatty acid synthesis in chick-embryo liver and stimulation of synthesis by exogenous glucose. *Biochim. Biophys. Acta* 248:34–40.

Dorsey, J. A. and Porter, J. W. 1968. The effect of palmityl coenzyme A on pigeon liver fatty acid synthetase. *J. Biol. Chem.* 243:3512–3516.

Dugan, R. E. and Porter, J. W. 1970. The binding of reduced nicotinamide adenine dinucleotide phosphate to mammalian and avian fatty acid synthetases. Number of binding sites and the effect of reagents and conditions on the binding of reduced nicotinamide adenine dinucleotide phosphate to enzyme. *J. Biol. Chem.* 245:2051–2059.

Dugan, R. E., Slakey, L. L., Briedis, A. V. and Porter, J. W. 1972. Factors affecting the diurnal variation in the level of β-hydroxy-β-methylglutaryl coenzyme A reductase and cholesterol-synthesizing activity in rat liver. *Arch. Biochem. Biophys.* 152:21–27.

Dugan, R. E., Ness, G. C., Lakshmanan, M. R., Nepokroeff, C. M. and Porter, J. W. 1974. Regulation of hepatic β-hydroxy-β-methylglutaryl coenzyme A reductase by the interplay of hormones. *Arch. Biochem. Biophys.* 161:499–504.

Easter, D. J. and Dils, R. 1968. Fatty acid biosynthesis. IV. Properties of acetyl-CoA carboxylase in lactating-rabbit mammary gland. *Biochim. Biophys. Acta* 152:653–668.

Edwards, P. A. 1973. Effect of adrenalectomy and hypophysectomy on the circadian rhythm of β-hydroxy-β-methylglutaryl coenzyme A reductase activity in rat liver. *J. Biol. Chem.* 248:2912–2917.

Edwards, P. A. 1975a. The influence of catecholamines on cyclic AMP on 3-hydroxy-3-methylglutaryl coenzyme A reductase activity and lipid biosynthesis in isolated rat hepatocytes. *Arch. Biochem. Biophys.* 170:188–203.

Edwards, P. A. 1975b. Effect on plasma lipoproteins and lecithin-cholesterol dispersions on the activity of 3-hydroxy-3-methylglutaryl-coenzyme A reductase of isolated rat hepatocytes. *Biochim. Biophys. Acta* 409: 39–50.

Edwards, P. A. and Gould, R. G. 1972. Turnover rate of hepatic 3-hydroxy-3-methylglutaryl coenzyme A reductase as determined by use of cycloheximide. *J. Biol. Chem.* 247:1520–1524.

Edwards, P. A. and Gould, R. G. 1974. Dependence of the circadian rhythm of hepatic β-hydroxy-β-methylglutaryl coenzyme A on ribonucleic acid synthesis. *J. Biol. Chem.* 249:2891–2896.

Edwards, P. A., Muroya, H. and Gould, R. G. 1972. *In vivo* demonstration of the circadian rhythm of cholesterol biosynthesis in the rat liver and intestine of the rat. *J. Lipid Res.* 13:396–401.

Edwards, P. A. Fogelman, A. M. and Popjak, G. 1976. A direct relationship between the amount of sterol lost from rat hepatocytes and the increase in activity of HMG-CoA reductase. *Biochem. Biophys. Res. Commun.* 68:64–69.

Elovson, J. and Vagelos, P. R. 1968. Acyl carrier protein. X. Acyl carrier protein synthetase. *J. Biol. Chem.* 243:3603–3611.

Elwood, J. C. and Morris, H. P. 1968. Lack of adaptation in lipogenesis by hepatoma 9121. *J. Lipid Res.* 9:337–341.

Emmer, M., De Crombrugghe, B., Pastan, I. and Perlman, R. 1970. Cyclic AMP receptor protein of *E. coli:* Its role in the synthesis of inducible enzymes. *Proc. Natl. Acad. Sci. U.S.A.* 66:480–487.

Erickson, S. K., Davison, A. M. and Gould, R. G. 1975. Correlation of rat liver chromatin-bound free and esterified cholesterol with the circadian rhythm of cholesterol biosynthesis in the rat. *Biochim. Biophys. Acta* 409:59–67.

Exton, J. H., Corgin, J. G. and Harper, S. C. 1972. Control of gluconeogenesis in liver. V. Effects of fasting, diabetes, and glucagon on lactate and endogenous metabolism in the perfused rat liver. *J. Biol. Chem.* 247:4996–5003.

Fain, J. N. 1964. Effects of dexamethasone and 2-deoxy-D-glucose on fructose and glucose metabolism by incubated adipose tissue. *J. Biol. Chem.* 239:958–962.

Fall, R. R. and Vagelos, P. R. 1972. Acetyl coenzyme A carboxylase. Molecular forms and subunit composition of biotin carboxyl carrier protein. *J. Biol. Chem.* 247:8005–8015.

Fall, R. R. and Vagelos, P. R. 1973. Acetyl coenzyme A carboxylase. Proteolytic modification of biotin carboxyl carrier protein. *J. Biol. Chem.* 248:2078–2088.

Fall, R. R., Nervi, A. M., Alberts, A. W. and Vagelos, P. R. 1971. Acetyl CoA carboxylase: Isolation and characterization of native biotin carboxyl carrier protein. *Proc. Natl. Acad. Sci. U.S.A.* 68:1512–1515.

Fischer, E. H., Pockes, A. and Sarri, J. 1970. The structure, function and control of glycogen phosphorylase. *Essays Biochem.* 6:23–68.

Fogelman, A. M., Edmond, J., Seager, J. and Popjak, G. 1975. Abnormal induction of 3-hydroxy-3-methylglutaryl coenzyme A reductase in leucocytes from subjects with heterozygous familial hypercholesterolemia. *J. Biol. Chem.* 250:2045–2055.

Frenkel, E. P. 1971. Studies on mechanism of the neural lesion of pernicious anemia. *J. Clin. Invest.* 50:33–34a.

Frenkel, E. P. 1972. Effect of propionate on fatty acid synthesis in normal and B_{12} deprived mice. *Clin. Res.* 20:77.

Frenkel, E. P., Kitchens, R. L. and Johnston, J. M. 1973. The effect of vitamin B_{12} deprivation on the enzymes of fatty acid synthesis. *J. Biol. Chem.* 248:7540–7546.

Frenkel, E. P., Kitchens, R. L., Johnston, J. M. and Frenkel, R. 1974. Effect of vitamin B_{12} deprivation on the rates of synthesis and degradation of rat liver fatty acid synthetase. *Arch. Biochem. Biophys.* 162:607–613.

Freychet, P., Laudat, M. H., Laudat, P., Rosselin, G., Kahn, C. R., Gorden, P. and Roth, J. 1972. Impairment of insulin binding to the fat cell plasma membrane in the obese hyperglycemic mouse. *FEBS Lett.* 25:339–342.

Ganguly, J. 1960. Studies on the mechanism of fatty acid synthesis. VII. Biosynthesis of fatty acids from malonyl CoA. *Biochim. Biophys. Acta* 40:110–118.

Geyer, R. P. 1967. Uptake and retention of fatty acids by tissue culture cells. In *Lipid metabolism in tissue culture cells*, eds. G. H. Rothblat and D. Kritchevsky, pp. 33–45. Philadelphia: Wistar Institute Press.

Geyer, R. P., Bennett, A. and Rohr, A. 1961. Fatty acids of the triglycerides and phospholipids of HeLa cells and strain L fibroblasts. *J. Lipid Res.* 3:80–83.

Gibson, D. M. and Hubbard, D. D. 1960. Incorporation of malonyl CoA into fatty acids by liver in starvation and alloxan-diabetes. *Biochem. Biophys. Res. Commun.* 3:531–535.

Gibson, D. M., Hicks, S. E. and Allmann, D. W. 1966. Adaptive enzyme formation during hyperlipogenesis. *Adv. Enzyme Regul.* 4:239–246.

Gibson, D. M., Lyons, R. T., Scott, D. F. and Muto, Y. 1972. Synthesis and degradation of the lipogenic enzymes of rat liver. *Adv. Enzyme Regul.* 10:187–204.

Goldberg, I. and Bloch, K. 1972. Fatty acid synthetases in *Euglena gracilis*. *J. Biol. Chem.* 247:7349–7357.

Goldberg, I., Shechter, I. and Bloch, K. 1973. Fatty acyl-coenzyme A elongation in brain of normal and quaking mice. *Science* 182:497–499.

Goldfarb, S. and Pitot, H. C. 1971. The regulation of β-hydroxy-β-methyl-glutaryl coenzyme A reductase in Morris hepatomas 5123C, 780, 9618A. *Cancer Res.* 31:1879–1882.

Goldfine, H., Ailhaud, G. P. and Vagelos, P. R. 1967. Involvement of acyl carrier protein in acylation of glycerol 3-phosphate in *Clostridium butyricum*. II. Evidence for the participation of acyl thioesters of acyl carrier protein. *J. Biol. Chem.* 242:4466–4475.

Goldstein, J. L. and Brown, M. S. 1973. Familial hypercholesterolemia: Identification of a defect in the regulation of 3-hydroxy-3-methyl-glutaryl coenzyme A reductase activity associated with overproduction of cholesterol. *Proc. Natl. Acad. Sci. U.S.A.* 70:2804–2808.

Goldstein, J. L. and Brown, M. S. 1974. Binding and degradation of low density lipoproteins by cultured human fibroblasts. *J. Biol. Chem.* 249:5153–5162.

Goldstein, J. L., Dana, S. E. and Brown, M. S. 1974. Esterification of low density lipoprotein cholesterol in human fibroblasts and its absence in homozygous familial hyper-cholesterolemia. *Proc. Natl. Acad. Sci. U.S.A.* 71:4288–4292.

Goodridge, A. G. 1972. Regulation of the activity of acetyl coenzyme A carboxylase by palmitoyl coenzyme A and citrate. *J. Biol. Chem.* 247:6946–6952.

Goodridge, A. G. 1973a. Regulation of fatty acid synthesis in isolated hepatocytes prepared from the livers of neonatal chicks. *J. Biol. Chem.* 248:1924–1931.

Goodridge, A. G. 1973b. On the relationship between fatty acid synthesis and the total activities of acetyl coenzyme A carboxylase and fatty acid synthetase in the liver of prenatal and early postnatal chicks. *J. Biol. Chem.* 248:1932–1938.

Goodridge, A. G. 1973c. Regulation of fatty acid synthesis in the liver of prenatal and early postnatal chicks. *J. Biol. Chem.* 248:1939–1945.

Goodridge, A. G. 1973d. Regulation of fatty acid synthesis in isolated hepatocytes. Evidence for a physiological role for long chain fatty acyl coenzyme A and citrate. *J. Biol. Chem.* 248:4318–4326.

Goodridge, A. G., Garay, A. and Silpananta, P. 1974. Regulations of lipogenesis and the total activities of lipogenic enzymes in a primary culture of hepatocytes from prenatal and early postnatal chicks. *J. Biol. Chem.* 249:1469–1475.

Goto, T., Ringelmann, E., Riedel, B. and Numa, S. 1967. Purification and crystallization of acetyl CoA carboxylase. *Life Sci.* 6(Part II):785–790.

Gould, R. G. and Popjak, G. 1957. Biosynthesis of cholesterol in vivo and in vitro from DL-β-hydroxy-β-methyl [2-^{14}C]valerolactone. *Biochem. J.* 66:51p.

Gould, R. G. and Swyryd, E. A. 1966. Sites of control of hepatic cholesterol biosynthesis. *J. Lipid Res.* 7:698–707.

Gould, R. G. and Taylor, C. B. 1950. Effect of dietary cholesterol on hepatic cholesterol synthesis. *Fed. Proc.* 9:179.

Greenbaum, A. L., Gumaa, K. A. and McLean, P. 1970. The distribution of hepatic metabolites and the control of the pathways of carbohydrate metabolism in animals of different dietary and hormonal status. *Arch. Biochem. Biophys.* 143:617–663.

Greengard, O. 1971. Enzymic differentiation in mammalian tissues. *Essays Biochem.* 7:159–205.

Gregolin, C., Ryder, E., Kleinschmidt, A. K., Warner, R. C. and Lane, M. D. 1966a. Molecular characteristics of liver acetyl CoA carboxylase. *Proc. Natl. Acad. Sci. U.S.A.* 56:148–155.

Gregolin, C., Ryder, E. Warner, R. C., Kleinschmidt, A. K. and Lane, M. D. 1966b. Liver acetyl CoA carboxylase: The dissociation-reassociation process and its relation to catalytic activity. *Proc. Natl. Acad. Sci. U.S.A.* 56:1751–1758.

Gregolin, C., Ryder, E. and Lane, M. D. 1968a. Liver acetyl coenzyme A carboxylase. I. Isolation and catalytic properties. *J. Biol. Chem.* 243:4227–4235.

Gregolin, C., Ryder, E., Warner, R. C., Kleinschmidt, A. K., Chang, H.-C. and Lane, M. D. 1968b. Liver acetyl coenzyme A carboxylase. II. Further molecular characterization. *J. Biol. Chem.* 243:4236–4245.

Guchhait, R. B. and Mukherjee, S. 1972. Effect of hepatic level of long-chain acyl CoA on fatty acid synthesis in starved rats. *Indian J. Biochem. Biophys.* 9:271–272.

Guchhait, R. B., Moss, J., Sokolski, W. and Lane, M. D. 1971. The carboxyl transferase component of acetyl CoA carboxylase: Structural evidence for inter-subunit translocation of the biotin prosthetic group. *Proc. Natl. Acad. Sci. U.S.A.* 68:653–657.

Guchhait, R. B., Polakis, S. E., Dimroth, P., Stoll, E., Moss, J. and Lane, M. D. 1974a. Acetyl coenzyme A carboxylase system of *Escherichia coli.*

Purification and properties of the biotin carboxylase, carboxyltransferase, and carboxyl carrier protein components. *J. Biol. Chem.* 249: 6633–6645.

Guchhait, R. B., Zwergel, E. E. and Lane, M. D. 1974b. Acetyl coenzyme A carboxylase. Subunit structure of the protomeric form of the avian liver enzyme. *J. Biol. Chem.* 249:4776–4780.

Guder, W., Nolte, I. and Wieland, O. 1968. The influence of thyroid hormones on β-hydroxy-β-methylglutaryl coenzyme A reductase in rat liver. *Eur. J. Biochem.* 4:273–278.

Guynn, R. W., Veloso, D. and Veech, R. I. 1972. The concentration of malonyl-coenzyme A and the control of fatty acid synthesis *in vivo*. *J. Biol. Chem.* 247:7325–7331.

Halperin, M. L., Robinson, B. H. and Fritz, I. B. 1972. Effects of palmitoyl-CoA on citrate and malate transport by rat liver mitochondria. *Proc. Natl. Acad. Sci. U.S.A.* 69:1003–1007.

Harris, R. A., Rivera, E. R., Villemez, C. L. and Quackenbush, F. W. 1967. Mechanism of suckling-rat hypercholesteremia. II. Cholesterol biosynthesis and cholic acid turnover studies. *Lipids* 2:137–142.

Harry, D. S., Morris, H. P. and McIntyre, N. J. 1971. Cholesterol biosynthesis in transplantable hepatomas: Evidence for impairment of uptake and storage of cholesterol. *J. Lipid Res.* 12:313–317.

Harry, D. S., Dini, M. and McIntyre, N. 1973. Effect of cholesterol feeding and biliary obstruction on hepatic cholesterol biosynthesis in the rat. *Biochim. Biophys. Acta* 296:209–220.

Hatch, M. D. and Stumpf, P. K. 1961. Fat metabolism in higher plants. XVI. Acetyl coenzyme A carboxylase and acetyl coenzyme A-malonyl coenzyme A transcarboxylase from wheat germ. *J. Biol. Chem.* 236:2879–2885.

Haugaard, E. S. and Stadie, W. C. 1953. The effect of hyperglycemic-glycogenolytic factor and epinephrine on fatty acid synthesis. *J. Biol. Chem.* 200:753–757.

Heller, R. A. and Gould, R. G. 1973. Solubilization and partial purification of hepatic 3-hydroxy-3-methylglutaryl coenzyme A reductase. *Biochem. Biophys. Res. Commun.* 50:859–865.

Heller, R. A. and Gould, R. G. 1974. Reversible cold inactivation of microsomal 3-hydroxy-3-methylglutaryl coenzyme A reductase from rat liver. *J. Biol. Chem.* 249:5254–5260.

Hers, H. G. and Kusaka, T. 1953. Le metabolisme du fructose-1 phosphate dans le foie. *Biochim Biophys. Acta* 11:427–437.

Hickman, P., Horton, B. J. and Sabine, J. R. 1972. Effect of adrenalectomy on the diurnal variation of hepatic cholesterogenesis in the rat. *J. Lipid Res.* 13:17–22.

Hicks, S. E., Allmann, D. W. and Gibson, D. M. 1965. Inhibition of hyperlipogenesis with puromycin or actinomycin D. *Biochim. Biophys. Acta* 106:441–444.

Higgins, M. and Rudney, H. 1973. Regulation of rat liver β-hydroxy-β-methylglutaryl-CoA reductase activity by cholesterol. *Nature New Biol.* 246:60–61.

Higgins, M., Kawanchi, T. and Rudney, H. 1971. The mechanism of the diurnal variation of hepatic HMG-CoA reductase activity in the rat. *Biochem. Biophys. Res. Commun.* 45:138–144.

Himes. R. H., Young, D. L., Ringelmann, E. and Lynen, F. 1963. The biochemical function of biotin. V. Further studies on methylcrotonyl CoA carboxylase. *Biochem. Z.* 337:48–61.

Howanitz, P. J. and Levy, H. R. 1965. Acetyl-CoA carboxylase and citrate cleavage enzyme in the rat mammary gland. *Biochim. Biophys. Acta* 106:430–433.

Howard, B. V. and Kritschevsky, D. 1969. The source of cellular lipid in the human diploid cell strain WI-38. *Biochim Biophys. Acta* 187:293–301.

Howard, B. V., Howard, W. J. and Bailey, J. M. 1974. Acetyl coenzyme A synthetase and the regulation of lipid synthesis from acetate in cultured cells. *J. Biol. Chem.* 249:7912–7921.

Hsu, R. Y. and Yun, S. L. 1970. Stabilization and physicochemical properties of the fatty acid synthetase of chicken liver. *Biochemistry* 9:239–245.

Hsu, R. Y., Wasson, G. and Porter, J. W. 1965. The purification and properties of the fatty acid synthetase of pigeon liver. *J. Biol. Chem.* 240:3736–3746.

Huber, J. and Hamprecht, B. 1972. Diurnal rhythm of hydroxymethylglutaryl-CoA reductase in rat liver. I. Change of the rhythm by shift of the light-dark phase. *Hoppe Seylers Z. Physiol. Chem.* 353:307–312.

Huber, J., Hamprecht, B., Muller, D. and Guder, W. 1972. Diurnal rhythm of hydroxymethylglutaryl-CoA reductase in rat liver. II. Rhythm of adrenalectomized animals. *Hoppe Seylers Z. Physiol. Chem.* 353:313–317.

Huber, J., Guder, W., Latzin, S. and Hamprecht, B. 1973. The influence of insulin and glucagon on hydroxymethylglutaryl coenzyme A reductase activity in rat liver. *Hoppe Seylers Z. Physiol. Chem.* 354:795–798.

Hynie, I. and Hahn, P. 1972. Changes in the activity of acetyl-CoA carboxylase in the intestinal mucosa of the rat during development. *J. Nutr.* 102:1311–1314.

Ingalls, A. M., Dickie, M. M. and Snell, G. O. 1950. Obese, a new mutation in the house mouse. *J. Hered.* 41:317–318.

Inoue, H. and Lowenstein, J. M. 1972. Acetyl coenzyme A carboxylase from rat liver. Purification and demonstration of different subunits. *J. Biol. Chem.* 247:4825–4832.

Jacob, E. J., Butterworth, P. H. W. and Porter, J. W. 1968. Studies on the substrate binding sites of the pigeon liver fatty acid synthetase. *Arch. Biochem. Biophys.* 124:392–400.

Jacobs, R. A. and Majerus, P. W. 1973. The regulation of fatty acid synthesis in human skin fibroblasts. Inhibition of fatty acid synthesis by free fatty acids. *J. Biol. Chem.* 248:8392–8401.

Jacobs, R., Kilburn, E. and Majerus, P. W. 1970. Acetyl coenzyme A carboxylase. The effects of biotin deficiency on enzyme in rat liver and adipose tissue. *J. Biol. Chem.* 245:6462–6467.

Jacobs, R. A. Sly, W. S. and Majerus, P. W. 1973. The regulation of fatty acid biosynthesis in human skin fibroblasts. *J. Biol. Chem.* 248:1268–1276.

Jost, J.-P. and Richenberg, H. V. 1971. Cyclic AMP. *Annu. Rev. Biochem.* 40:741–774.

Kahn, C. R., Neville, D. M., Jr. and Roth, J. 1973. Insulin-receptor interaction in the obese-hyperglycemic mouse. A model of insulin resistance. *J. Biol. Chem.* 248:244–250.

Kanangara, C. G. and Stumpf, P. K. 1972. Fat metabolism in higher plants. LIV. A procaryotic type acetyl CoA carboxylase in spinach chloroplasts. *Arch. Biochem. Biophys.* 152:83–91.

Kandutsch, A. A. and Chen, H. W. 1973. Inhibition of sterol synthesis in cultured mouse cells by 7α-hydroxycholesterol,7β-hydroxycholesterol, and 7-ketocholesterol. *J. Biol. Chem.* 248:8408–8417.

Kandutsch, A. A. and Chen, H. W. 1974. Inhibition of sterol synthesis in cultured mouse cells by cholesterol derivatives oxygenated in the side chain. *J. Biol. Chem.* 249:6057–6061.

Kandutsch, A. A. and Chen, H. W. 1975. Regulation of sterol synthesis in cultured cells by oxygenated derivatives in cholesterol. *J. Cell. Physiol.* 85:415–424.

Kandutsch, A. A. and Hancock, R. L. 1971. Regulation of the rate of sterol synthesis and the level of β-hydroxy-β-methylglutaryl coenzyme A reductase activity in mouse liver and hepatomas. *Cancer Res.* 31:1396–1401.

Kandutsch, A. A. and Saucier, S. E. 1969a. Prevention of cyclic and triton-induced increases in hydroxymethylglutaryl coenzyme A reductase and sterol synthesis by puromycin. *J. Biol. Chem.* 244:2299–2305.

Kandutsch, A. A. and Saucier, S. E. 1969b. Regulation of sterol synthesis in developing brains of normal and jimpy mice. *Arch. Biochem. Biophys.* 135:201–208.

Kandutsch, A. A. and Saucier, S. E. 1972. Sterol and fatty acid synthesis in developing brains of three myelin-deficient mouse mutants. *Biochim. Biophys. Acta* 260:26–34.

Katzen, H. M. and Schimke, R. T. 1965. Multiple forms of hexokinase in the rat: Tissue distribution, age dependency, and properties. *Proc. Natl. Acad. Sci. U.S.A.* 54:1218–1225.

Kaul, L. and Berdanier, C. D. 1972. Diurnal rhythms of serum insulin and hepatic NADP-linked dehydrogenases in meal-fed rats. *Fed. Proc.* 31:669.

Kelley, R. E., Jr. and Joel, C. D. 1973. The activity of acetyl-coenzyme A carboxylase in rat brain. *Biochem. Soc. Trans.* 1:467–469.

Kirsten, E. S. and Watson, J. A. 1974. Regulation of 3-hydroxy-3-methylglutaryl coenzyme A reductase in hepatoma tissue culture cells by serum lipoproteins. *J. Biol. Chem.* 249:6104–6109.

Kishimoto, Y., Williams, M., Moser, H. W., Hignite, C. and Biemann, K. 1973. Branched chain and odd-numbered fatty acids and aldehydes in the nervous system of a patient with deranged vitamin B_{12} metabolism. *J. Lipid Res.* 14:69–77.

Klain, G. J. and Meikle, A. W. 1974. Mannoheptulose and fatty acid synthesis in the rat. *J. Nutr.* 104:473–477.

Klain, G. J. and Weiser, P. C. 1973. Changes in hepatic fatty acid synthesis following glucagon injections *in vivo*. *Biochem. Biophys. Res. Commun.* 55:76–83.

Kleinschmidt, A. K., Moss, J. and Lane, M. D. 1969. Acetyl coenzyme A carboxylase: Filamentous nature of the animal enzymes. *Science* 166:1276–1278.

Knappe, J., Ringelman, E. and Lynen, F. 1961. On the biochemical function of biotin. III. The chemical structure of enzymatically formed carboxyl-biotins. *Biochem. Z.* 335:168–176.

Knappe, J., Wenger, G. and Wiegard, V. 1963. On the structure of carboxylated β-methylcrotonyl carboxylase (CO_2 biotin enzyme). *Biochem. Z.* 337:232–246.

Knoche, H. W. and Koths, K. E. 1973. Characterization of a fatty acid synthetase from *Corynebacterium diptheriae*. *J. Biol. Chem.* 248:3517–3519.

Knoche, H., Esders, T. W., Koths, K. and Bloch, K. 1973. Palmityl coenzyme A inhibition of fatty acid synthesis. Relief by bovine serum albumin and mycobacterial polysaccharides. *J. Biol. Chem.* 248:2317–2322.

Knudsen, J. 1972. Fatty acid synthetase from cow mammary gland tissue cells. *Biochim. Biophys. Acta* 280:408–414.

Korchak, H. M. and Masoro, E. J. 1962. Changes in the level of the fatty acid synthesizing enzymes during starvation. *Biochim. Biophys. Acta* 58:354–356.

Kornacker, M. S. and Lowenstein, J. M. 1964. Citrate cleavage enzyme in livers of obese and nonobese mice. *Science* 144:1027–1028.

Kuhn, L., Castorph, H. and Schweizer, E. 1972. Gene linkage and gene-enzyme relations in the fatty-acid-synthetase system of *Saccharomyces cerevisiae*. *Eur. J. Biochem.* 24:492–497.

Kumar, S. and Porter, J. W. 1971. The effects of reduced nicotinamide adenine dinucleotide phosphate, its structural analogues, and coenzyme A and its derivatives on the rate of dissociation, conformation, and enzyme activity of the pigeon liver fatty acid synthetase complex. *J. Biol. Chem.* 246:7780–7789.

Kumar, S., Dorsey, J. A., Muesing, R. A. and Porter, J. W. 1970. Comparative studies of the pigeon liver fatty acid synthetase complex and its subunits. Kinetics of partial reactions and the number of binding sites of acetyl and malonyl groups. *J. Biol. Chem.* 245:4732–4744.

Kumar, S., Muesing, R. A. and Porter, J. W. 1972. Conformational changes, inactivation, and dissociation of pigeon liver fatty acid synthetase complex. Effects of ionic strength, pH, and temperature. *J. Biol. Chem.* 247:4749–4762.

Kusunose, M., Kusunose, E., Kowa, Y. and Yamamura, Y. 1959. Carbon dioxide fixation into malonate in *Mycobacterium avium*. *J. Biochem. (Tokyo)* 46:525–527.

Lakshmanan, M. R., Nepokroeff, C. M. and Porter, J. W. 1972. Control of the synthesis of fatty-acid synthetase in rat liver by insulin, glucagon, and adenosine 3′,5′ cyclic monophosphate. *Proc. Natl. Acad. Sci. U.S.A.* 69:3516–3519.

Lakshmanan, M. R., Nepokroeff, C. M., Ness, G. C., Dugan, R. E. and Porter, J. W. 1973. Stimulation by insulin of rat liver β-hydroxy-β-methylglutaryl coenzyme A reductase and cholesterol-synthesizing activities. *Biochem. Biophys. Res. Commun.* 50:704–710.

Lakshmanan, M. R., Dugan, R. E., Nepokroeff, C. M., Ness, G. C. and Porter, J. W. 1975a. Regulation of rat liver β-hydroxy-β-methylglutaryl coenzyme A reductase activity and cholesterol levels of serum and liver in various dietary and hormonal states. *Arch. Biochem. Biophys.* 168:89–95.

Lakshmanan, M. R., Nepokroeff, C. M., Kim, M. and Porter, J. W. 1975b. Adaptive synthesis of fatty acid synthetase and acetyl-CoA carboxylase by isolated rat liver cells. *Arch. Biochem. Biophys.* 169:737–745.

Landman, A. D. and Dakshinamurti, K. 1973. Isolation of acetyl CoA apocarboxylase by Sepharose-avidin affinity chromatography. *Anal. Biochem.* 56:191–195.

Landman, A. D. and Dakshinamurti, K. 1975. Acetyl-coenzyme A carboxylase. Role of the prosthetic group in enzyme polymerization. *Biochem. J.* 145:545–548.

Lane, M. D., Edwards, J., Stoll, E. and Moss, J. 1970. Tricarboxylic acid activator-induced changes at the active site of acetyl-CoA carboxylase. *Vitam. Horm.* 28:345–363.

Lane, M. D., Moss, J., Ryder, E. and Stoll, E. 1971. The activation of acetyl CoA carboxylase by tricarboxylic acids. *Adv. Enzyme Regul.* 9:237–251.

Lane, M. D., Moss, J. and Polakis, S. E. 1974. Acetyl coenzyme A carboxylase. In *Current topics in cellular regulation*, eds. B. L. Horecker and E. R. Stadtman, pp. 139–195. New York: Academic Press.

Lee, K. H., Thrall, T. and Kim, K.-H. 1973. Hormonal regulation of acetyl CoA carboxylase. Effect of insulin and epinephrine. *Biochem. Biophys. Res. Commun.* 54:1133–1140.

Leuthardt, F. and Testa, E. 1951. Die phosphorylierung der fructose in der leber. II. (Mitteilung). *Helv. Chim. Acta* 34:931–938.

Lin, C. Y. and Kumar, S. 1971. Primer specificity of mammary fatty acid synthetase and the role of the soluble β-oxidative enzymes. *J. Biol. Chem.* 246:3284–3290.

Lin, C. Y. and Kumar, S. 1972. Pathway for the synthesis of fatty acids in mammalian tissues. *J. Biol. Chem.* 247:604–606.

Linn, T. C. 1967. The effect of cholesterol feeding and fasting upon β-hydroxy-β-methylglutaryl coenzyme A reductase. *J. Biol. Chem.* 242:990–993.

Linn, T. L., Pettit, F. H. and Reed, L. J. 1969. α-Keto acid dehydrogenase complexes. X. Regulation of the activity of the pyruvate dehydrogenase complex from beef kidney mitochondria by phosphorylation and dephosphorylation. *Proc. Natl. Acad. Sci. U.S.A.* 62:234–241.

Liou, G. I. and Donaldson, W. E. 1973. Relative activities of acetyl-CoA carboxylase and fatty acid synthetase in chick liver: Effects of dietary fat. *Can. J. Biochem.* 51:1029–1033.

Lockwood, E. A., Bailey, E. and Taylor, C. B. 1970. Factors involved in changes in hepatic lipogenesis during development of the rat. *Biochem. J.* 118:155–162.

Lombardi, B., Pani, P. and Schlunk, F. F. 1968. Choline-deficiency fatty liver: Impaired release of hepatic triglycerides. *J. Lipid Res.* 9:437–446.

Lornitzo, F. A., Qureshi, A. A. and Porter, J. W. 1974. Separation of the half-molecular-weight nonidentical subunits of pigeon liver fatty acid synthetase by affinity chromatography. *J. Biol. Chem.* 249:1654–1656.

Lynen, F. 1961. Biosynthesis of saturated fatty acids. *Fed. Proc.* 20:941–951.

Lynen, F. 1967. The role of biotin-dependent carboxylations in biosynthetic reactions. *Biochem. J.* 102:381–400.

Lynen, F. 1969. Yeast fatty acid synthetase. *Methods Enzymol.* 14:17–33.

Lynen, F. and Rominger, K. L. 1963. Formation of acetyl-CoA carboxylase from its apocarboxylase. *Fed. Proc.* 22:537.

Lynen, F., Knappe, J., Lorch, E., Jutting, G., Ringelmann, E. and Lachance, J.-P. 1961. Zur biochemischen Funktion des Biotins. II. Reinigung und Wirkungsweise der β-Methylcrotonyl-Carboxylase. *Biochem. Z.* 335:123–167.

Lynen, F., Hopper-Kessel, I. and Eggerer, H. 1964. Zur biosynthese der fettsauren. 3. Die fettsaurensynthetase der hefe und die bildung enzymegebundener acetessigsaure. *Biochem. Z.* 340:95–124.

Maitra, S. K. and Kumar, S. 1974a. Crotonyl coenzyme A reductase activity of bovine mammary fatty acid synthetase. *J. Biol. Chem.* 249:111–117.

Maitra, S. K. and Kumar, S. 1974b. Physiochemical properties of bovine mammary fatty acid synthetase. *J. Biol. Chem.* 249:118–125.

Majerus, P. W. and Kilburn, E. 1969. Acetyl coenzyme A carboxylase. The roles of synthesis and degradation in regulation of enzyme levels in rat liver. *J. Biol. Chem.* 244:6254–6262.

Majerus, P. W. and Vagelos, P. R. 1967. Fatty acid biosynthesis and the role of the acyl carrier protein. *Adv. Lipid Res.* 5:1–33.

Majerus, P. W., Alberts, A. W. and Vagelos, P. R. 1964. The acyl carrier protein of fatty acid synthesis: Purification, physical properties, and substrate binding site. *Proc. Natl. Acad. Sci. U.S.A.* 51:1231–1238.

Majerus, P. W., Alberts, A. W. and Vagelos, P. R. 1965a. Acyl carrier protein. IV. The identification of 4'-phosphopantetheine as the prosthetic group of the acyl carrier protein. *Proc. Natl. Acad. Sci. U.S.A.* 53:410–417.

Majerus, P. W., Alberts, A. W. and Vagelos, P. R. 1965b. Acyl carrier protein. VII. The primary structure of the substrate binding site. *J. Biol. Chem.* 240:4723–4726.

Majerus, P. W., Jacobs, R., Smith, M. B. and Morris, H. P. 1968. The regulation of fatty acid biosynthesis in rat hepatomas. *J. Biol. Chem.* 243:3588–3595.

Maragoudakis, M. E. 1969. Inhibition of hepatic acetyl coenzyme A carboxylase by hypolipidemic agents. *J. Biol. Chem.* 244:5005–5013.

Maragoudakis, M. E. 1970a. On the mode of action of lipid-lowering agents. II. *In vitro* inhibition of acetyl coenzyme A carboxylase by a hypolipidemic drug. *Biochemistry* 9:413–417.

Maragoudakis, M. E. 1970b. On the mode of action of lipid-lowering agents. III. Kinetics of activation and inhibition of acetyl-coenzyme A carboxylase. *J. Biol. Chem.* 245:4136–4140.

Maragoudakis, M. E. 1971. On the mode of action of lipid-lowering agents. VI. Inhibition of lipogenesis in rat mammary gland cell culture. *J. Biol. Chem.* 246:4046–4052.

Maragoudakis, M. E. and Hankin, H. 1971. On the mode of action of lipid-lowering agents. V. Kinetics of the inhibition *in vitro* of rat acetyl coenzyme A carboxylase. *J. Biol. Chem.* 246:348–358.

Maragoudakis, M. E., Hankin, H. and Wasvary, J. M. 1972. On the mode of action of lipid-lowering agents. VII. *In vivo* inhibition and reversible binding of hepatic acetyl enzyme A carboxylase by hypolipidemic drugs. *J. Biol. Chem.* 247:342–347.

Maragoudakis, M. E., Hankin, H. and Kalinsky, H. 1974. Adaptive response of hepatic acetyl-CoA carboxylase to dietary alterations in genetically obese mice and their lean controls. *Biochim. Biophys. Acta* 343:590–597.

Margolis, S. and Baum, H. 1966. The association of acetyl-coenzyme A carboxylase with the microsomal fraction of pigeon liver. *Arch. Biochem. Biophys.* 114:445–451.

Martin, D. B. and Vagelos, P. R. 1962. The mechanism of tricarboxylic acid cycle regulation of fatty acid synthesis. *J. Biol. Chem.* 237:1787–1792.

Mason, J. V. and Donaldson, W. E. 1972. Fatty acid synthesizing systems in chick liver: Influence of biotin deficiency and dietary fat. *J. Nutr.* 102:667–672.

Matsuhashi, M., Matsuhashi, S. and Lynen, F. 1964a. Zur biosynthese der fettsauren IV. Acetyl-CoA carboxylase aus hefe. *Biochem. Z.* 340:243–262.

Matsuhashi, M., Matsuhashi, S. and Lynen, F. 1964b. Zur biosynthese der fettsauren. V. Die Acetyl-CoA carboxylase aus rattenleber und ihre aktivierung durch citronensaure. *Biochem. Z.* 340:263–289.

Matsumara, S. 1970. Conformation of acyl carrier protein from *Mycobacterium phlei. Biochem. Biophys. Res. Commun.* 38:238–243.

McGee, R. and Spector, A. A. 1974. Short-term effects of free fatty acids on the regulation of fatty acid biosynthesis in Ehrlich ascites tumor cells. *Cancer Res.* 34:3355–3362.

McLean, P., Brown, J., Greenslade, K. and Brew, E. 1966. Effect of alloxan-diabetes on the glucose-ATP phosphotransferase activity of adipose tissue. *Biochem. Biophys. Res. Commun.* 23:117–121.

McNamara, D. J. and Rodwell, V. W. 1975. Regulation of hepatic 3-hydroxy-3-methylglutaryl coenzyme A reductase: *In vitro* inhibition by a protein present in bile. *Arch. Biochem. Biophys.* 168:378–385.

McNamara, D. J., Quackenbush, F. W. and Rodwell, V. W. 1972. Regulation of hepatic 3-hydroxy-3-methylglutaryl coenzyme A: Developmental pattern. *J. Biol. Chem.* 247:5805–5810.

Meikle, A. W., Klain, G. J. and Hannon, J. P. 1973. Inhibition of glucose oxidation and fatty acid synthesis in liver slices from fed, fasted and fasted-refed rats by glucagon, epinephrine, and cyclic adenosine-3',5'-monophosphate. *Proc. Soc. Exp. Biol. Med.* 143:379–381.

Mellenberger, R. W. and Bauman, D. E. 1974. Metabolic adaptations during lactogenesis. Fatty acid synthesis in rabbit mammary tissue during pregnancy and lactation. *Biochem. J.* 138:373–379.

Menahan, I. A. and Wieland, O. 1969. The role of endogenous lipid in gluconeogenesis and ketogenesis of perfused rat liver. *Eur. J. Biochem.* 9:182–188.

Merrifield, R. B. 1963. Solid phase peptide synthesis. I. The synthesis of a tetrapeptide. *J. Am. Chem. Soc.* 85:2149–2154.

Middleton, B. 1973. The oxoacyl-coenzyme A thiolases of animal tissues. *Biochem. J.* 132:717–730.

Mildvan, A. S., Scrutton, M. C. and Utter, M. F. 1966. Pyruvate carboxylase. VII. A possible role for tightly bound manganese. *J. Biol. Chem.* 241:3488–3498.

Miller, A. L. and Levy, H. R. 1969. Rat mammary acetyl-coenzyme A carboxylase. I. Isolation and characterization. *J. Biol. Chem.* 244:2334–2342.

Mookerjea, S. 1971. Action of choline in lipoprotein metabolism. *Fed. Proc.* 30:143–150.

Moss, J. and Lane, M. D. 1972a. Acetyl coenzyme A carboxylase. III. Further studies on the relation of catalytic activity to polymeric state. *J. Biol. Chem.* 247:4944–4951.

Moss, J. and Lane, M. D. 1972b. Acetyl coenzyme A carboxylase. IV. Biotinyl prosthetic group-independent malonyl coenzyme A decarboxylation and carboxyl transfer: Generalization to other biotin enzymes. *J. Biol. Chem.* 247:4952–4959.

Moss, J., Yamagishi, M., Kleinschmidt, A. K. and Lane, M. D. 1972. Acetyl coenzyme A carboxylase. Purification and properties of the bovine adipose tissue enzyme. *Biochemistry* 11:3779–3786.

Muesing, R. A., Lornitzo, F. A., Kumar, S. and Porter, J. W. 1975. Factors affecting the reassociation and reactivation of the half-molecular weight nonidentical subunits of pigeon liver fatty acid synthetase. *J. Biol. Chem.* 250:1814–1823.

Munck, A. 1971. Glucocorticoid inhibition of glucose uptake by peripheral tissues: Old and new evidence, molecular mechanisms and physiological significance. *Perspect. Biol. Med.* 14:265–269.

Murthy, V. K. and Steiner, G. 1972. Hepatic acetic thiokinase: Possible regulatory step in lipogenesis. *Metabolism* 21:213–221.

Muto, Y. and Gibson, D. M. 1970. Selective dampening of lipogenic enzymes of liver by exogenous polyunsaturated fatty acids. *Biochem. Biophys. Res. Commun.* 38:9–15.

Nakanishi, S. and Numa, S. 1970. Purification of rat liver acetyl-coenzyme A carboxylase and immunochemical studies on its synthesis and degradation. *Eur. J. Biochem.* 16:161–173.

Nakanishi, S. and Numa, S. 1971. Synthesis and degradation of liver acetyl coenzyme A carboxylase in genetically obese mice. *Proc. Natl. Acad. Sci. U.S.A.* 68:2288–2292.

Nandedkar, A. K. N. and Kumar, S. 1969. Biosynthesis of fatty acids in mammary tissue. II. Synthesis of butyrate in lactating rabbit mammary supernatant fraction by the reversal of β-oxidation. *Arch. Biochem. Biophys.* 134:563–571.

Nath, K. and Koch, A. L. 1970. Protein degradation in *Escherichia coli*. I. Measurement of rapidly and slowly decaying components. *J. Biol. Chem.* 245:2889–2900.

Nath, K. and Koch, A. L. 1971. Protein degradation in *Escherichia coli*. II. Strain differences in the degradation of protein and nucleic acid resulting from starvation. *J. Biol. Chem.* 246:6956–6967.

Nelson, P. G. 1975. Nerve and muscle cells in culture. *Physiol Rev.* 55:1–61.

Nepokroeff, C. M., Lakshmanan, M. R., Ness, G. C., Muesing, R. A., Kleinsek, D. A. and Porter, J. W. 1974. Coordinate control of rat liver lipogenic enzymes by insulin. *Arch. Biochem. Biophys.* 162:340–344.

Nervi, A. M., Alberts, A. W. and Vagelos, P. R. 1971. Acetyl CoA carboxylase. III. Purification and properties of a biotin carboxyl carrier protein. *Arch. Biochem. Biophys.* 143:401–411.

Ness, G. C., Dugan, R. E., Lakshmanan, M. R., Nepokvoeff, C. M. and Porter, J. W. 1973. Stimulation of hepatic β-hydroxy-β-methylglutaryl coenzyme A reductase activity in hypophysectomized rats by L-tri-iodothyronine. *Proc. Natl. Acad. Sci. U.S.A.* 70:3839–3842.

Nishikori, K., Iritani, N. and Numa, S. 1973. Levels of acetyl-coenzyme A carboxylase and its effectors in rat liver after short-term fat-free refeeding. *FEBS Lett.* 32:19–21.

Numa, S., Matsuhashi, M. and Lynen, F. 1961. Zur storung der fettsaure-synthese bei hunger und alloxan-diabetes. I. Fettsauresynthese in der leber normaler und hungernder ratten. *Biochem. Z.* 334:203–217.

Numa, S., Ringelmann, E. and Lynen, F. 1964. Zur biochemischen funktion des biotins. VIII. Die bindung der kohlensaure in der carboxylierten acetyl-CoA-carboxylase. *Biochem. Z.* 340:228–242.

Numa, S., Bortz, W. M. and Lynen, F. 1965a. Regulation of fatty acid synthesis at the acetyl-CoA carboxylation step. *Adv. Enzyme Regul.* 3:407–423.

Numa, S., Ringelmann, E. and Lynen, F. 1965b. Zur hemmung der acetyl-CoA-carboxylase durch fettsaure-coenzyme A-verbindungen. *Biochem. Z.* 343:243–257.

Numa, S., Ringlemann, E. and Riedel, B. 1966. Further evidence for polymeric structure of liver acetyl CoA carboxylase. *Biochem. Biophys. Res. Commun.* 24:750–757.

Numa, S., Nakanishi, S., Hashimoto, T., Iritani, N. and Okazaki, T. 1970. Role of acetyl coenzyme A carboxylase in the control of fatty acid synthesis. *Vitam. Horm.* 28:213–243.

Pearce, J. 1968. The effect of dietary fat on lipogenic enzymes in the liver of the domestic fowl. *Biochem. J.* 109:702–704.

Pine, M. J. 1965. Heterogeneity of protein turnover in *Escherichia coli*. *Biochim. Biophys. Acta* 104:439–456.

Plate, C. A., Joshi, V. C., Sedgwick, B. and Wakil, S. J. 1968. Studies on the mechanism of fatty acid synthesis. XXI. The role of fructose 1,6-diphosphate in the stimulation of the fatty acid synthetase from pigeon liver. *J. Biol. Chem.* 243:5439–5445.

Polakis, S. E., Guchhait, R. B., Zwergel, E. E., Lane, M. D. and Cooper, T. G. 1974. Acetyl coenzyme A carboxylase system of *Escherichia coli.* Studies on the mechanisms of the biotin carboxylase- and carboxyltransferase-catalyzed reactions. *J. Biol. Chem.* 249:6657–6667.

Porter, J. W., Kumar, S. and Dugan, R. E. 1971. Synthesis of fatty acids by enzymes of avian and mammalian species. *Prog. Biochem. Pharmacol.* 6:1–101.

Powell, G. L., Elovson, J. and Vagelos, P. R. 1969. Acyl carrier protein. XII. Synthesis and turnover of the prosthetic group of acyl carrier protein *in vivo. J. Biol. Chem.* 244:5616–5624.

Powell, G. L., Bauza, M. and Larrabee, A. R. 1973. The stability of acyl carrier protein in *Escherichia coli. J. Biol. Chem.* 248:4461–4466.

Prescott, D. J. and Vagelos, P. R. 1972. Acyl carrier protein. *Adv. Enzymol.* 36:269–311.

Prescott, D. J., Elovson, J. and Vagelos, P. R. 1969. Acyl carrier protein XI. The specificity of acyl carrier protein synthetase. *J. Biol. Chem.* 244:4517–4521.

Pugh, E. L. and Wakil, S. J. 1965. Studies on the mechanism of fatty acid synthesis. XIV. The prosthetic group of acyl carrier protein and the mode of its attachment to the protein. *J. Biol. Chem.* 240:4727–4733.

Qureshi, A. A., Lornitzo, F. A. and Porter, J. W. 1974. The isolation of acyl carrier protein from the pigeon liver fatty acid synthetase complex II. *Biochem. Biophys. Res. Commun.* 60:158–165.

Qureshi, A. A., Jenik, R. A., Kim, M., Lornitzo, F. A. and Porter, J. W. 1975a. Separation of two active forms (holo-*a* and holo-*b*) of pigeon liver fatty acid synthetase and their interconversion by phosphorylation and dephosphorylation. *Biochem. Biophys. Res. Commun.* 66:344–351.

Qureshi, A. A., Kim, M., Lornitzo, A., Jenik, R. A. and Porter, J. W. 1975b. Separation of pigeon liver apo-holo-fatty acid synthetases by affinity chromatography. *Biochem. Biophys. Res. Commun.* 64:836–844.

Raff, R. A. 1970. Induction of fatty acid synthesis in cultured mammalian cells: Effects of cycloheximide and X-rays. *J. Cell Physiol.* 75:341–352.

Raskin, P., McGarry, J. D. and Foster, D. W. 1974. Independence of cholesterol and fatty acid biosynthesis from cyclic adenosine monophosphate concentration in the perfused rat liver. *J. Biol. Chem.* 249:6029–6032.

Regen, D. M. and Terrell, E. B. 1968. Effects of glucagon and fasting on acetate metabolism in perfused rat liver. *Biochim. Biophys. Acta* 170:95–111.

Robinson, C. A., Butcher, R. W. and Sutherland, E. W. 1971. *Cyclic AMP.* New York: Academic Press.

Robinson, J. D., Brady, R. O. and Bradley, R. M. 1963. Biosynthesis of fatty acids. IV. Studies with inhibitors. *J. Lipid Res.* 4:144–150.

Rodwell, V. W., McNamara, D. J. and Shapiro, D. J. 1973. Regulation of hepatic 3-hydroxy-3-methylglutaryl coenzyme A reductase. *Adv. Enzymol.* 38:373–412.

Roncari, D. A. K. 1974a. Mammalian acyl carrier protein. Dissociation of the acyl carrier protein subunit from dog liver fatty acid synthetase complex. *J. Biol. Chem.* 249:7035–7037.

Roncari, D. A. K. 1974b. Mammalian fatty acid synthetase. I. Purification and properties of human liver complex. *Can. J. Biochem.* 52:221–230.

Roncari, D. A. K. 1975. Mammalian fatty acid synthetase. II. Modification of purified human liver complex activity. *Can. J. Biochem.* 53:135–142.

Roncari, D. A. K., Bradshaw, R. A. and Vagelos, P. R. 1972. Acyl carrier protein. XIX. Amino acid sequence of liver fatty acid synthetase peptides containing 4′-phosphopantetheine. *J. Biol. Chem.* 247:6234–6242.

Rosenfeld, B. 1973. Regulation by dietary choline of hepatic fatty acid synthetase in the rat. *J. Lipid Res.* 14:557–562.

Rothblat, G. H. and Buchko, M. K. 1971. Effect of exogenous steroids on sterol synthesis in L-cell mouse fibroblasts. *J. Lipid Res.* 12:647–652.

Rothblat, G. H., Boyd, R. and Deal, C. 1971. Cholesterol biosynthesis in W1-38 and W1-38 VA 13A tissue culture cells. *Exp. Cell Res.* 67:436–440.

Rous, S. 1970. Effect of dibutyryl cAMP on the enzymes of fatty acid synthesis and of glycogen metabolism. *FEBS Lett.* 12:45–48.

Rous, S. 1974. Search for phosphorylated forms of fatty acid synthesis enzymes in the living animal. *FEBS Lett.* 44:55–58.

Rudack, D., Davie, B. and Holten, D. 1971. Regulation of rat liver glucose 6-phosphate dehydrogenase levels by adenosine 3′-5′-monophosphate. *J. Biol. Chem.* 246:7823–7824.

Ryder, E. 1970. Effect of development on chicken liver acetyl-coenzyme A carboxylase. *Biochem. J.* 119:929–930.

Ryder, E., Gregolin, C., Chang, H.-C. and Lane, M. D. 1967. Liver acetyl CoA carboxylase: Insight into the mechanism of activation by tricarboxylic acids and acetyl CoA. *Proc. Natl. Acad. Sci. U.S.A.* 57:1455–1462.

Sabine, J. R. 1969. Control of cholesterol synthesis in hepatomas. The effect of bile salts. *Biochim. Biophys. Acta* 176:600–604.

Sabine, J. R., Abraham, S. and Morris, H. P. 1968. Defective dietary control of fatty acid metabolism in four transplantable rat hepatomas: Numbers 5123 C, 7793, 7795, and 7800. *Cancer Res.* 28:46–51.

Saggerson, E. D. and Greenbaum, A. L. 1970. The regulation of triglyceride synthesis and fatty acid synthesis in rat epididymal adipose tissue. Effects of altered dietary and hormonal conditions. *Biochem. J.* 119:221–242.

Scallen, T. J., Seetharam, B., Srikantaiah, M. V., Hansbury, E. and Lewis, M. K. 1975. Sterol carrier protein hypothesis: Requirement for three substrate-specific soluble proteins in liver cholesterol biosynthesis. *Life Sci.* 16:853–874.

Schacht, U. and Granzer, E. 1970. On the effect of the hypolipidaemic phenyl ether CH-13-437 on the liver metabolism of the rat. *Biochem. Pharmacol.* 19:2963–2971.

Schimke, R. T. and Doyle, D. 1970. Control of enzyme levels in animal tissues. *Annu. Rev. Biochem.* 39:929–976.

Schneider, W. C., Striebish, M. J. and Hogeboom, G. H. 1956. Cytochemical studies. VII. Localization of endogenous citrate in rat liver fractions. *J. Biol. Chem.* 222:969–977.

Schweizer, E. and Golling, H. 1970. A *Saccharomyces cerevisiae* mutant defective in saturated fatty acid biosynthesis. *Proc. Natl. Acad. Sci. U.S.A.* 67:660–666.

Schweizer, E. F., Piccinnini, F., Duba, C., Gunther, S., Ritter, E. and Lynen, F. 1970. Die Malonyl-Bindungestellen des Fettsauresynthetase-komplexes aus Hefe. *Eur. J. Biochem.* 15:483–499.

Schweizer, E., Kuhn, L. and Castorph, H. 1971. A new gene cluster in yeast: The fatty acid synthetase system. *Hoppe Seylers Z. Physiol. Chem.* 352:377–384.

Schweizer, E., Kniep, B., Castorph, H. and Holzner, U. 1973. Pantetheine-free mutants of the yeast fatty-acid-synthetase complex. *Eur. J. Biochem.* 39:353–362.

Seidman, I. A., Horland, A. A. and Teebor, G. W. 1967. Hepatic glycolytic and gluconeogenic enzymes of the obese-hyperglycemic mouse. *Biochim. Biophys. Acta* 146:600–603.

Seidman, I. A., Horland, A. A. and Teebor, G. W. 1970. Glycolytic and gluconeogenic enzyme activities in the hereditary obese-hyperglycemic syndrome and in acquired obesity. *Diabetologia* 6:313–316.

Shah, S. N. 1973. Regulation of hepatic cholesterol synthesis from mevalonate in suckling and weaned rats. *Lipids* 8:284–288.

Shapiro, D. J. and Rodwell, V. W. 1969. Diurnal variation and cholesterol regulation of hepatic HMG-CoA reductase activity. *Biochem. Biophys. Res. Commun.* 37:867–872.

Shapiro, D. J. and Rodwell, V. W. 1971. Regulation of hepatic 3-hydroxy-3-methylglutaryl coenzyme A reductase and cholesterol synthesis. *J. Biol. Chem.* 246:3210–3216.

Shapiro, D. J. and Rodwell, V. W. 1972. Fine structure of the cyclic rhythm of 3-hydroxy-3-methylglutaryl coenzyme A reductase: Differential effects of cholesterol feeding and fasting. *Biochemistry* 11:1042–1045.

Shapiro, D. J., Taylor, J. M., McKnight, G. S., Palacios, R., Gonzalez, C., Kiely, M. and Schimke, R. T. 1974. Isolation of hen oviduct ovalbumin and rat liver albumin polysomes by indirect immunoprecipitation. *J. Biol. Chem.* 249:3665–3671.

Siegel, L., Foote, J. L. and Coon, M. J. 1965. The enzymatic synthesis of propionyl coenzyme A holocarboxylase from d-biotinyl 5′-adenylate and the apocarboxylase. *J. Biol. Chem.* 240:1025–1031.

Sillero, M. A. G., Sillero, A. G. and Sols, A. 1969. Enzymes involved in fructose metabolism in liver and the glyceraldehyde metabolic crossroads. *Eur. J. Biochem.* 10:345–350.

Silpananta, P. and Goodridge, A. G. 1971. Synthesis and degradation of malic enzyme in chick liver. *J. Biol. Chem.* 246:5754–5761.

Simoni, R. O., Criddle, R. S. and Stumpf, P. K. 1967. Fat metabolism in higher plants. XXXI. Purification and properties of plant and bacterial acyl carrier proteins. *J. Biol. Chem.* 242:573–581.

Siperstein, M. D. and Fagan, V. M. 1964. Deletion of the cholesterol-negative feedback system in liver tumors. *Cancer Res.* 24:1108–1115.

Siperstein, M. D. and Fagan, V. M. 1966. Feedback control of mevalonate synthesis by dietary cholesterol. *J. Biol. Chem.* 241:602–609.

Siperstein, M. D. and Guest, M. J. 1960. Studies on the site of the feedback control of cholesterol synthesis. *J. Clin. Invest.* 39:642–652.

Siperstein, M. D., Fagan, V. M. and Morris, H. P. 1966. Further studies on the deletion of the cholesterol feedback system in hepatomas. *Cancer Res.* 26:7–11.

Siperstein, M. D., Gyda, A. M. and Morris, H. P. 1971. Loss of feedback control of hydroxymethylglutaryl coenzyme A reductase in hepatomas. *Proc. Natl. Acad. Sci. U.S.A.* 68:315–317.

Slakey, L. L., Craig, M. C., Beytia, E., Briedis, A., Feldbruegge, D. H., Dugan, R. E., Qureshi, A. A., Subbarayan, C. and Porter, J. W. 1972. The effects of fasting, refeeding, and time of day on the levels of enzymes effecting the conversion of β-hydroxy-β-methylglutaryl-coenzyme A to squalene. *J. Biol. Chem.* 247:3014–3022.

Smith, S. and Abraham, S. 1970a. Fatty acid synthesis in developing mouse liver. *Arch. Biochem. Biophys.* 136:112–121.

Smith, S. and Abraham, S. 1970b. Fatty acid synthetase from lactating rat mammary gland. I. Isolation and properties. *J. Biol. Chem.* 245:3209-3217.

Smith, S. and Abraham, S. 1971. Fatty acid synthetase from lactating rat mammary gland. II. Studies on the termination sequence. *J. Biol. Chem.* 246:2537-2542.

Spector, A. A. 1972. Fatty acid, glyceride and phospholipid metabolism. In *Growth, nutrition and metabolism of cells in culture,* eds. G. H. Rothblat and V. J. Cristofalo, pp. 257-296. New York: Academic Press.

Spector, A. A., John, K. and Fletcher, J. E. 1969. Binding of long-chain fatty acids to bovine serum albumin. *J. Lipid Res.* 10:56-67.

Spencer, A. F. and Lowenstein, J. M. 1967. Citrate content of liver and kidney of rat in various metabolic states and in fluoroacetate poisoning. *Biochem. J.* 103:342-348.

Spiro, R. G. and Hastings, A. B. 1958. Studies of carbohydrate metabolism in rat liver slices. XI. Effect of prolonged insulin administration to the alloxan-diabetic animal. *J. Biol. Chem.* 230:751-759.

Stauffacher, W. and Renold, A. E. 1969. Effect of insulin *in vivo* on diaphragm and adipose tissue of obese mice. *Am. J. Physiol.* 216:90-105.

Stauffacher, W., Orci, L., Cameron, D. P., Burr, I. M. and Renold, A. E. 1971. Spontaneous hyperglycemia and/or obesity in laboratory rodents: An example of the possible usefulness of animal disease models with both genetic and environmental components. *Recent Progr. Horm. Res.* 27:41-95.

Steiner, G. and Cahill, G. F. 1966. Fatty acid synthesis and control in brown adipose tissue homogenates. *Can. J. Biochem.* 44:1587-1596.

Stoops, J., Arslanian, M., Oh, Y. H., Aune, K. D., Vanaman, T. C. and Wakil, S. J. 1975. Evidence for two polypeptide chains comprising the enzymes of fatty acid synthetase complex. *Fed. Proc.* 34:644.

Strauss, A., Alberts, A. W., Hennessy, S. and Vagelos, P. R. 1976. Regulation of the synthesis of hepatic fatty acid synthetase: Quantification using polysomal translation in a cell-free system. *Proc. Natl. Acad. Sci. U.S.A.* 72:4366-4370.

Strong, C. R. and Dils, R. 1972. The fatty acid synthetase complex of lactating guinea-pig mammary gland. *Int. J. Biochem.* 3:369-377.

Sugiyama, T., Clinkenbeard, K., Moss, J. and Lane, M. D. 1972. Multiple cytosolic forms of hepatic β-hydroxy-β-methylglutaryl CoA synthase: Possible regulatory role in cholesterol synthesis. *Biochem. Biophys. Res. Commun.* 48:255-261.

Sullivan, A. C., Hamilton, J. G., Miller, D. N. and Wheatley, V. R. 1972. Inhibition of lipogenesis in rat liver by (−)hydroxycitrate. *Arch. Biochem. Biophys.* 150:183-190.

Takeda, Y., Inoue, H., Honjo, K., Tanioka, H. and Daikuhara, Y. 1967. Dietary response of various key enzymes related to glucose metabolism in normal and diabetic rat liver. *Biochem. Biophys. Acta* 136:214-222.

Taketa, K. and Pogell, B. M. 1966. The effect of palmityl coenzyme A on glucose 6-phosphate dehydrogenase and other enzymes. *J. Biol. Chem.* 241:720-726.

Tanabe, T., Wada, K., Ozaki, T. and Numa, S. 1975. Acetyl-coenzyme A-carboxylase from rat liver. Subunit structure and proteolytic modification. *Eur. J. Biochem.* 57:15-24.

Taylor, C. B., Bailey, E. and Bartley, W. 1967. Changes in hepatic lipogenesis during development of the rat. *Biochem. J.* 105:717-722.

Taylor, J. M. and Schimke, R. T. 1973. Synthesis of rat liver albumin in a rabbit reticulocyte cell-free protein-synthesizing system. *J. Biol. Chem.* 248:7661-7668.

Taylor, J. M. and Schimke, R. T. 1974. Specific binding of albumin antibody to rat liver polysomes. *J. Biol. Chem.* 249:3597–3601.

Tepperman, H. M. and Tepperman, J. 1972. Mechanism of inhibition of lipogenesis by 3′,5′ cyclic AMP. In *Insulin action,* ed. I. B. Fritz, pp. 543–569. New York: Academic Press.

Teraoka, H. and Numa, S. 1975. Content, synthesis and degradation of acetyl-coenzyme A carboxylase in the liver of growing chicks. *Eur. J. Biochem.* 53:465–470.

Tormanen, C. D., Redd, W. L., Srikantaiah, M. V. and Scallen, T. J. 1976. Purification of 3-hydroxy-3-methylglutaryl coenzyme A reductase. *Biochem. Biophys. Res. Commun.* 68:754–762.

Tsutsumi, E. and Takenaka, F. 1969. Inhibition of pyruvate kinase by free fatty acids in rat heart muscle. *Biochim. Biophys. Acta* 117:355–357.

Tubbs, P. K. and Garland, P. B. 1963. Fatty acyl thioesters of coenzyme A: Inhibition of fatty acid synthesis *in vitro* and determination of levels in normal, fasted, and fat- or sugar-fed rats. *Biochem. J.* 89:25P.

Tubbs, P. K. and Garland, P. B. 1964. Variations in tissue contents of coenzyme A thioesters and possible metabolic implications. *Biochem. J.* 93:550–557.

Tweto, J. and Larrabee, A. R. 1972. The effect of fasting on synthesis and 4′-phosphopantetheine exchange in rat liver fatty acid synthetase. *J. Biol. Chem.* 247:4900–4904.

Tweto, J., Liberati, M. and Larrabee, A. R. 1971. Protein turnover and 4′-phosphopantetheine exchange in rat liver fatty acid synthetase. *J. Biol. Chem.* 246:2468–2471.

Tweto, J., Dehlinger, P. and Larrabee, A. R. 1972. Relative turnover rates of subunits of rat liver fatty acid synthetase. *Biochem. Biophys. Res. Commun.* 48:1371–1377.

Unger, R. H., Eisentraut, A. M. and Madison, L. L. 1963. The effects of total starvation upon the levels of the circulating glucagon and insulin in man. *J. Clin. Invest.* 42:1031–1039.

Ureta, T., Radojkovic, J. and Niemeyer, H. 1970. Inhibition by catecholamines of the induction of rat liver glucokinase. *J. Biol. Chem.* 245:4819–4824.

Vagelos, P. R. and Larrabee, A. R. 1967. Acyl carrier protein. IX. Acyl carrier protein hydrolase. *J. Biol. Chem.* 242:1776–1781.

Vagelos, P. R., Alberts, A. W. and Martin, D. B. 1962. Activation of acetyl-CoA carboxylase and associated alteration of sedimentation characteristics of the enzyme. *Biochem. Biophys. Res. Commun.* 8:4–8.

Vagelos, P. R., Alberts, A. W. and Martin, D. B. 1963. Studies on the mechanism of activation of acetyl coenzyme A carboxylase by citrate. *J. Biol. Chem.* 238:533–540.

Vagelos, P. R., Majerus, P. W., Alberts, A. W. and Ailhaud, G. 1966. Structure and function of the acyl carrier protein. *Fed. Proc.* 25:1485–1494.

Van Den Bosch, H. and Vagelos, P. R. 1970. Fatty acyl-CoA and fatty acyl-acyl carrier protein as acyl donors in the synthesis of lysophosphatidate and phosphatidate in *Escherichia coli. Biochim. Biophys. Acta* 218:233–248.

Van Den Bosch, H., Williamson, J. R. and Vagelos, P. R. 1970. Localization of acyl carrier protein in *Escherichia coli. Nature (Lond.)* 228:338–341.

Vanaman, T. C., Wakil, S. J. and Hill, R. L. 1968a. The preparation of tryptic, peptic, thermolysin, and cyanogen bromide peptides from the acyl carrier protein of *Escherichia coli. J. Biol. Chem.* 243:6409–6419.

Vanaman, T. C., Wakil, S. J. and Hill, R. L. 1968b. The complete amino acid sequence of the acyl carrier protein of *Escherichia coli. J. Biol. Chem.* 243:6420–6431.

Vance, D. E., Mitsuhashi, O. and Bloch, K. 1973. Purification and properties of the fatty acid synthetase from *Mycobacterium phlei. J. Biol. Chem.* 248:2303–2309.

Volpe, J. J. and Kishimoto, Y. 1972. Fatty acid synthetase of brain: Development, influence of nutritional and hormonal factors and comparison with liver enzyme. *J. Neurochem.* 19:737–753.

Volpe, J. J. and Marasa, J. C. 1975a. Hormonal regulation of fatty acid synthetase, acetyl-CoA carboxylase and fatty acid synthesis in mammalian adipose tissue and liver. *Biochim. Biophys. Acta* 380:454–472.

Volpe, J. J. and Marasa, J. C. 1975b. Regulation of palmitic acid synthesis in cultured glial cells: Effects of lipid on fatty acid synthetase, acetyl-CoA carboxylase, fatty acid and sterol synthesis. *J. Neurochem.* 25:333–340.

Volpe, J. J. and Marasa, J. C. 1975c. Regulation of hepatic fatty acid synthetase in the obese-hyperglycemic mutant mouse. *Biochim. Biophys. Acta* 409:235–248.

Volpe, J. J. and Marasa, J. C. 1976a. Regulation of palmitic acid synthesis in cultured glial cells: Effects of glucocorticoid on fatty acid synthetase, acetyl-CoA carboxylase, fatty acid and sterol synthesis. *J. Neurochem.* 27:841–845.

Volpe, J. J. and Marasa, J. C. 1976b. Long term regulation by theophylline of fatty acid synthetase, acetyl-CoA carboxylase and lipid synthesis in cultured glial cells. *Biochim. Biophys. Acta* 431:195–205.

Volpe, J. J. and Marasa, J. C. 1977. Short-term regulation of fatty acid synthesis in cultured glial and neuronal cells. *Brain Res.,* in press.

Volpe, J. J. and Vagelos, P. R. 1973a. Fatty acid synthetase of mammalian brain, liver and adipose tissue: Regulation by prosthetic group turnover. *Biochim. Biophys. Acta* 326:293–304.

Volpe, J. J. and Vagelos, P. R. 1973b. Saturated fatty acid biosynthesis and its regulation. *Annu. Rev. Biochem.* 42:21–60.

Volpe, J. J. and Vagelos, P. R. 1974. Regulation of mammalian fatty acid synthetase. The roles of carbohydrate and insulin. *Proc. Natl. Acad. Sci. U.S.A.* 71:889–893.

Volpe, J. J. and Vagelos, P. R. 1976. Mechanisms and regulation of biosynthesis of saturated fatty acids. *Physiol. Rev.* 56:340–417.

Volpe, J. J., Lyles, T. O., Roncari, D. A. K. and Vagelos, P. R. 1973. Fatty acid synthetase of developing brain and liver. Content, synthesis, and degradation during development. *J. Biol. Chem.* 248:2502–2513.

Waite, M. and Wakil, S. J. 1962. Studies on the mechanism of fatty acid synthesis. XII. Acetyl coenzyme A carboxylase. *J. Biol. Chem.* 237:2750–2757.

Wakil, S. J. 1961. Mechanism of fatty acid synthesis. *J. Lipid Res.* 2:1–24.

Wakil, S. J. and Ganguly, J. 1959. On the mechanism of fatty acid synthesis. *J. Am. Chem. Soc.* 41:2597–2598.

Wakil, S. J., Pugh, E. L. and Sauer, F. 1964. The mechanism of fatty acid synthesis. *Proc. Natl. Acad. Sci. U.S.A.* 52:106–114.

Wakil, S. J., Goldman, J. K., Williamson, I. P. and Toomey, R. E. 1966. Stimulation of fatty acid biosynthesis by phosphorylated sugars. *Proc. Natl. Acad. Sci. U.S.A.* 55:880–887.

Wakil, S. J., Mizugaki, M., Shapiro, M. and Weeks, G. 1968. The fatty acid system of *Escherichia coli.* In *Membrane models and the formation of biological membranes,* eds. L. Bolis and B. A. Pethica, pp. 122–137. Amsterdam: North-Holland.

Watson, J. A. 1972. Regulation of lipid metabolism in *in vitro* cultured minimal deviation hepatoma 7288C. *Lipids* 7:146–155.

White, L. W. 1971. Regulation of hepatic cholesterol biosynthesis by clofibrate administration. *J. Pharmacol. Exp. Ther.* 178:361–370.

White, L. W. and Rudney, H. 1970. Regulation of 3-hydroxy-3-methylglutarate and mevalonate biosynthesis by rat liver homogenates: Effects of fasting, cholesterol feeding, and triton administration. *Biochemistry* 9:2725–2731.

Wiegand, R. D., Rao, G. A. and Reiser, R. 1973. Dietary regulation of fatty acid synthetase and microsomal glycerophosphate acyltransferase activities in rat liver. *J. Nutr.* 103:1414–1424.

Wieland, O. and Siess, E. 1970. Interconversion of phospho- and dephosphoforms of pig heart pyruvate dehydrogenase. *Proc. Natl. Acad. Sci. U.S.A.* 65:947–954.

Wieland, O., Neufeldt, I., Numa, S. and Lynen, F. 1963. Zur storung der fettsauresynthese bei hunger und alloxandiabetes. II. Fettsauresynthese in der leber alloxandiabetischer ratten. *Biochem. Z.* 336:455–459.

Williamson, D. H., Bates, M. W. and Krebs, H. A. 1968. Activity and intracellular distribution of enzymes of ketone-body metabolism in rat liver. *Biochem. J.* 108:353–361.

Williamson, I. P., Goldman, J. K. and Wakil, S. J. 1966. Studies on the fatty acid synthesizing system from pigeon liver. *Fed. Proc.* 25:340.

Windmueller, H. G. 1964. An orotic acid-induced, adenine-reversed inhibition of hepatic lipoprotein secretion in the rat. *J. Biol. Chem.* 239:530–537.

Yang, P. C., Bock, R. M., Hsu, R. Y. and Porter, J. W. 1965. Physiochemical studies of fatty acid synthetase. A multi-enzyme complex from pigeon liver. *Biochem. Biophys. Acta* 110:608–615.

Yang, P. C., Butterworth, P. H. W., Bock, R. M. and Porter, J. W. 1967. Further studies on the properties of the pigeon liver fatty acid synthetase. *J. Biol. Chem.* 242:3501–3507.

Yeh, Y. Y. and Leveille, G. A. 1971. *In vitro* and *in vivo* restoration of hepatic lipogenesis in fasted chicks. *J. Nutr.* 101:803–810.

Yen, T. T. and Steinmetz, J. A. 1972. Lipolysis of genetically obese and/or hyperglycemic mice with reference to insulin response of adipose tissue. *Horm. Metab. Res.* 4:331–337.

Yu, H. L. and Burton, D. N. 1974a. Studies on the adaptive synthesis of rat liver fatty acid synthetase. *Arch. Biochem. Biophys.* 161:297–305.

Yu, H. L. and Burton, D. N. 1974b. Adaptive synthesis of rat liver fatty acid synthetase: Evidence for *in vitro* formation of active enzyme from inactive protein precursors and 4'-phosphopantetheine. *Biochem. Biophys. Res. Commun.* 61:433–438.

Yun, S.-L. and Hsu, R. Y. 1972. Fatty acid synthetase of chicken liver. Reversible dissociation into two nonidentical subcomplexes of similar size. *J. Biol. Chem.* 247:2689–2698.

Zakim, D. and Ho, W. 1970. The acetyl-CoA carboxylase and fatty acid synthetase activities of rat intestinal mucosa. *Biochim. Biophys. Acta* 222:558–559.

Zakim, D., Pardini, R. S., Herman, R. H. and Sauberlich, H. E. 1967. Mechanism for the differential effects of high carbohydrate diets on lipogenesis in rat liver. *Biochim. Biophys. Acta* 144:242–251.

Zakim, D., Pardini, R. S. and Herman, R. H. 1970. Effect of clofibrate (ethylchlorophenoxyisobutyrate) feeding on glycolytic and lipogenic enzymes and hepatic glycogen synthesis in the rat. *Biochem. Pharmacol.* 19:305–310.

Zubay, G., Schwartz, D. and Beckwith, J. 1970. Mechanism of activation of catabolite-sensitive genes: A positive control system. *Proc. Natl. Acad. Sci. U.S.A.* 66:104–110.

Chapter 4

LIPIDS AND LIPOPROTEINS IN DIABETES MELLITUS

Dana E. Wilson
Department of Medicine
College of Medicine
University of Utah
Salt Lake City, Utah

W. Virgil Brown
Department of Medicine
School of Medicine
University of California, San Diego,
La Jolla, California

INTRODUCTION

The primary objectives of this chapter are (1) to provide a succinct, up-to-date review of normal lipoprotein physiology and biochemistry; (2) to review the available data describing lipoprotein abnormalities and their pathogenesis in diabetic humans; and (3) to examine in some detail the biochemistry, physiology, and endocrine regulation of lipoprotein lipase (LPL). Although LPL, with the rare exception of familial hyperchylomicronemia, is in a sense an "enzyme in search of a disease," much evidence points to the conclusion that this important lipoprotein catabolic enzyme may be altered in diabetic humans and may contribute to the pathogenesis of hyperlipidemia. Recent discoveries in lipoprotein physiology and new information about the biochemistry of LPL and techniques for its measurement, we feel, justify the emphasis of our review.

In related areas, which are to be covered in depth by other contributors to this volume, we have chosen to cite review articles and to present generally accepted conclusions without exhaustive documentation by original experimental data. The reader who wishes to pursue studies on lipoprotein structure and metabolism in greater detail should consult the excellent reviews by Eisenberg and Levy (1975) and Jackson et al. (1976).

THE LIPOPROTEINS

Synthesis

Role of the intestine. Approximately 100 g of triglyceride (TG) and 0.5 g of cholesterol (mainly as cholesterol ester) are consumed in the diet each day. After emulsification with bile salts and phospholipids in the small bowel, the triglycerides are hydrolyzed to free fatty acids (FFA) and 2-monoglycerides by pancreatic lipase (Hofmann and Borgstrom, 1964). Mixed micelles of bile salts, phospholipids, fatty acids, and monoglycerides interact with the intestinal epithelial cell membrane and, by mechanisms not clearly understood, fatty acids and monoglycerides are transferred into the cell. Uptake of dietary fat is virtually complete in the jejunum. Bile salts are mainly retained in the lumen of the intestine, to be reabsorbed later in the distal ileum (Wilson and Dietschy, 1972; Hofmann and Mekhjian, 1973). Transport of the FFA from the microvillus membrane through the cytoplasm of the epithelial cell is facilitated by (and possibly dependent on) a low-molecular-weight (12,000) protein (Ockner et al., 1972). This soluble intracellular protein has a high affinity for long-chain unsaturated fatty acids and a low affinity for medium-chain-length (C_8 to C_{12}) fatty acids.

After delivery to the smooth endoplasmic reticulum, the fatty acid is activated by conversion to an acyl coenzyme A (CoA) derivative (Brindley and Hubscher, 1966). It is in the smooth endoplasmic reticulum of the absorptive cell that fatty acyl CoA is converted by transacylation to more complex lipids—primarily triglycerides and phospholipids (Rao and Johnston, 1966). Fatty acids of 12 carbons or less enter the portal vein without activation or transacylation (Greenberger et al., 1966). This is due in part to a low affinity for the transport protein as well as to the substrate specificity of the thiokinase for longer-chain fatty acid derivatives of CoA. Thus, it is primarily the long-chain fatty acids that are incorporated into the lipids of intestinal lipoproteins.

During fat absorption, lipid droplets rapidly appear in the vesicles of the endoplasmic reticulum, accumulate in the cisternae of the Golgi apparatus, and are soon visible by electron microscopy in the intercellular spaces (Cardell et al., 1967). These particles are usually greater than 1,000 Å in diameter (range 800–10,000 Å) and are called "chylomicrons" following the original description of the lipid particles seen by light microscopy in the blood after a meal (Gage and Fish, 1924). These particles reach the bloodstream only after entering the villous lacteal, to pass through the mesenteric lymphatic channels and the thoracic duct and finally join the venous plasma in the neck.

The chylomicron structure is believed to be a lipid droplet composed of TG and small amounts of cholesterol ester surrounded by a single layer of polar lipids and protein. This outer "hydrophilic membrane" contains phospholipids (primarily phosphatidylcholine and sphingomyelin), unesterified cholesterol, and several different apolipoproteins (Table 1). At least two of these apolipoproteins originate in the gut epithelial cell (Windmueller et al., 1973). One is apparently identical to the major apolipoprotein of high-density lipoprotein (HDL), apo AI, and the second identical to that of low-density lipoprotein (LDL), apo B. There is considerable evidence that the presence of the apolipoproteins is essential for chylomicron synthesis and secretion. Patients with abetalipoproteinemia whose plasma contains no detectable apo B do not produce chylomicrons despite absorption of the fatty acids and resynthesis of TG by the intestinal epithelium (Gotto et al., 1971). Inhibition of protein synthesis by puromycin markedly reduced lipid absorption (Sabesin and Isselbacher, 1965). Later studies using partial inhibition of protein synthesis with acetohexamide demonstrated a marked shift in the chylomicron size distribution to larger particles. Since the ratio of surface to core material decreases as the diameter increases, synthesis of larger particles allows fat absorption to proceed despite reduction in the supply of surface protein components (Glickman and Kirsch, 1973).

A third group of proteins present in lymphatic TG-rich lipoproteins has been referred to collectively as the C apolipoproteins (Table 2). They consist of three polypeptides: apo CI (6,000 daltons), apo CII (10,000 daltons), and apo CIII (8,700 daltons). Apo CII is a required cofactor for the lipolytic action of adipose tissue (LaRosa et al., 1970: Havel et al., 1970b) and myocardial LPLs (Havel et al., 1973a), enzymes responsible for the uptake of triglyceride into these tissues. Recently, another lipolytic enzyme in post-heparin plasma has been described which requires apo CI for full activity (Ganesan and Bass, 1975). The source and function of this enzyme are not yet established (Ganesan and Bradford, 1971). Apo CI has also been found to facilitate the activity of lecithin:cholesterol acyltransferase *in vitro*. The function of apo CIII is not known. This most abundant of the C apoproteins carries a strong negative charge, due in part to its content of sialic acid. Through providing a surface charge, apo CIII may prevent self-aggregation of lipoproteins and reduce nonspecific interactions with cell surfaces.

Little, if any, of the C apoproteins is synthesized in the gut, yet these constitute the major portion of the protein mass of lymph chylomicrons. It is currently believed that the liver is the principal source of these small apolipoproteins and that they enter the plasma as components of hepatic VLDL and HDL. A rapidly exchanging plasma pool is thus formed which involves chylomicron, VLDL, and HDL (Eisenberg and Levy, 1975). Newly synthesized chylomicrons receive C apolipoproteins in the lymph, primarily through transfer from HDL (Havel, et al., 1973b). They later return to HDL during the hydrolysis of chylomicron lipid by lipoprotein lipase. These apolipoproteins are thus reutilized many times in TG transport, saving much of the metabolic energy that would otherwise be required to synthesize each of the proteins necessary for a completed chylomicron.

It should be noted that TG-rich lipoproteins are produced in the bowel

TABLE 1 Properties of Human Plasma Lipoproteins[a]

Property	Chylomicrons	VLDL	IDL	LDL	HDL
Diameter Å	800–10,000	280–800	Unknown	200–250	90–120
Density, g/ml	0.95	0.95–1.006	1.006–1.019	1.019–1.063	1.063–1.21
Electrophoretic mobility	Origin	"pre-β" or α z	β	β	α
Lipid content, %	95–99	80–95	75–85	75	45–55
Triglyceride	80–95	55–80	10–50	5–10	5–10
Cholesterol + ester	2–7	5–15	20–40	60–75	25–35
Phospholipid	3–9	10–20	15–25	25–30	50–60
Apolipoproteins					
Major	Apo B	Apo B	Apo B	Apo B	Apo AI
	Apo CI	Apo CI	Apo E		Apo AII
	Apo CII	Apo CII			
	Apo CIII	Apo CIII			
		Apo E			
Minor	Apo AI	Apo D	Apo CI		Apo CI
	Apo AII	Apo AI	Apo CII		Apo CII
		Apo AII	Apo CIII		Apo CIII
					Apo D
					Apo E

[a]Data are from Fredrickson et al., 1972; Eisenberg and Levy, 1975; Jackson et al., 1976. The data on intermediate-density lipoprotein are less well documented than those on the other lipoproteins.

TABLE 2 Proteins of Human Plasma Lipoproteins

Apolipoprotein		Lipoprotein[a]	C-terminal amino acid	N-terminal amino acid	Molecular weight
Preferred title	Alternate title				
AI	apoGln-I	HDL, chylomicrons	Glutamine	Aspartic acid	28,000
AII	apoGln-II	HDL, chylomicrons	Glutamine	Pyrrolidone Carboxylic acid	17,000
B	apo-LDL	LDL, IDL, VLDL, chylomicrons	Blocked?	Glutamic acid	(see below)
CI	apo-Ser	Chylomicrons, VLDL, HDL	Serine	Threonine	7,000
CII	apo-Glu	Chylomicrons, VLDL, HDL	Glutamic acid	Threonine	10,000
CIII	apo-Ala	Chylomicrons, VLDL, HDL	Alanine	Serine	8,764
D	apo AIII "Thin-line peptide"	HDL	?	?	?20,000
E	arginine-rich protein (ARP)	IDL, HDL, VLDL	Alanine	Lysine	~40,000

[a]Lipoproteins are listed in decreasing order of the percentage of protein contributed by the apolipoprotein(s).

in the absence of dietary fat. These are usually less than 800 Å in diameter and have the size and ultracentrifugal characteristics of VLDL (Baxter, 1966; Ockner and Jones, 1970). It seems likely that these are the result of the reabsorption of lipids from the bile and from the degradation of gut mucosal cells. Neither *de novo* synthesis of fatty acids nor their uptakes from plasma appears to provide significant substrate for gut VLDL synthesis and secretion (Gangl and Ockner, 1975). The magnitude of VLDL efflux from the gut during the fasting state is not known but is probably much less than from the liver.

There is clear evidence for HDL production by the gut (Windmueller and Spaeth, 1972). These contain the major apoprotein of plasma HDL (apo AI) but little quantitative information regarding the structure or relative amounts of this lipoprotein has appeared. Although gut perfusion studies with radiolabeled amino acids result in labeled apolipoproteins in VLDL and HDL, no labeling of LDL was found. Similar results with liver perfusion studies have contributed to the concept of LDL as a catabolic product of VLDL rather than a product of direct intracellular synthesis (Noel and Rubinstein, 1974; Marsh, 1974).

Role of the liver. Triglyceride secretion from the liver occurs primarily in VLDL. These are spherical particles, 300-800 Å in diameter. The major lipid constituent is TG (50-75% by mass), which, as in chylomicrons, is thought to exist as an inner core with cholesterol ester (5-10%). Phospholipid (10-20%), unesterified cholesterol (5-10%), and protein (5-15%) are more abundant than in chylomicrons, consistent with the larger surface volume ratio in the smaller VLDL particles. Production of TG is dependent on the availability of fatty acid for synthesis of more complex lipids in a manner similar to that for the gut epithelial cell. This has been demonstrated in *in vitro* liver perfusion studies in which the fatty acid content of the perfusate is altered (Alcindor et al., 1970: Heimberg and Wilcox, 1972). In the fasting state approximately 1 g/hr of TG is put out by the liver in VLDL, a rate of secretion which is about four times that estimated from the bowel under similar conditions (Havel, 1971). Thus, the liver is the major source of plasma VLDL and of TG in postabsorptive humans.

Free fatty acids for TG synthesis by the liver must come from one of three sources: (1) synthesis by fatty acid synthetase from acetyl CoA and thus from a variety of lipid and nonlipid precursors, (2) mobilization of stored hepatic TG, or (3) free fatty acids arising from extrahepatic tissues, primarily adipose tissue. Studies in normal humans indicate that the third source is of major importance (Havel et al., 1970a). Thus, factors that affect rates of FFA mobilization can be expected to affect TG secretion in a similar direction. This does not mean that other substrates for hepatic metabolism, such as glycerol or amino acids, are unimportant in VLDL production, but that their impact is primarily through the sparing of FFA taken up from plasma, allowing a larger fraction to enter the pathways of TG synthesis (Nestel,

1967). A variety of hormones, including catecholamines, glucagon, and growth hormone, can stimulate fatty acid mobilization, whereas insulin plays an important counterregulatory role by suppressing the intracellular hormone-sensitive lipase of adipose tissue and reducing fatty acid flux from this source. The imbalance of these hormonal factors can produce marked derangements in lipid metabolism, such as those observed in diabetes mellitus (a subject discussed in detail later).

On entry into the liver, free fatty acids may be resynthesized into triglycerides and phospholipids by esterification with α-glycerophosphate, or they may enter the mitochondria for β-oxidation to acetyl CoA. In a recent review, the case has been made that the major determinant of the fate of the fatty acid is the rate of entry into the mitochondrion, a rate probably determined by activity of the long-chain fatty acyl-carnitine transferase reaction at the mitochondrial membrane (McGarry and Foster, 1972). The acetyl CoA formed by β-oxidation may be utilized in the tricarboxylic acid cycle with generation of ATP, CO_2, and water; resynthesized into fatty acids by fatty acid synthetase; or converted into ketones. In livers of normal animals ketone production is very low and the flux of acetyl CoA has been found to be divided approximately equally between pathways of fatty acid synthesis and of oxidation. In states of insulin deficiency, acetoacetate and β-hydroxybutyrate production increase at the expense of the fatty acid and triglyceride synthetic pathways, with very little effect on the flow of acetyl CoA into the tricarboxylic acid cycle. Thus, control mechanisms must be operative in the pathways of *de novo* TG synthesis from acetyl CoA. It should be noted that although plasma FFAs are the only appreciable source of VLDL triglyceride fatty acids during most circumstances, carbohydrate carbon is significantly incorporated into hepatic TG during feeding of very high carbohydrate diets (Volpe and Vagelos, 1974).

Electron microscopic studies have given a clearer understanding of the mechanism of synthesis and secretion of VLDL from the liver cell. On perfusing the liver with FFA-containing solutions, osmiophilic particles begin to develop in the smooth endoplasmic reticulum and accumulate in the Golgi apparatus (Jones et al., 1967; Stein and Stein, 1967). Finally, they are seen in the space of Disse and in the hepatic sinusoids. Inhibitors of protein synthesis or secretion block this sequence of events and triglycerides accumulate in the liver (Bar-On et al., 1973; LeMarchand et al., 1973; Stein and Stein, 1973). Isolated particles from the Golgi apparatus contain approximately 75% of the protein mass found in plasma VLDL (Hamilton, 1972). This protein contains apo B, apo C, and apo E (Table 2). It has been suggested by Hamilton (1972) that the SER is synthesized by the rough endoplasmic reticulum containing the apo B as a part of the biliary membrane. Nonpolar lipids are then deposited in the membrane in association with apo B to result in a spherical particle recognizable as VLDL. The concept of a pool of apo B awaiting addition of TG is consistent with the observation that VLDL secretion from the perfused rat liver continued for up to 1 hr after administration of cyclohexamide (Bar-On et al., 1973) and that these lipoproteins contained all the immunochemical characteristics of those secreted before addition of the inhibitor. This also agrees with data showing the presence of apo B in the gut epithelial cell and a reduction in its content during postprandial formation of chylomicrons (Rachmilewitz et al., 1976).

Addition of sugars to the apolipoproteins of VLDL occurs before their secretion. Specific roles for these sugars are not known, but it has been suggested that they may be important in the secretion of VLDL since inhibition of this secretion by orotic acid feeding was associated with the failure of glycosylation of apo CIII in the rat (Pottenger et al., 1973).

As noted above, the Golgi VLDL contains less protein than is found on the same lipoproteins in plasma. There is now much evidence for transfer of apoproteins from plasma HDL to VLDL and chylomicrons, thus completing their surface coats in the lymph and plasma compartments. This is indicated by the rapid equilibration of ^{125}I-labeled C apolipoproteins between HDL and VLDL *in vitro* (Eisenberg et al., 1972) and *in vivo* (Eisenberg and Rachmilewitz, 1973) and the loss of the lipoprotein lipase activator from HDL during fat absorption with a concomitant gain in the activator by chylomicrons (Havel et al., 1973b).

High-density lipoprotein has also been found in Golgi apparatus from liver (Hamilton, 1972). This nascent HDL differs from plasma HDL in several characteristics. With electron microscopy it appears as a disk 45 Å thick and approximately 200 Å in diameter. It contains little cholesterol ester and is rich in phospholipid, protein, and free cholesterol. The apolipoprotein fraction contains more apo E and less apo AI than the circulating plasma HDL (Felker et al., 1976). It has been suggested that the enzyme lecithin:cholesterol acyltransferase (LCAT) produces a spherical particle by esterifying the free cholesterol in nascent HDL with a resultant transfer of nonpolar lipid into the central core. HDL similar to that described as nascent HDL from liver perfusion studies is found in patients with genetic LCAT deficiency (Forte et al., 1974). On incubation of these lipoproteins with LCAT from normal individuals, spherical particles similar to normal HDL particles are generated.

Examination of material from the Golgi apparatus from both liver and gut has failed to reveal evidence for the independent synthesis of LDL. Kinetic studies in normal subjects with ^{125}I-labeled VLDL in the apolipoprotein moieties also suggest that all of the plasma LDL results from the degradation of triglyceride-rich lipoproteins containing apo B—that is, chylomicrons and VLDL (Bilheimer et al., 1972; Eisenberg et al., 1973).

Lipoprotein Catabolism

Lipoprotein lipase. This triglyceride lipase was initially described by Korn (1955a, 1955b) in studies of rat heart and adipose tissue. It was characterized by the requirement of a lipoprotein cofactor for full activity and by inhibition when assayed in the presence of protamine or high concentrations of salt (e.g., 1 M sodium chloride). The enzyme is of major importance in the degradation of TG in plasma lipoproteins, facilitating its uptake by a variety of tissues. Quantitatively most important in this process are adipose tissue and muscle. This enzyme can also be found in mammary gland, lung, kidney, spleen, skin, and intestine (Robinson, ,1970). Lipoprotein lipase is thought to be localized along the capillary endothelial cell membrane, from which it can be released by heparin injected intravascularly. The enzyme has been highly purified from rat (Fielding et al., 1974) and human plasma (Fielding, 1970; Augustin et al., 1976); from bovine milk (Egelrud and Olivecrona, 1972); from adipose tissue of chicken (Kompiang et al., 1976), rat (Greten and Walter, 1973), and pig (Bensadoun et al., 1974); and from swine and human heart (Ehnholm et al., 1975; Twu et al., 1976). Molecular weights have been determined in several studies. A value of 60,000–70,000 has been found in each instance, with the exception of the rat plasma enzyme, which had a molecular weight of approximately 37,000 (Fielding et al., 1974). Some controversy exists with regard to its positional specificity. Preference for the 1 and equal preference for the 1 and 3 positions of TG have been reported (Nilsson-Ehle et al., 1973; Morley et al., 1975).

The requirement for apo CII as an activator for the purified enzyme has been found by most investigators; however, one group has reported the purification of a second form of LPL activated by apo CI (Ganesan and Bass, 1975, 1976). The definition of the tissue source of this enzyme and its metabolic role need further study. The mechanism of the apolipoprotein activation of these lipases is unclear. Brockerhoff (1973) has suggested that the protein may function as a surface-active component, binding at the lipid-water interface, thereby providing proper orientation of the enzyme for cleavage of the lipid-ester bond.

Intravenous injection of protamine in the experimental animal inhibits the enzyme markedly and results in rapid accumulation of TG-rich lipoproteins (Spitzer, 1953). Recently, a more elegant and specific demonstration of the effects of blocking LPL action, utilizing antisera prepared against enzyme purified from chicken adipose tissue, has been reported (Kompiang et al., 1976). On injection of the antiserum into the bloodstream of the cockerel, clearance of radiolabeled VLDL was virtually eliminated and the plasma TG mass accumulated at its calculated rate of production. The importance of LPL in human lipoprotein metabolism is clearly demonstrated by the existence of type I hyperlipoproteinemia, a form of hyperchylomicronemia in which the enzyme is markedly deficient, both in postheparin plasma (Havel and Gordon, 1960; Ehnholm et al., 1974b) and in the tissues (Harlan et al., 1967). Inverse relationships between the plasma TG level and the level of the enzyme in both adipose tissue and postheparin plasma have been found in normal subjects (Huttunen et al., 1976; Persson, 1973).

Assay of lipoprotein lipase in postheparin plasma proved problematical until it was recognized that a second triglyceride hydrolase was simultaneously released by heparin injection (LaRosa et al., 1972; Krauss et al., 1974). This enzyme resides in liver, and when measured in human postheparin plasma, its activity is approximately equal to that of LPL. It differs from LPL in that it shows no increase in activity in the presence of lipoproteins or apolipoproteins and is not inhibited by protamine sulfate (Greten et al., 1972; Ehnholm et al., 1974a) or by solutions of high ionic strength (Ehnholm et al., 1975a, 1975b). When judged against TG-hydrolyzing ability, the hepatic enzyme is more active as a phospholipase (W. V. Brown et al., 1975) or a thioesterase (against palmitoyl CoA) than is LPL (Jansen and Hulsman, 1974; Baginsky and Brown, 1977). Utilizing their differing affinities for heparin (bound covalently to Sepharose beads), the two enzymes have been separated and highly purified. Amino acid composition, terminal group analysis, and tryptic peptide mapping studies have revealed no differences. Therefore, it is currently believed that they may share a common peptide backbone and differ only in their carbohydrate side chains (Augustin et al., 1976). This difference is sufficient for production of antisera that are specific for the enzymes. These antisera have been used in an assay which, after selective immunoprecipitation, allows the individual determination of hepatic triglyceride lipase or lipoprotein lipase. In type I hyperlipoproteinemia, the virtual absence of LPL has been confirmed by these assays, whereas the hepatic form of the enzyme is present. Currently, the role of the hepatic TG lipase in lipoprotein catabolism is unknown.

Chylomicron catabolism. In normal individuals chylomicrons are rapidly cleared from the plasma with a half-life of ½ hr or less. The initial phase of this clearance occurs in the extrahepatic tissues with binding of the chylomicron to the capillary endothelial cell membrane, followed by the hydrolytic action of lipoprotein lipase on the inner core of triglyceride (Scow et al., 1976). The process is extremely rapid, with studies in rat adipose tissue indicating uptake of the major portion of the triglyceride within 1-2 min after attachment of the chylomicron to the capillary endothelial cell (Stein et al., 1970). A portion of the phospholipid and the major part of the cholesterol ester of chylomicrons are not taken up by extrahepatic tissue, but are released for uptake into the liver as the so-called "chylomicron remnant" (Noel et al., 1975; Mjos et al., 1975). Specificity of uptake by the liver is supported by the continued circulation of these remnants in the hepatectomized rat and by liver perfusion studies in which removal from the medium suggests the existence of a saturable high-affinity binding process (Sherrill and Dietschy, 1976). In the intact rat, over 80% of the cholesterol ester of chylomicrons is taken up by the liver. With regard to the proteins of the chylomicron, the fate of apo AI and apo B are not known. Apo CII and apo CIII are apparently returned to plasma HDL, as noted above.

VLDL catabolism. It is currently believed that the degradation of very low density lipoprotein follows a pathway very similar to that described previously for chylomicrons. Because of the lack of elegant electron microscopic studies, less is known about its interaction at the capillary endothelial surface, but several studies utilizing isotopically labeled VLDL have given extensive data on the kinetics of turnover of both protein and lipid components (Eisenberg et al., 1972; Eisenberg and Rachmilewitz, 1973; Quarfordt et al., 1970; Nikkila and Kekki, 1971). Observations in patients with hyperlipoproteinemia suggest that VLDL and chylomicrons share a common saturable route of degradation, presumably at the LPL step. After VLDL is isolated, protein components are labeled with ^{125}I, and the lipoprotein is reinjected, the C apolipoproteins rapidly equilibrate with those in HDL. Radiolabeled apo B appears in the density range 1.006–1.019 (intermediate-density lipoprotein) and in the low-density range (1.019–1.063). Monitoring of these fractions generates curves of increasing radioactivity followed by a decline. Mathematical analyses of these data indicate that in normal individuals almost all apo B in VLDL ultimately enters the LDL range after a transient existence as intermediate-density lipoprotein (IDL). It has been calculated that the VLDL source is adequate to provide for the entire turnover of apo B in LDL. In hyperlipoproteinemics, more apo B is removed from the VLDL than can be accounted for by the calculated synthetic rate of LDL. For this reason, mathematical models have been constructed that suggest clearance of a portion of the apo B in VLDL (and IDL) without final conversion to LDL (Phair et al., 1972). In the rat, the major portion of apo B in IDL is removed directly by the liver without appearing in LDL (Eisenberg and Rachmilewitz, 1973). The apparent discrete steps of conversion of VLDL apo B to that of IDL and then LDL may be an illusion generated by current methodology, which uses specific density ranges for definition. It is quite possible that many small steps of interconversion are involved as triglyceride and phospholipid molecules are removed in the peripheral tissues. In fact, there is evidence for interconversion of large VLDL particles to smaller ones (Barter and Nestel, 1972).

LDL catabolism. In normal individuals low-density lipoproteins have a half-life of approximately 3 days, and in some forms of hypercholesterolemia this may be markedly prolonged (Langer et al., 1972). The tissues responsible for the uptake of LDL are not known, but studies in hepatectomized animals suggest that extrahepatic tissues are capable of playing the major role in removal. This is compatible with studies indicating a specific cell-surface receptor for LDL in fibroblasts (Brown et al., 1975b), smooth muscle cells (Bierman et al., 1974), and lymphocytes (Fogelman et al., 1975; Ho et al., 1976). After binding to this receptor, LDL particles are taken into the cell by endocytosis, followed by lysosomal hydrolysis of the protein by peptidases (Goldstein and Brown, 1974) and of the cholesterol ester by acid cholesterol esterase (Brown et al., 1975a). Free cholesterol then inhibits the synthesis of HMG-CoA reductase, the key regulatory enzyme of *de novo* cholesterol synthesis. Finally, an acyl-CoA cholesterol acyltransferase is stimulated, possibly by the intracellular cholesterol, resulting in its storage as cholesterol ester. If the exogenous source of lipoprotein is withdrawn, the intracellular cholesterol ester stores are hydrolyzed, providing for synthesis of cell components. In addition, the number of binding sites for LDL on the surface of the cell increases markedly; and HMG-CoA reductase activity rises to provide for the endogenous synthesis of cholesterol. The system thus allows for proper cellular levels of intracellular cholesterol, either from exogenous or endogenous sources, yet it protects against abnormal intracellular accumulation of the sterol (Goldstein and Brown, 1975a). Functional deficiency of LDL receptors has been found in subjects with familial type II hyperlipoproteinemia (familial hypercholesterolemia). Some patients with the homozygous form of this disorder appear to have a total lack of receptors and fail to bind or take up the lipoprotein through the high-affinity mechanism (Goldstein and Brown, 1975b; Anderson et al., 1976). LDL is taken up at a reduced rate by these cells through nonspecific pinocytotic vesicles, but the sterol contained therein fails to suppress endogenous cholesterol synthesis. As a result, these cells may be in danger of cholesterol overload when grown in the presence of high levels of LDL. Subjects who are heterozygous for this disorder appear to have approximately half the normal number of binding sites and are therefore less efficient in the uptake of LDL from the surrounding medium (Goldstein and Brown, 1975b). Heterogeneity has already appeared in this system, since some patients who are clinically homozygous for type II hyperlipoproteinemia demonstrate some specific binding of LDL, although they are severely deficient compared to normal individuals (Goldstein et al., 1975).

HDL catabolism. Newly synthesized HDL contains very little cholesterol ester, being rich in phospholipid, unesterified cholesterol, and protein (Hamilton, 1972). The protein components in nascent HDL differ in their source. Those from the liver contain apo A, apo C, and apo E (Felker et al., 1976), whereas the gut-generated particles contain only apo A, with particular enrichment of apo AI (Windmueller and Spaeth, 1972). These differences in nascent HDL structure may explain in part the heterogeneity noted in circulating plasma HDL. As implied by the name, these are the most dense of the plasma lipoproteins and are the smallest in size, with a diameter of about 100 Å. Approximately half the mass is protein and the remainder is divided equally between phospholipid and cholesterol (both ester and free). A very small amount of triglyceride is found in HDL from normal subjects (Table 1). These lipoproteins are clearly heterogeneous as they circulate in plasma and have been divided into HDL_2 and HDL_3, according to increasing density. The major apolipoproteins apo AI and apo AII exist in varying proportions in these different density ranges, from nearly equimolar in the heavier HDL_3 range to a preponderance of apo AI in the less dense HDL_2 range (Borut and Aladjem, 1971; Kostner et al., 1974). When isotopically labeled plasma HDL is reinjected *in vitro,* decay curves for the two apolipoproteins are identical. This suggests that the clearance mechanisms operate with very similar rates on the lipoproteins containing this variety of apo AI/apo AII ratios. It has been reported that isotopically labeled HDL is taken up by rat hepatocytes and degraded by lysosomal enzymes therein (Rachmilewitz et al., 1972; Roheim et al., 1971).

In normal fasting individuals, the major portion of the circulating C apolipoproteins is present in HDL. These may be bound to the surface of particles containing apo AI and apo AII or exist on separate lipoprotein species (Alaupovic, 1971; Alaupovic et al., 1972). These apo C proteins in HDL act as a reservoir for completing the surface coat of nascent chylomicrons and VLDL, thereby providing the activator protein (apo CII) for lipoprotein lipase.

It has been stated above that most of the LDL may be cleared by extrahepatic tissues, thus transporting large amounts of cholesterol into cells that have no capacity to degrade the sterol nucleus. Others have suggested that the return of cholesterol to the liver may be greatly facilitated by transport within HDL. After uptake by the hepatocyte, HDL cholesterol can be returned to plasma in newly synthesized lipoproteins or secreted in the bile as neutral sterol or bile acids. The circulating enzyme LCAT may play an important role in cholesterol transport by converting the HDL surface cholesterol to cholesterol ester (Glomset, 1968; Glomset and Norum, 1973). Migration to an internal position of the less polar lipid should then provide additional space on the surface of HDL for cholesterol transfer from extrahepatic cells. Apolipoproteins of HDL appear to activate the LCAT reaction *in vitro,* but controversy currently exists as to whether this activation is a function of the apo AI, apo CI, or apo D. The last has been proposed as a separate lipoprotein family, existing in small quantities in the HDL range (McConathy and Alaupovic, 1973; Köstner, 1974).

The accumulation of cholesterol ester in the tissues of subjects with familial HDL deficiency, Tangier disease (Fredrickson et al., 1972), and the negative correlation of arteriosclerotic disease with plasma HDL levels (Rhoads et al., 1976) are observations that appear to fit well with the proposed function of HDL in cholesterol transport.

PLASMA LIPIDS AND LIPOPROTEINS IN DIABETES

Classification of Plasma Lipoprotein Disorders

Prior to the 1960s, the disorders of lipid transport were classified mainly from the gross morphology of xanthomas, the appearance of the plasma, the plasma concentrations of cholesterol and triglycerides, and associations with other disease states (Thannhauser, 1947, 1950, 1958; Thannhauser and Magendantz, 1938). Quantitative lipoprotein measurement was largely limited to the research laboratory, although ultracentrifugal lipoprotein analyses provided the basis for the application of simpler techniques to greater numbers of patients (Gofman et al., 1954). The broad outlines of several more-or-less discrete clinical syndromes were defined, but the situation was unsatisfactory from a number of standpoints. Terminology was cumbersome and uninformative with regard to underlying biochemical and pathophysiological events. More seriously, this framework failed to suggest testable hypotheses for clinical investigation.

In the latter part of the 1960s, there was a surge in the interest of investigators in lipoprotein physiology and metabolism. The realization that lipoproteins could be regarded as structures with their own metabolic "pathways" led to testable hypotheses about the origin, fate, and control of lipoprotein concentrations in plasma. A decade later, a number of these questions have been answered with important clinical and therapeutic consequences.

The clinician began to think in terms of lipoproteins during this same period. This was greatly stimulated by certain easily applicable laboratory techniques. In 1963, Lees and Hatch reported that, with minor modifications, the standard system for serum protein electrophoresis could be used to identify the major lipoprotein species in plasma. In 1967, Fredrickson, et al. described a new classification based on semiquantitative electrophoretic analysis of the plasma lipoproteins. They interpreted available data within this scheme and studied relatively large numbers of selected hyperlipoproteinemic individuals and their families. One of the great advantages of the system seemed to be the clear familial aggregation of the individual phenotypes. In instances in which other disease states did not appear to underlie the lipid elevations, the pattern of inheritance was often consistent with a major gene defect. Second, the response or lack thereof to a given therapy was more consistent within the phenotypic groupings. The fundamental soundness of this approach was supported by the initial physiologic observations, such as lipoprotein turnover studies performed with selected small groups of subjects of a given phenotype. Pathogenetic models have been more informative and consistent with observed data when they have been based on hololipoprotein metabolism rather than postulated defects in the metabolism of individual lipoprotein lipids. Fredrickson and his co-workers have been careful to point out, however, that the classification system does not necessarily imply that the hyperlipoproteinemias result from mutations arising at loci regulating the structure or metabolism of the individual lipoproteins and that this working classification, while it has stimulated new physiological insights, is still basically descriptive. It must eventually be replaced by an etiologic classification (Fredrickson and Levy, 1972).

More recently, this classification has been challenged, particularly with respect to its usefulness in the daily practice of medicine. The objections that have been raised are valid ones and merit scrutiny, in our opinion. It was not surprising that this system, developed in a population referred to the Clinical

Center at the National Institutes of Health, began to experience difficulties when applied to less selected groupings. First, it became quite clear that there are major discrepancies between certain phenotypes and presumed genotypes (Goldstein et al., 1973b; Motulsky, 1976). The commonest phenotypes (IIB, IV, and IIA) have not been genetically homogeneous within pedigrees. Single pedigrees often exhibit two or more phenotypes, patients may "convert to different phenotypes" under a variety of environmental situations, and presumably noninherited phenocopies are widely prevalent. Recent evidence suggests that even among kindreds in which the phenotype characteristic of type II hyperlipoproteinemia (familial hypercholesterolemia) appears to be consistent in affected relatives, there are at least two cellular defects conferring different responses to therapy (Breslow et al., 1975; Goldstein et al., 1975). Thus, alternative proposals, based on plasma lipid concentrations combined with pedigree examination, have been introduced to provide consistent genetic models for the major hyperlipidemic disorders.

Despite refinements in lipoprotein electrophoresis and improved resolution of lipoprotein classes, there are reasons for dissatisfaction with the phenotyping methodology as well. The diagnosis of familial dyslipoproteinemia (type III, floating β disease) is most safely made with ancillary ultracentrifugation, a procedure that entails considerable expense and has a very low yield (Wood et al., 1972). The laboratory report, "compatible with hyperlipoproteinemia type IIB, III, or IV," is frustratingly familiar to clinicians. Moreover, whether or not elevated β- or pre-β lipoproteins are reported has often depended on measured cholesterol and triglyceride concentrations rather than independent interpretation of the electrophoresis pattern!

Recently, attempts have been made to base diagnostic and therapeutic strategies solely on fasting cholesterol and triglyceride values along with inspection of the plasma or serum (an important step that is often ignored). There are a number of advantages to this approach: (1) it is pedagogically convenient; (2) lipoprotein electrophoresis rarely offers significant additional information; and (3) the cumulative cost of lipoprotein electrophoresis in screening for hyperlipidemia becomes enormous.

We feel, however, that there has been some confusion in reaching this view and that if it were implemented fully in our approach to the diagnosis and treatment of hyperlipidemias, it would be a step backward. Dissatisfaction with lipoprotein phenotyping reflects, to a large degree, inadequacies in laboratory technology and the semiquantitative interpretation of electrophoretic patterns. Description of the hyperlipoproteinemias only in terms of plasma lipid concentrations obscures valuable information and ignores important physiological concepts. Although hypercholesterolemia is the best epidemiological predictor of coronary risk, such information cannot be applied meaningfully in individual situations. For example, the consequences of a 50 mg/dl increase in serum total cholesterol appear to be vastly different if the cholesterol is carried in chylomicrons, LDL, or HDL (Rhoads et al., 1976).

While satisfactory laboratory methods for quantitative lipoprotein measurements are not in widespread use and any phenotypic classification will need modification as new genetic and etiologic discoveries are made, the concept of lipoproteins as metabolically respectable structures remains an invaluable one. Questions such as the utility of measuring HDL before beginning treatment of moderate hypercholesterolemia may be answered positively in the near future and result in the pendulum swinging back toward partial lipoprotein quantification. Meanwhile, to inspect the plasma and measure plasma lipids, but to think "lipoproteins," seems to be a prudent compromise (Havel, 1970, 1975; Fredrickson, 1975). These considerations apply both to the routine management of diabetic patients and to hyperlipoproteinemic individuals in general.

Review of Lipoprotein Phenotypes

The lipoprotein phenotyping scheme has been presented in many publications and has been modified with the advent of new information (Fredrickson and Levy, 1972). For the convenience of the reader, the salient features of the phenotypic designations are given in Tables 3 and 4. This system is based on the electrophoretic mobilities of the major lipoprotein groupings, β, pre-β, and α, which are named for their comigration with the plasma globulins. Chylomicrons do not leave the origin in the supporting media commonly used for this purpose. Although simple, inexpensive, and efficient, the electrophoretic systems do not provide quantitative data without elaborate adaptations. Since lipoprotein levels in hyperlipoproteinemia lie at the upper end of a continuous distribution, the importance of quantitation has become increasingly obvious.

A density class designation has arisen from ultracentrifugal analysis and isolation of lipoproteins. The great practical usefulness of this instrument

TABLE 3   Clinical Features of the Six Hyperlipoproteinemias

Phenotype	CAD[a]	Xanthomas[b]	Clinical features
I	0	EX	Fat intolerance, lipoprotein lipase deficiency
IIA	3	TEND, TUB, XE	LDL receptor abnormality
IIB	2–3	TEND, TUB, XE	
III	3	TEND, TUB, XE TE, P	Obesity
IV	2	±	Hyperuricemia
V	±	EX	Carbohydrate intolerance

[a]Relative atherogenic risk for the various phenotypes, ranging from minimal (0) to marked (3).

[b]EX, eruptive; TEND, tendinous; TUB, tuberous; XE, xanthelasma; TE, tuberoeruptive; and P, plane. Most hyperlipoproteinemic individuals do not show xanthomatosis.

TABLE 4   Lipoprotein Phenotyping System[a]

Phenotype[b] (WHO classification)	Lipoprotein species increased	
	Lipoprotein Density class	Electrophoretic nomenclature
I	Chylomicrons	Chylomicrons
IIA	LDL	Beta
IIB	LDL + VLDL	Beta + pre-beta
III	IDL	"Floating-beta"
IV	VLDL	Pre-beta
V	Chylomicrons + VLDL	Chylomicrons + pre-beta

[a]Beaumont et al., 1970.

[b]The definition of type III was modified since the first classification when the unique characteristics of IDL were recognized. The type II phenotype was subdivided into IIA and IIB.

for investigative work with lipoproteins has resulted in the continued use of density class nomenclature for physical, biochemical, and physiological experiments. For these reasons, the density class nomenclature is now to be preferred. Table 5 compares the genetic and lipoprotein phenotyping designations. Phenotypic heterogeneity within the genetically defined hyperlipidemias is apparent.

Lipid and Lipoprotein Abnormalities in Diabetes Mellitus

Xanthomatosis. The history of the lipoprotein transport disorders began years ago with the report of several patients with xanthomatosis by Addison and Gull (1851). They described a 27-yr-old patient, John Sheriff, who presented with a 6 month history of polyuria. A year after the onset of symptoms of diabetes he developed an eruption over the arms, legs, trunk,

TABLE 5   Comparison of Genetic and Phenotypic Classifications of the Major Familial Hyperlipoproteinemias[a]

Genetic designation	Phenotypes	Genetic mechanism	Frequency in population (%)
Familial hypercholesterolemia	IIA or IIB	Autosomal dominant	0.1–0.5
Polygenic hypercholesterolemia	IIA or IIB	Polygenic	5
Familial hypertriglyceridemia	IV (V)	Autosomal dominant	1
Familial combined hyperlipidemia	IIA, IIB, IV (rarely V)	Autosomal dominant	1.5

[a]Adapted from Motulsky (1976) and the data of Hazzard et al. (1973).

face, and scalp. It consisted of "scattered tubercles of various sizes, some being as large as a small pea. They were of a yellowish colour, mottled with a deepish rose-tint. . . ."

In the following 50 yr the major morphologic types of xanthomatosis were described, and eventually the relationship between these lesions and hyperlipidemia was recognized. Throughout this period, reports of secondary xanthomatosis associated with diabetes mellitus and hepatobiliary or renal disease predominated (Jensen, 1967).

Lipid abnormalities in diabetes. "In severe diabetes high degrees of hyperlipemia is a rare symptom, a moderate or slight hyperlipemia a relatively frequent one. . . . Higher degrees of hyperlipemia were found only in connection with marked acidosis . . . In mild and moderate cases above 50 years of age is not seldom found some degrees of hyperlipemia or hypercholesterinemia, which appears independent of active symptoms and probably owns another significance than the hyperlipemia found in younger ages."

These inferences were made by Blix in 1926, from "cholesterin" measurements and inspection of plasma. For the most part, they hold true today. Only a few points will be made here since the plasma lipid abnormalities in diabetes have been described elsewhere in this volume. A review of carbohydrate, lipid, and lipoprotein abnormalities in diabetic nonhuman primates has been published recently (Howard, 1975).

Definitions. "Lipemia" and "hyperlipemia" imply the presence of opalescent or milky serum and thus increased VLDL, IDL, or chylomicron concentrations, since these TG-rich lipoproteins are large enough to produce light-scattering. "Hyperlipidemia" is a more general term, which includes not only the lipemias but also any abnormal elevation of the other plasma lipids. Thus, familial hypercholesterolemia (IIA) is "hyperlipoproteinemia" (LDL increased) or "hyperlipidemia" (cholesterol increased) but not "lipemia" (since the plasma is clear).

With full appreciation for the nosologic nightmare that may be perpetuated, we have preserved two terms already in the literature. The "diabetic-hyperlipemic syndrome" refers to any overtly lipemic state in diabetes (Nikkila and Kekki, 1973). "Diabetic lipemia" has been given a more specific meaning by Bagdade et al. (1967). This rare situation implies the presence of a removal defect for dietary fat. Thus, diabetic lipemia is a special form of the diabetic-hyperlipemic syndrome.

Finally, any conclusion about the prevalence and interactions of diabetes and hyperlipoproteinemia must be qualified with the confession that the diagnoses of these conditions are imprecise. Since pathognomonic manifestions are infrequent in diabetic or hyperlipidemic individuals, biochemical criteria have been proposed for the diagnosis of these conditions. Lipid values prevalent in atherosclerosis-prone populations have been used to define "normal" blood lipid concentrations. Similarly, diabetes has been diagnosed on the basis of oral glucose tolerance. Siperstein (1975) has concluded that "the great majority of patients who are diagnosed as having diabetes mellitus on the basis of the currently accepted standards for abnormal GTT's do not have and will not develop the disease." For these reasons, our concepts of these two disorders and their interactions must be considered tentative until genotypically affected and normal individuals can be distinguished more accurately.

Insulin-Dependent Diabetes. In insulin-dependent diabetes with ketoacidosis, plasma triglyceride and free fatty acid concentrations are often markedly elevated, whereas cholesterol concentrations are only modestly elevated (Man and Peters, 1934; Nikkila and Kekki, 1973). If one calculates the approximate serum triglyceride concentration from Man and Peters' data for nonphospholipid fatty acids for their 15 patients with ketoacidosis (assuming a plasma FFA concentration of 3 meq/liter), about three-quarters were hypertriglyceridemic (>200 mg/dl). One-quarter were sufficiently so to have had lipemic plasma (>400 mg/dl). In the ten patients in whom cholesterol values were reported initially, the mean was 241 mg/dl; half had total cholesterol values, corrected for hemoconcentration, of more than 250 mg/dl. In a prospective study of short-term withdrawal of insulin therapy in insulin-dependent diabetics, there was a small but consistent rise in fasting triglyceride and FFA concentrations (Bagdade et al., 1968). Elevation of triglyceride to abnormal concentrations was unusual in this latter setting.

An extreme situation occurs in diabetic lipemia, a rare manifestation of uncontrolled diabetes that is characterized by its prolonged evolution, ketonuria, and massive hypertriglyceridemia. Fully developed ketoacidosis is not a feature of this disorder. Eruptive xanthomatosis may or may not be present. Some patients with diabetic lipemia have normal plasma triglycerides after treatment with insulin, while others do not (E. L. Bierman, personal communication). Their lipemia depends on dietary fat intake, chronic insulin deprivation, and defective lipase-mediated triglyceride removal (Bagdade et al., 1967, 1968). Addison and Gull's original patient appears to have had this syndrome.

Adult-Onset Diabetes. Serum lipid concentrations in nonketosis-prone maturity-onset diabetes have been studied exhaustively. The pioneering observations in this area were again made by Man, Peters, Albrink, and collaborators (Man and Peters, 1935; Albrink et al., 1963). Since then, a number of large epidemiologic investigations have contributed to our appreciation of the frequent association between diabetes mellitus and hyperlipidemia. An exhaustive review of this extensive literature is beyond the scope of this summary.

In comparison to normal populations, both serum cholesterol and triglyceride concentrations have been elevated in diabetic populations. Triglyceride and cholesterol concentrations are shifted toward higher values in diabetics with vascular complications compared to those without (Santen et al., 1972; Albrink et al., 1963). In the Framingham study (Garcia et al., 1974), diabetics were found to have higher cholesterol and Sf 20–400 lipoproteins than the general population. Elevated serum triglycerides may be a better predictor of vascular disease (particularly microangiopathy) than serum cholesterol (Martin and Warne, 1975). Although there is not complete uniformity among them, most studies have shown that basal insulin levels and body weight have been positively correlated with plasma triglyceride concentrations (Santen et al., 1972; Wilson et al., 1970; Ford et al., 1969; Bergqvist, 1970; Rodger and Du, 1973). These interrelationships have been more clear-cut in diabetic individuals with vascular disease than those without (Albrink et al., 1963; Ahuja et al., 1969).

Serum lipid concentrations, therefore, are altered in the major clinical types of diabetes. In juvenile-onset ketosis-prone diabetes, hypertriglyceridemia and hypercholesterolemia are resolved with insulin therapy. In maturity-onset diabetes, hypercholesterolemia and hypertriglyceridemia are frequent and persist despite therapy. They are closely related to the presence of adiposity and, less certainly, to hyperglycemia. Rarely, slowly evolving ketonuric diabetes results in massive hypertriglyceridemia and xanthomatosis. These latter patients often fail to become normolipidemic on therapy for diabetes alone.

Lipoprotein abnormalities in diabetes mellitus (Tables 6 and 7). There have been surprisingly few systematic studies of the prevalence and characteristics of the hyperlipoproteinemias in diabetes (Table 6). Most studies fail to include data from matched control populations. Comparisons of the prevalence of hyperlipoproteinemia in diabetic populations with published figures for normals are suspect since (1) few quantitative lipoprotein analyses have been made; (2) diabetic populations may carry selection bias for microvascular and macrovascular complications; and (3) there has been little uniformity in chosen "normal limits" among various studies.

Chance et al. (1969) reported serum lipid concentrations and qualitative lipoprotein electrophoretic patterns for 135 newly diagnosed juvenile diabetics, some of whom were in ketoacidosis. Over three-quarters had abnormal lipoprotein electrophoreses. Of these, 4% were reported to have type IIA, 18% type IIB (according to current nomenclature), 43% type IV, and 12% type V hyperlipoproteinemia. Thus, nearly three-quarters of these children had elevated pre-β lipoprotein (VLDL) concentrations and one-quarter had elevated LDL concentrations.

In a recent study of 40 juvenile diabetics, Chase and Glasgow (1976) found elevated cholesterol, triglyceride, and LDL and depressed HDL concentrations in comparison to 48 control children. Over half of the diabetic children were hypercholesterolemic, hypertriglyceridemic, or both. These observations are of special concern since all but three of the diabetic children were considered to be in good clinical control. Moreover, these authors noted a significant inverse correlation between HDL and LDL concentrations, both of which appear to have independent effects on the atherogenic diathesis.

A few studies of the prevalence and characteristics of hyperlipopro-

TABLE 6 Prevalence of the Lipoprotein Phenotypes in Adult-Onset Diabetic Populations and in Three Free-Living Adult Populations

N	Age (mean ± SD or range)	Lipoprotein phenotype (% of total)					Normal limits (Chol/TG)	Reference
		Normal	Type II	Type III	Type IV	Type V		
				Normal				
207	20–64	79.2	18.4		2.4		275/	Leren and Haabrekke, 1971[a]
1,118	48 (13)	87.3	3.7	0.2	8.6	0.2	275/200	Wood et al, 1972[b]
92	50	92.4	3.3 (IIA)		4.3		299/261[c]	Hedstrand and Vessby, 1976
		73.9	14.1 (10.8 IIA) (3.3 IIB)		12.0		278/211[d]	
				Diabetics				
98	61 (12)	68	12 (8 IIA) (4 IIB)		20		300/150	Wilson et al., 1970
53	16–63	45	9 (2 IIA) (7 IIB)[e]	6	36	4		Nikkila and Kekki, 1973
97	55 (13)	73	12 (IIA)		14		200[f]/200	Schonfeld et al., 1974
270	13 (2)	76	11		10	3	230[g]/140	Kaufmann et al., 1975

[a]Leren and Haabrekke's study was in Scandinavia; subjects were considerably younger than those in the diabetic groups.
[b]Wood et al.'s study was in the United States.
[c]95th percentile.
[d]85th percentile.
[e]The author's designation "pseudo III" was assumed to represent type IIB hyperlipoproteinemia.
[f]An LDL-cholesterol concentration of 200 mg/dl was used as the cut-off point in this study.
[g]90% upper limit from Fredrickson and Levy, 1972.

TABLE 7   Summary Tabulation of the Most Commonly
Reported Lipoprotein Abnormalities in Diabetes Mellitus[a]

Diabetic status	Lipoproteins	Phenotype
Juvenile-onset/ketosis prone		
Well-controlled	Usually normal	Normal
Ketoacidosis	↑ VLDL	IV
(+ removal defect)	↑ VLDL and chylos	V
Maturity-onset		
Well-controlled	Normal	Normal
	↑ VLDL	IV
	↑ LDL	IIA
	↑ VLDL and LDL	IIB
Diabetic-hyperlipemic syndrome		
Typical	↑↑ VLDL	IV
(+ removal defect, "diabetic lipemia")[b]	↑↑ VLDL and chylos	V

[a]See also Table 6.

[b]Diabetic lipemia is a rare form of the diabetic-hyper-lipemic syndrome in which there is an overt defect in the removal of dietary fat.

teinemia in maturity-onset diabetes have been reported (Table 6). In adult diabetic clinic populations, elevated VLDL and, less often, elevated LDL concentrations have been found. In general, patients with abnormalities in VLDL have been more obese and more hyperglycemic than those with the IIA phenotype or those without lipoprotein abnormalities.

Schonfeld and co-workers (1974) published a careful study of the prevalence of hyperlipoproteinemia in 97 diabetic outpatients and 72 non-diabetic hyperlipoproteinemic adults of roughly similar age, sex, and weight. In their study, increased LDL was associated with insulin therapy, a finding that could have been related to differences in dietary adherence by the insulin-treated patients. Nikkila and Kekki (1973) published lipoprotein phenotyping data as part of their larger study. In tabulating these data, we have excluded ketonuric patients but included patients with the "diabetic-hyperlipemic" syndrome. It was not clear in their report whether or not the type III designation had been based on ultracentrifugation. The increased prevalence and diversity of hyperlipoproteinemia in this study is likely to have been due to more severe diabetes, since the patients were all admitted to the hospital for treatment.

The data in Table 6 are consistent with the idea that LDL abnormalities are two or three times more frequent among diabetics in comparison with the normal American population. This conclusion must be tempered by the reservations outlined above.

In 1951, Barr et al. noted that α lipoprotein cholesterol was both absolutely and relatively decreased in patients with premature atherosclerosis. The filtration theory of atherogenesis and the discovery that LDL carries the majority of plasma cholesterol under normal circumstances led to primary investigative emphasis on LDL metabolism in atherogenesis. In comparison, the role of HDL in atherogenesis was given little attention for the next two decades. In the past several years the idea that HDL are antiatherogenic has enjoyed renewed popularity. A variety of lines of clinical and epidemiological evidence have converged to support the idea that low HDL concentrations are atherogenic, independently of changes in VLDL and LDL, and, conversely, that high HDL levels are associated with longevity.

To cite but a few of these recent studies: In a cooperative study of several thousand subjects, Castelli et al. (1975) found lower HDL cholesterol levels in subjects with coronary heart disease (CAD) than those without. HDL cholesterol was inversely related to CAD prevalence but this relationship was essentially independent of total or LDL cholesterol. In a study of Japanese men in Hawaii, the prevalence of CAD was inversely related to HDL cholesterol and independent of LDL cholesterol, obesity, or hypertriglyceridemia (Rhoads et al., 1976).

There are few data available for HDL in diabetic humans. In the aforementioned study by Barr et al. (1951), HDL concentrations were strikingly depressed in some atherosclerotic adult-onset diabetic patients. This has been notable in other data (e.g., Furman et al., 1961).

Schonfeld et al. (1974) found small but statistically significant differences in the composition of LDL and HDL in diabetes. Both lipoprotein classes were enriched with triglyceride, independent of effects of blood sugar, age, sex, race, and adiposity. Since there is a progressive loss of TG from chylomicrons, VLDL, and IDL during their catabolism to LDL, these authors speculated that the compositional changes in LDL and HDL might reflect abnormalities in lipoprotein catabolic pathways in diabetes. Their data also showed a modest depression in plasma HDL concentrations in normolipidemic adult diabetics. These and other scattered data suggest that HDL concentrations may be abnormally low in at least some diabetic individuals.

An isolated report of hyper-α-lipoproteinemia in three adult-onset diabetic patients is of interest (Willie and Aarseth, 1973) in view of the recent findings that kindreds with familial elevations of HDL have an elongated life expectancy (Glueck et al., 1975). All three diabetic patients were hypercholesterolemic and one had premature CHD. From this anecdotal information it is tempting to speculate that the antiatherogenicity of HDL was nullified by other factors in the milieu of diabetes. In the streptozotocin-diabetic rat, all three lipoprotein classes (VLDL, LDL, and HDL) have been increased. HDL elevations were particularly striking in rats with diabetes of longer duration (Bar-On et al., 1976). Differences between the changes in lipoproteins in diabetic rats and humans may be related to differences in pathways of lipoprotein catabolism in these two species (Eisenberg and Rachmilewitz, 1973). These observations point out the need for additional descriptive studies of the plasma HDL concentration in diabetic humans and its relationship to other lipoprotein abnormalities.

Relationships between Carbohydrate and Lipid Abnormalities

Despite the common-sense impression that diabetes, hyperlipidemia, and obesity are closely interrelated conditions, the basis for their coexistence has not been defined. This has been due, in part, to the lack of satisfactory methods for the diagnosis of genetic diabetes and the interpretation of abnormal glucose tolerance tests (Siperstein, 1975).

An association between familial hyperlipoproteinemia and carbohydrate intolerance was noted in the initial experience of the National Institutes of Health group. Glueck et al. (1969) reported insulin and glucose values after an oral glucose load (OGTT) for patients with types II, III, IV, and V hyperlipoproteinemia. The patients were selected in such a manner as to exclude patients with overt diabetes mellitus who required therapy with sulfonylureas or insulin. The occurrence of glucose intolerance in those with type II hyperlipoproteinemia was not much different from that in their normal control population (33% versus 28%). In type III, carbohydrate intolerance occurred in 39%, in type IV 52%, and in type V 77% of patients. Insulin responses were variable. Although no significant correlations within the groups were noted between the degree of adiposity and hypertriglyceridemia or carbohydrate intolerance, the type III, IV, and V patients as a group were more obese than either the control subjects or the type II patients. Conversely, in an important recent paper, Kyner and associates (1976) reported studies of control subjects and the offspring of two diabetic parents. In concordance with previously cited data, both VLDL and LDL elevations were more common in men genetically predisposed to diabetes, whether or not oral glucose tolerance was abnormal (chemical diabetes). In this study, fasting TG concentrations correlated positively with glucose-stimulated insulin secretion in normal and prediabetic subjects (normal OGTT) and with blood glucose in genetically predisposed subjects.

Several possible explanations for these associations must be considered.

1. Diabetes mellitus and hyperlipoproteinemia (particularly IV and V) are due to closely linked but separate genes.
2. Hyperlipoproteinemia (or a biochemically related phenomenon such as accelerated FFA flux) interferes with glucose assimilation and leads to carbohydrate intolerance and, ultimately, overt diabetes mellitus (Felber and Vanotti, 1964).
3. Diabetes or the diabetic genotype lead to familial hyperlipo-proteinemia.

4. Both hyperlipoproteinemia and glucose intolerance are the result of a more fundamental inherited or environmental defect such as fat cell hypertrophy (Albrink and Davidson, 1966).
5. Hyperlipoproteinemia and glucose intolerance are independently inherited defects. Their coexistence is due to coincidence, unrecognized selection bias, or synergistic interactions between the two defects that facilitate case recognition.

Data supporting the last of these possibilities has been published by Brunzell et al. (1975a). They selected index patients with genetic hypertriglyceridemia with or without diabetes mellitus defined as being on treatment with insulin or sulfonylureas for fasting hyperglycemia. The incidence of diabetes in the index patients was 27%. The frequency of diabetes in their first-degree relatives was nearly identical, whether or not hypertriglyceridemia was present. In the diabetic index patients with familial hypertriglyceridemia, diabetic therapy failed to restore triglycerides to normal, whereas it did so in sporadic (nonfamilial) cases. These studies provide support for the concept that diabetes and hyperlipoproteinemia are genetically independent.

In the absence of pedigree data, an empirical approach to the problem of distinguishing primary from secondary hyperlipoproteinemia in the presence of glucose intolerance has been to treat the diabetes first. If, after optimal therapy, hyperlipoproteinemia persists, then one may conclude that the hyperlipidemia is primary. Although the foregoing study supports such an approach, further verification is needed.

A central issue in sorting out the genetic and environmental factors responsible for the apparent relationship between carbohydrate intolerance and endogenous hyperlipoproteinemia has to do with the roles of obesity and hyperinsulinemia (Bierman and Porte, 1968). A unifying hypothesis for these relationships is shown in Fig. 1. Correlations have been sought for a number of the component factors: serum immunoreactive insulin (IRI) with TG concentrations or VLDL secretion; serum FFA and TG concentrations with glucose tolerance, adiposity, insulin, triglyceride, glucose, and FFA concentrations and FFA turnover. Plasma triglyceride concentrations have been found to correlate with adult-onset adiposity and recent weight gain (Albrink and Meigs, 1964), serum IRI (Reaven et al., 1967; Kuo and Feng, 1970), and ILA (Kuo and Feng, 1970). In some studies, plasma TG has correlated with hyperglycemia (Ford et al., 1969), but other studies have failed to show any such relationship (Carlson and Wahlberg, 1966). From their data, Kyner et al. (1976) have suggested that the emergence of the diabetic phenotype is accompanied by a shift of the normal situation in which there is a correlation between insulin response and plasma TG concentration to a situation in which a glucose-to-triglyceride correlation appears.

A direct effect of insulin on hepatic TG production was suggested (Reaven et al., 1967) on the basis of stimulation of hepatic FFA uptake

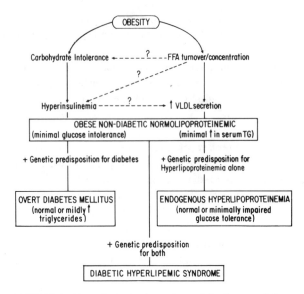

FIGURE 1 Hypothetical scheme to explain the associations between diabetes, hyperlipoproteinemia, and obesity. The broken lines indicate the possible interactions between carbohydrate and lipid metabolism discussed in the text. This scheme probably does not apply to ketoacidotic diabetes.

(Shoemaker et al., 1962). More recent studies with rat liver perfused *ex vivo* have shown that insulin decreases fatty acid oxidation and increases fatty acid esterification and the secretion of VLDL. The effects of increased substrate (fructose) and insulin were additive (Topping and Mayes, 1972). In an analogous manner, hyperinsulinemia and hyperglycemia in the obese diabetic may lead to augmented VLDL synthesis and hypertriglyceridemia.

It is doubtful whether FFA and TG themselves interfere with glucose assimilation *in vivo* (Randle, 1966). Insulin antagonism by FFA in muscle is of uncertain significance in humans (Eder et al., 1970). Infusion of FFA in dogs increases plasma insulin abruptly. Under these conditions glucose falls, although more slowly than one would expect from the immediate rise in insulin (Crespin et al., 1972). These acute studies do not support the idea that elevated FFA would lead to hyperglycemia. Recent studies have failed to demonstrate any substantial effect of elevated plasma TG on carbohydrate assimilation (Felber and Vanotti, 1964; Gibson et al., 1974).

The proposal outlined in Figs. 1 and 2 reconciles lack of cosegregation of familial hyperlipidemia and genetic diabetes with the foregoing clinical observations. Obesity or fat cell enlargement (and probably other insulin-antagonistic events) are associated with basal or glucose-stimulated hyper-insulinemia, hyperglycemia, and accelerated FFA mobilization (Ostrander,

1974; Bernstein et al., 1975; Stern et al., 1973; Girolamo et al., 1974). Likewise, plasma TG concentration is elevated in the presence of overweight (Ostrander, 1974; Nestel and Whyte, 1968). Thus, modest hyperlipidemia and carbohydrate intolerance may both occur as a consequence of adiposity. Frank hyperlipidemia, clinically overt diabetes, and the diabetic-hyperlipemic syndrome develop only in the presence of major genes for diabetes and hyperlipoproteinemia. To explain the observed frequencies of all forms of hyperlipidemia in diabetes, both genes or sets of genes would need to be relatively common in the population. The abnormal genes controlling plasma TG concentration could be those regulating either synthetic or catabolic pathways.

Might known inherited forms of hyperlipoproteinemia explain the occurrence of diabetic-hyperlipemic syndromes? Or, to ask this question differently, could there be a genetic basis for severe "acquired" hyperlipoproteinemia?

As noted earlier, the first established instance of hyperlipoproteinemia due to LPL deficiency was in the homozygotic condition, familial hyperchylomicronemia (type I). Harlan and his co-workers (1967) examined the parents of these probands and found that lipoprotein lipase activity (LPLA) in adipose tissue was decreased to approximately half of normal values. Thus, in this situation, the heterozygous "carrier" state can be identified.

If we were to assume that the homozygous condition occurred once in every million live births, the gene frequency (q) would be 0.001 and the

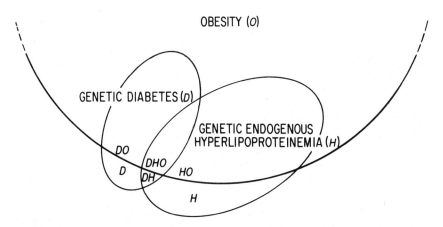

FIGURE 2 Venn diagram of the disease sets of diabetes, hyperlipidemia, and obesity based on the hypothesis that coexistence of the genes for hyperlipoproteinemia and diabetes is necessary for the appearance of the diabetic-hyperlipemic syndrome and that obesity (genetic component unspecified) is a common factor in the expression of both genes. The relative areas of the sets would apply if the prevalences for obesity, endogenous hyperlipoproteinemia, and diabetes in the population were 20, 8, and 4%, respectively (Feinstein, 1963).

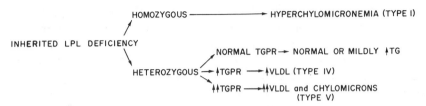

FIGURE 3 Proposed role for heterozygous LPL deficiency in the pathogenesis of severe "acquired" hypertriglyceridemia.

population frequency of the heterozygous condition would be 0.002.[1] In a very gross manner this does not seem to be out of line with the frequency of massive lipemia in individuals with other disorders that might increase TG production, such as uncontrolled diabetes (see below).

In Fig. 3 we propose that genes for LPL deficiency exist in the general population. Under rare circumstances, matings of heterozygotes produce offspring with familial hyperchylomicronemia. Heterozygotes with normal TG production rates might have normal TG concentrations or have values at the upper end of the lognormal distribution of normal TGs. When stressed by factors that increase triglyceride production rates (TGPRs), however, plasma concentrations would rise. With markedly increased TG production rates, both VLDL and chylomicrons might accumulate in the plasma.

An alternative genetic basis for massive "acquired" hypertriglyceridemia could be the coexistence of homozygous familial hypertriglyceridemia (homozygous type IV) and poorly controlled diabetes. If we assume that the prevalence estimate of Wood et al. (1972) for type IV hyperlipoproteinemia is comprised entirely of hypertriglyceridemia due to a major autosomal dominant gene, the Hardy-Weinberg equilibrium allows us to calculate the following. The population frequency of the abnormal allele, q, is 0.0408. The probability of the heterozygous state, $2pq$, would be 0.078 and that of the homozygous state would be 0.0017. The latter figure is remarkably close to our armchair estimate of the frequency of the heterozygous LPL-deficient state.[2] The existence of a homozygous form of familial hypertriglyceridemia has not been established. Nevertheless, these speculations afford a hypothetical genetic scheme to explain massive acquired hypertriglyceridemia.

---

[1] From the Hardy-Weinberg equilibrium, the population frequencies for normal and LPL-deficient genes are p and q, respectively. If the frequency of the homozygous condition, q^2, were 0.000001, then q would be 0.001. Since the population genotypic frequencies are $p^2 + 2pq + q^2$, and since p is very close to 1, the estimated frequency of the heterozygous state is $2q$, or 0.002.

[2] Note, however, that Motulsky's estimate of the prevalence of autosomal dominant familial hypertriglyceridemia was only 1% (Table 5). The calculated frequency of the homozygous form of familial hypertriglyceridemia would then be much smaller (2.5×10^{-5}).

PATHOPHYSIOLOGY

A great deal is known about changes in TG and TG-rich lipoprotein metabolism in acute and chronic diabetic states. The broad outlines of this subject will be summarized here. The reader who wishes to pursue the subject in greater depth is referred to exhaustive reviews (Nikkila, 1969, 1973). Much less is known about LDL and HDL metabolism in diabetes, although there is some evidence that the synthetic or degradative processes that maintain the composition and concentration of these plasma lipoproteins are abnormal.

Ketosis-Prone Diabetes

In insulinopenic (ketosis-prone) diabetes, lipolysis of TG stored in the adipocyte is unchecked by insulin and therefore FFA is released and the plasma FFA concentration rises. Plasma FFA concentrations parallel FFA turnover. In addition to the loss of the antilipolytic effect of insulin, other hormones such as glucagon (Pozza et al., 1971; Schade and Eaton, 1975), growth hormone (Fineberg and Merimee, 1974; Luft and Guillemin, 1974; Nikkila and Pelkonen, 1975), and catecholamines (Vaughan and Steinberg, 1963; Steinberg, 1966) may further stimulate the release of FFA. Circulating fatty acids are bound to albumin during transport through the vascular compartment. Net uptake of FFA by the liver is in direct proportion to FFA concentration in portal venous blood (Nikkila, 1973).

The metabolic options for FFA in the liver are: (1) ketone body formation, (2) oxidation, (3) reesterification to form triglyceride, and/or (4) reesterification to form phospholipid and other lipid esters. *De novo* fatty acid synthesis in the liver is depressed in acutely diabetic experimental animals (Nikkila, 1969) but the importance of this effect in insulinopenic humans is not known. Experiments with rat liver slices suggest that increased hepatic glucagon and cyclic AMP levels suppress *de novo* lipogenesis (Meikle et al., 1973). In juvenile diabetics with ketoacidosis, triglyceride (VLDL) secretory rates are increased and there is a significant correlation between the production rate and plasma levels of TG (Nikkila and Kekki, 1973).

The role of decreased clearance of TG-rich lipoproteins in this setting is not entirely clear. The plasma TG pool is expanded because of the increased rate of entry of endogenous lipoprotein (VLDL) . Since VLDL and chylomicrons appear to share a common removal mechanism, the half-life and fractional decay of chylomicrons or artificial fat emulsions are prolonged in proportion to the fasting (endogenous) TG concentration (Nestel, 1964). Nikkila and Kekki (1973) have examined the fractional removal of an artificial fat emulsion in diabetic and nondiabetic subjects by the intravenous administration of Intralipid. They found a hyperbolic relationship between fractional removal of exogenous fat and the initial fasting plasma TG concentration. Diabetics did not appear substantially different from control subjects when basal TG concentrations were taken into account. Triglyceride turnover for their group of ten ketotic subjects was elevated three-fold above controls. Plasma TG concentration was positively correlated with TG turnover. The relationship between turnover rate and plasma TG concentration failed to show any defect in TG removal efficiency. These data, *in toto,* indicate that the major factor in the pathogenesis of hyperlipoproteinemia in the insulin-dependent diabetic is augmented endogenous synthesis and secretion of lipoprotein. They also suggest that "removal defects" in exogenous fat metabolism may occur as a consequence of an expanded pool of VLDL. In this sense, delayed clearance of chylomicrons can be a consequence of competition with VLDL for a shared removal pathway, and need not necessarily be due to an intrinsic defect in the pathway.

Maturity-Onset Diabetes

Obese maturity-onset diabetics have elevated FFA turnover (Nestel and Whyte, 1968; Birkenhäger and Tjabbes, 1969; Miller et al., 1968). In patients with endogenous hypertriglyceridemia, basal and stimulated lipolysis *in vitro* are increased and the inhibition of catecholamine-stimulated lipolysis by insulin is blunted, regardless of adipocyte size (Bjorntorp and Hood, 1966; Kuo et al., 1966). Other workers have noted the coexistence of endogenous hypertriglyceridemia, hyperinsulinemia, and adipocyte enlargement without clinical diabetes or obesity (Albrink and Davidson, 1966; Bernstein et al., 1975; Eaton and Nye, 1973). One wonders whether adipocyte enlargement might exist in some lean individuals and initiate the series of events that lead to endogenous hyperlipoproteinemia in the absence of obesity.

These phenomena can be compared with the exaggerated lipolytic stimulus of absolute insulinopenia. Kinetic studies in humans have demonstrated increased TG turnover with plasma TG concentrations appropriate to the measured turnover (Nikkila and Kekki, 1973). A few older obese patients with the diabetic-hyperlipemic syndrome have had higher plasma TG concentrations than one would predict from the "on line" relationship between TG concentration and turnover, suggesting that there was a true defect in lipoprotein removal (Nikkila and Kekki, 1973).

Postheparin Lipolytic Activity

Methods. The role of lipoprotein lipase in idiopathic hyperlipemia (type I, familial hyperchylomicronemia) was uncovered by Havel and Gordon (1960), who showed that these patients had delayed chylomicron clearance and diminished postheparin lipolytic activity (PHLA). An assay based on titration of FFA released from a coconut oil emulsion (Ediol) by the lipases in postheparin plasma was used in virtually all clinical studies for the next decade (Fredrickson et al., 1963). The assay, however, has now been recognized to have two major drawbacks in addition to tedium and lack of sensitivity: (1) It does not distinguish between the several triglyceride and partial glyceride hydrolases in postheparin plasma. These are now known to have different physiological significance and to vary independently under several circumstances (Ehnholm et al., 1975a, 1975b; Faergeman and Damgaard-Pedersen, 1973). Ediol contains large amounts of monoglyceride and so provides substrate for monoglyceride as well as triglyceride hydrolase activities (Nilsson-Ehle and Belfrage, 1972; Greten et al., 1969). (2) Artificial substrates, in particular those which contain partial glycerides, phospholipids, and detergents, may behave quite differently from the natural substrates, VLDL or chylomicrons. Huttunen and Nikkila (1973) compared Intralipid (a soybean oil emulsion), with VLDL and chylomicrons as substrates for human PHLA. Activities for chylomicrons and VLDL correlated well with each other, but neither correlated with activity against Intralipid. They found a significant negative correlation between fasting TG concentration and PHLA against endogenous substrates but not against the artificial emulsion.

These observations underscore the hazards in drawing physiological conclusions from earlier studies of PHLA in humans and argue for further investigations with methods that circumvent these methodological problems (Greten et al., 1976; Huttunen et al., 1975).

PHLA in diabetic animals. In contrast to the large number of studies of tissue LPL activity in animals, only a few studies of PHLA in experimental diabetic animal models have been reported. O'Connor and Schnatz (1968) examined PHLA and serum TG concentrations in rabbits made chronically diabetic with alloxan. Despite marked hyperlipemia and hyperpre-beta-lipoproteinemia, PHLA against an artificial TG emulsion was normal and there was no chylomicronemia. Elkeles and Williams (1974) measured PHLA, heart and adipose tissue LPL, and TG concentrations in rats 2 days after alloxanization. The diabetic animals had hypertriglyceridemia but PHLA was not substantially different from that in control animals. Thus, in short-term experimental diabetes in animals, hypertriglyceridemia is not accompanied by depression of total PHLA.

Jansen and Hülsman (1975) have examined hepatic and extrahepatic lipase activities in postheparin plasma from diabetic rats. These authors have presented evidence for the identity of hepatic TG hydrolase and palmitoyl-CoA hydrolase activities in postheparin plasma. In their experiments strepto-zotocin diabetic rats showed an increase in TG hydrolase activity but a reduction in palmitoyl-CoA hydrolase activity compared with control animals. They interpreted these data as indicating that hepatic lipase is decreased and extrahepatic lipase activity increased in diabetes mellitus. Changes in lipase activities in this direction do not suggest the presence of a removal block in the diabetic animal, since the extrahepatic enzyme is thought to be the important one in VLDL and chylomicron assimilation (Ehnholm et al., 1975c).

PHLA in diabetic humans. In humans, PHLA abnormalities are related to the duration, severity, and type of diabetes, as well as to the presence of diabetic complications such as uremia or nephrotic syndrome. Schnatz and

O'Connor (1967) reported subnormal PHLA in 18 ketoacidotic patients and found a significant negative correlation between PHLA and serum TG concentration. Jones et al. (1966) found no detectable differences in PHLA (against an artificial substrate) in insulin-dependent, stable "insulin independent," or ketoacidotic-hyperlipidemic patients.

Bagdade and co-workers (1967, 1968) described a distinct subgroup of diabetics in whom PHLA seems to be affected with regularity. In diabetic lipemia, PHLA is depressed and returns to normal following institution of insulin therapy. These same authors (1968) studied seven juvenile diabetics on insulin withdrawal and found a substantial decrease in PHLA in five patients after 48 hr. Fasting plasma TG rises were small in all but one despite *ad libitum* feeding during the insulinopenic period. The basis for the discrepancy between these sets of data is not clear.

An indirect mechanism for depletion of tissue LPL may contribute to abnormalities in PHLA in lipemia. Shafrir and Biale (1960) infused Intralipid or VLDL into rats. They observed a marked decrease in adipose tissue LPL and an increase in heart LPL activities. Serum lipase activity, measured in the absence of prior heparin adminstration, was markedly decreased. They suggested that adipose tissue LPL may be "leached" from the tissues by hypertriglyceridemic states. Huttunen et al. (1976) cited unpublished observations that infusion of fat emulsions intravenously does not diminish heparin-reieasable TGLA in humans. Whether such a phenomenon contributes to the pathogenesis of diabetic lipemia has not been determined. The more widely accepted postulate, that LPL protein synthesis and LPL secretion are impaired in lipemia, is discussed below.

Steiner (1968) studied a nondiabetic patient with alcoholism, abdominal pain and fat-induced (type V) hyperlipoproteinemia. Postheparin plasma from this patient showed normal PHLA against Ediol but no activity against chylomicron preparations. PHLA inhibitors were not present. A similar defect in two nondiabetic siblings has been thought to represent either a mutant gene for an LPL with unusual substrate specificities, or an inherited LPL deficiency with a compensatory increase in another TG hydrolase(s) (Schreibman et al., 1973). Five patients who had had the diabetic-hyperlipemic syndrome, however, showed comparable PHLA against artificial fat emulsions and human chylomicrons (Wilson et al., 1969). Thus, there is no reason to suspect that there is a qualitative defect in PHLA against natural substrate in patients with the diabetic-hyperlipemic syndrome.

Recently, several laboratories have studied PHLA during prolonged heparin infusion. By analogy with the insulin response to glucose infusion, early- and late-phase PHLA responses have been described. Huttunen et al. (1975) have used this technique, along with specific immunoprecipitation of hepatic triglyceride lipase (HTGL), to examine the relationship between postheparin triglyceride concentration and exogenous fat removal in hyperlipoproteinemia. They found a significant inverse correlation between the early

LPL (extrahepatic lipoprotein lipase) response and basal TG concentration as well as a significant positive correlation with the removal of intravenously administered Intralipid. These data support the idea that rapidly released LPL reflects the enzyme pool responsible for the removal of VLDL and chylomicrons. Its early release suggested that it was the rapidly mobilizable pool associated with capillary endothelium (Bezman et al., 1962; Chajek et al., 1975). Neither the early or late hepatic lipase nor the late LPL response correlated with basal TG. The late-phase release of HTGL correlated significantly with the Intralipid removal rate, but the physiological relevance of this finding is unknown. Fasting abolished the acute phase response, but the late response was similar to that seen in the fed state. Intralipid removal was slightly increased during fasting. Huttunen et al. (1975) concluded that fasting may change the pathways of TG removal without impairing removal efficiency.

Brunzell et al. (1975b) have applied a heparin infusion technique to study diabetic and hypertriglyceridemic subjects. Total late-phase PHLA was depressed in 12 untreated diabetic subjects in comparison to normal and nondiabetic hypertriglyceridemic controls. Early-phase PHLA was the same in all groups. Two patients with subnormal PHLA had deficient early- and late-phase responses. Early-phase response was corrected rapidly by antidiabetic therapy, whereas late-phase abnormalities did not become normal for weeks or months. These and the foregoing data cannot be compared directly since HTGL and LPL were not measured individually in the latter study. They do suggest that the readily releasable pool of LPL, which is rate-determining in VLDL and chylomicron removal, is usually normal in untreated diabetes, despite subnormal late-phase release. The late-phase release may be deficient in diabetes because it depends on protein synthesis or subsequent energy-dependent steps (see below).

Lipoprotein lipase and plasma TG concentration. Several lines of evidence support the idea that LPL is a determinant of plasma TG and VLDL concentrations, both in normal and in some hypertriglyceridemic individuals. Until recently, the only unassailable example of LPL deficiency has been familial hyperchylomicronemia (type I) (Havel and Gordon, 1960). Even in the presence of the florid homozygotic syndrome, PHLA has been measurable. Attempts to correlate PHLA with other forms of hyperlipoproteinemia (types IV and V) or with basal plasma TG in normal individuals have led to conflicting results (see Robinson, 1970).

The recent demonstration that PHLA consists of two or more distinct activities that have different physiological significance has resolved some of these difficulties. In the case of type I, for example, PHLA in plasma was accounted for by HTGL. LPL levels have been extremely low or unmeasurable. Type V patients, in general, have had normal HTGL and deficient LPLA, whereas total PHLA has not been depressed with any regularity (Greten et al., 1976; Huttunen et al., 1976). Systematic studies of postheparin plasma LPLA in diabetes have not yet been done.

The importance of LPL in endogenous VLDL removal has now been demonstrated directly in experimental animals (Kompiang et al., 1976). Antibody to purified chicken LPL was made in rabbits. Anti-LPL sera were injected intravenously into cockerels. This completely eliminated VLDL removal and led to an immediate and progressive rise in serum TG. The lipoproteins that accumulated in plasma were characteristic of newly secreted VLDL. These observations establish the importance of LPL in VLDL catabolism and show that under some conditions, deficient or inhibited LPL may produce increased plasma VLDL.

More direct evidence in humans is available. Adipose tissue LPL activities (LPLA) have shown an inverse correlation between LPLA and plasma TG concentration in normal subjects (Persson, 1972) and in some hyperlipoproteinemic states (Pykalisto et al., 1976). Huttunen et al. (1975, 1976) have used HTGL antibody to distinguish LPL and HTGL. They tested 82 normal individuals and 20 hyperlipoproteinemic patients and, in some, also measured endogenous TG kinetics. In normal subjects (TG < 200 mg/dl) LPL activity was inversely correlated with fasting TG concentration. LPLA was higher in women, a finding consistent with their lower plasma TG concentration but TG production rates that are similar to those of men ("more efficient removal"). LPLA fell with age, whereas TG increased with age in women. LPLA also correlated with Intralipid removal rate (at normal fasting TG levels) and the fractional removal of endogenous TG.

Finally, LPL was abnormal in endogenous hyperlipoproteinemia. In 17 men with type IV or type IIB hyperlipoproteinemia, the mean LPL was depressed about 25 percent ($p < 0.005$). There was considerable overlap in these values, however. When their data were recalculated, only two of the 17 had LPL values 2 standard deviations below the normal mean, and there was no correlation between LPLA and fasting serum TG concentration in hyperlipidemia. All three type V subjects had LPL values 2 SD below the mean normal value. These results are in accord with the suggestion that endogenous hyperlipoproteinemia is a kinetically mixed defect and that both overproduction and underremoval of VLDL are involved in its pathogenesis. They also suggest that there may be considerable heterogeneity in LPL in normolipidemic individuals, who might become hypertriglyceridemic were they to have increased triglyceride production rates. Studies of LPLA in diabetes with similar methods will be of great interest.

TISSUE LIPOPROTEIN LIPASE

In this section, we will examine some of the details of LPL action at the cellular level, the endocrine regulation of LPL synthesis and activity, and abnormalities in these processes in diabetes. The interested reader is referred to an encyclopedic review for details of earlier studies (Robinson, 1970).

Robinson has suggested that LPL plays a directive role in determining the pattern of triglyceride fatty acid uptake by the extrahepatic tissues. Enzyme activities in specific tissues are known to vary in opposite directions in particular physiological situations and to correlate with the uptake of triglyceride fatty acids (TGFA) by these tissues. For example, LPL activity increases in muscle but falls in adipose tissue during starvation. Similar changes may occur in uncontrolled diabetes. Thus, even if major differences in the kinetics of removal of TG-rich lipoproteins do not exist in the majority of diabetics, it is still possible that there are important differences in the distribution of TGFA at the tissue level.

Site of LPL Action

Electron micrographs of adipose tissue from animals fed lipid-rich diets or perfused with chylomicrons have shown chylomicrons within the capillary lumen and attached to the luminal endothelium. Chylomicrons, which are larger than 1,000 Å in diameter, do not penetrate the endothelial barrier (Blanchette-Mackie and Scow, 1971). The initial steps in TGFA assimilation by adipose tissue must occur at the endothelial-intravascular surface. It has been suspected for many years from electron microscopic studies and the very rapid appearance of PHLA in the blood after heparin administration that LPL is bound to superficial sites (Ballard et al., 1971). As noted above, lipoprotein lipase from a variety of sources and the hepatic triglyceride lipase bind strongly to heparin *in vitro*.

Blood vessels contain acidic mucopolysaccharides, notably chondroitin sulfate, heparin sulfate, and dermatan sulfate (Kumar et al., 1967; Olivecrona et al., 1976). It is assumed that LPL binds to these highly anionic compounds on the endothelial surface where displacement by exogenously administered heparin occurs (Olivecrona et al., 1976). Moreover, the distribution space of heparin closely approximates the plasma volume (Chen et al., 1975), suggesting that heparin releases LPL from the plasma-endothelial interface. Light microscopy with histochemical techniques capable of demonstrating lipase activity against endogenous blood chylomicrons has shown that triglyceride hydrolytic products in mesenteric adipose tissue are confined to capillaries. In mice fasted 6 days, this activity is lost (Moskowitz and Moskowitz, 1965). During their assimilation, intact chylomicrons are seen partially enveloped by the luminal surface of the capillary endothelium. If tissue is incubated under conditions where insoluble Ca-Pb soaps are formed, electron-opaque precipitates are seen within vacuoles and microvesicles of the capillary endothelium and in the subendothelial space. These observations, as well as experiments with isolated fat cells (Schotz et al., 1969), have been the basis for the idea that initial hydrolysis of the TG-rich lipoproteins occurs at the capillary endothelial surfaces, and the fatty acids and partial glycerides are taken into vacuoles and vesicles in the endothelial cell, where further hydrolysis occurs. The contents of the vacuoles are released into the subendothelial space and, ultimately, TGFA enter the adipocyte, where they are reesterified and stored as TG.

Lipoprotein Lipase Synthesis and Secretion (Fig. 4)

The uptake of lipoprotein TGFA by adipose tissue is a direct function of its lipoprotein lipase activity (Bezman et al., 1962; Garfinkel et al., 1967). Lipoprotein lipase activity in fasted animals is drastically reduced. Cunningham and Robinson (1969) found that LPL activity in adipose tissue from fed rats falls rapidly with incubation at $37°C$ in the absence of glucose and insulin. The initial low LPL levels in adipose tissue from starved animals do not decrease further under these conditions. They concluded that adipose tissue from fed rats must contain two forms of LPL. An unstable form accounts for the major proportion of the total activity in fed animals. A second, stable form predominates in adipose tissue from starved animals.

Schotz and Garfinkel (1965), Eagle and Robinson (1964), and Wing and Robinson (1968) investigated the effects of inhibitors of protein synthesis on the increase in adipose tissue LPL from starved rats after refeeding or *in vitro* incubation with glucose. Both groups noted that recovery of normal fed LPL levels was abolished by puromycin. Wing et al. (1967) injected rats with cyclohexamide and determined LPL activities of adipose tissue, muscle, and heart. In each tissue, LPL declined in an exponential fashion with a half-life of approximately 3 hr. Patten (1970) demonstrated rapid loss of LPL activity in isolated fat cells incubated with cyclohexamide. These data suggest that either the enzyme itself or another protein necessary for LPL activity is normally synthesized and degraded at a rapid rate. Together, these data show that LPL activity in adipose tissue is under dynamic control and, furthermore,

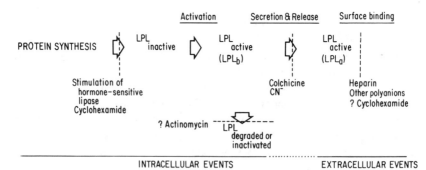

FIGURE 4 Model of LPL synthesis, activation, secretion, and endothelial binding. The evidence for this scheme, which has been adapted from publications of several authors, is discussed in the text. LPL is synthesized within the adipocyte. A pool of inactive LPL becomes activated and becomes the major intracellular form, LPL_b. Energy-dependent activation and transport result in the secretion of LPL, which is bound as LPL_a by the capillary endothelium. The hydrolysis of chylomicron and VLDL triglyceride fatty acid is initiated at the endothelial surface.

that there are two or more forms of the enzyme. Paradoxically, actinomycin D increases adipose tissue LPL. This increase in LPL is most simply explained by postulating a differential effect of actinomycin D on an LPL-degrading enzyme (or enzymes) (Garfinkel et al., 1967; Wing and Robinson, 1968).

Garfinkel and Schotz (1972) were able to separate two species of lipoprotein lipase (LPL$_a$ and LPL$_b$) on the basis of differences in apparent molecular weight. Subsequently, a third species (LPL$_i$) has been identified (Nilsson-Ehle, 1976). In postheparin plasma only the larger species are found (LPL$_a$ and LPL$_i$). In isolated fat cells nearly all of the LPL present is the smaller species (LPL$_b$). Similar findings were reported for heart LPL. These data implied that the major intracellular species is LPL$_b$, and that LPL$_a$ is bound outside the adipocyte but is releasable by heparin.

During incubation of isolated fat cells in the presence of heparin and glucose, consistently more LPL is released into the incubation medium than is present in the fat cells at the beginning of the incubation period (Stewart and Schotz, 1974). To determine whether new protein synthesis is involved, workers have examined the effects of cyclohexamide in this system (Stewart and Schotz, 1971; Cryer et al., 1975a; Stewart et al., 1969). With cyclohexamide present in the medium, the amount of LPL activity released into the medium was not changed. Thus, the heparin-stimulated release of LPL from isolated fat cells appears to be independent of new protein synthesis. Other experiments (Stewart and Schotz, 1974; Schotz et al., 1969) have shown that the release of LPL can be inhibited by cyanide. These data imply that the secretion-release phenomenon is energy-dependent.

Chajek et al. (1975) and Cryer et al. (1975b) have shown that colchicine, which inhibits secretion of a variety of other proteins by cells by interfering with the microtubular transport system, inhibits the heparin-stimulated release of LPL from isolated adipocytes or PHLA in the intact rat. Although effects of colchicine at sites other than the microtubular system have not been excluded (see Chajek et al., 1975), these data suggest that LPL shares this common secretory mechanism for proteins. Borensztajn et al. (1975) have confirmed these findings in rat heart.

Endocrine Regulation of Adipose Tissue LPL

Methods for analysis of adipose tissue LPL. Several different approaches to the measurement of adipose tissue LPL activity have been used. Defatted acetone:ether powders of adipose tissue have been used to measure total LPLA. Since rates of TGFA uptake by tissue appear to correlate best with the heparin-releasable fraction, other investigators have first incubated adipose tissue with heparin-containing buffer and then measured LPLA in the eluate. Since activation and secretion of LPL occur during incubation, heparin eluates contain more LPL activity than is present in acetone:ether powders (Pykalisto et al., 1975c). Finally, LPL activity has been measured by incubation of whole tissue fragments. Although the latter technique may provide some idea of the net result of all of the processes shown in Fig. 4, interpretation of the results is very complex (Guy-Grand and Bigorie, 1973).

The manner in which adipose tissue LPL activities are expressed is critical to the interpretation of published data and has major consequences for our understanding of the control of LPL in tissue. Since adipocyte enlargement is an important feature of the metabolic derangements that underlie maturity-onset (obesity-associated) diabetes, the relationships between fat cell geometry and LPL content must be considered. In order to examine these relationships and to clarify the assumptions on which various experimental approaches are based, we have illustrated the theoretical relationships among LPL content, fat cell diameter, surface area, and volume (Fig. 5). In Fig. 5, A

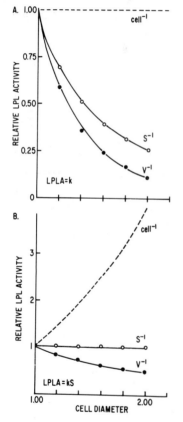
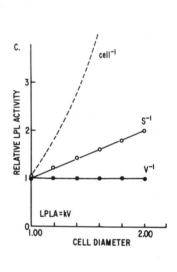

FIGURE 5 Relative LPL activity per cell (cell^{-1}), per unit surface area (S^{-1}), and per unit volume (V^{-1}) for three possible relationships between cellular lipoprotein lipase activity with adipocyte enlargement. Relative values have been calculated for cell surface area and volume over a twofold increase in cell diameter. (A) LPL activity (LPLA) is assumed to be constant (LPLA = k). (B) LPLA is assumed to be directly proportional to cell surface area (LPLA = kS). (C) LPLA is assumed to be a function of cell volume (LPLA = kV).

to C, we have shown the results of three different algebraic models for adipocyte LPL content. In the first, LPL is assumed to be constant, regardless of adipocyte size (Fig. 5A). In this case, LPL expressed on the basis of either adipocyte volume or surface area decreases with increasing adipocyte diameter. In Fig. 5B, LPLA is assumed to be a function of membrane surface area. In this case, as adipocyte diameter doubles LPLA per cell increases, whereas LPLA expressed as a function of volume falls to half its initial value. In Fig. 5C, LPLA is assumed to increase in direct proportion to adipocyte volume; thus activity of LPLA per cell or unit surface area increases.

In Fig. 6, A and B, these relationships are shown for LPLA per tissue mass and LPLA per cell, respectively. In these calculations we have assumed that tissue mass is directly related to the volume of its adipocytes. These two

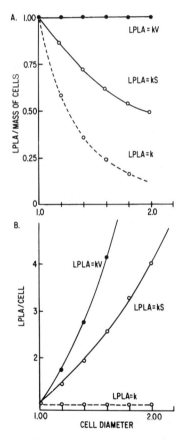

FIGURE 6 Changes in lipoprotein lipase activity per cell and per mass of cells for each of the three relationships describing LPL activity in the fat cell in Fig. 5.

methods for expressing LPL data, whichever of the three relationships for adipocyte LPL content is chosen, give strikingly different results. If, for example, LPL is a function of cell (or cytosol) volume, LPLA per tissue mass is constant regardless of cell diameter, whereas LPLA per cell increases dramatically.

In order to extrapolate results of *in vitro* studies of adipose tissue LPL content to the *in vivo* situation and to draw even tentative hypotheses about rates of TGFA assimilation in adipose tissue, one needs to know the critical parameter(s) of TGFA hydrolysis. *A priori,* there does not seem to be much reason to choose between the three alternative models; that is, whether LPL per cell, LPL per unit adipocyte surface area, or the LPL concentration within the cell is the most critical factor in maintaining homeostasis of plasma lipoprotein TGFA uptake. *In vivo,* the situation is undoubtedly even more complicated since TGFA hydrolysis and assimilation occur at the capillary endothelial surface and depend on LPL secretion by the adipocyte and its subsequent binding. Satisfactory geometrical models would, therefore, need to take into account changes in adipose tissue vascularity as well as cell size with enlargement of the adipose organ.

Hormonal regulation of LPL activity in different tissues. The concept that lipoprotein lipase may play a directive role in TGFA assimilation has arisen from the work of Robinson and co-workers (1970). This idea was the outgrowth of observations that hormones have had different, often opposite, effects on lipoprotein lipases from different tissues. Most recently, this concept has been developed for adipose tissue and heart lipoprotein lipases by Borensztajn et al. (1972), who examined the effects of insulin in fed and starved rats. During starvation LPLA in adipose tissue fell, while there was reciprocal increase in heart LPLA. Administration of insulin or tolbutamide to starved animals produced an increase in adipose tissue LPLA to levels similar to LPLA in fed animals, but did not decrease heart enzyme activity.

In other experiments, insulin injection into fed rats prevented the decline in adipose tissue LPLA on subsequent starvation. It did not, however, prevent the rise of heart LPLA. These *in vivo* experiments indicate that insulin plays an important role in regulating adipose tissue LPL. Single injections of insulin, which led to physiological levels of circulating hormone, increased adipose tissue LPL within 3 hr and maintained it at those levels for at least another 3 hr, despite an only transient increase in plasma insulin above basal concentrations. The failure of insulin to modify heart LPLA in this system suggests that either LPLA in the two tissues is controlled by different hormones or cellular mechanisms (for example, the hormone receptors) are radically different in these tissues. A third, but less likely, possibility is that the heart LPL and adipose tissue LPL are, in fact, different enzymes. Experimental data with purified enzymes from heart and adipose tissue have shown that the enzymes have similar properties and molecular weights (Twu et al., 1976; Bensadoun et al., 1974).

Recently Garfinkel et al. (1976) have found that insulin treatment of fasted rats increases whole adipose tissue, but not isolated fat cell LPLA. Both LPL_a and a smaller species, thought to be LPL_b, were increased. These data conflicted with the earlier postulate that LPL_a was the extracellular and LPL_b the intracellular enzyme. Subsequent experiments have shown that the smaller species was LPL_i and not LPL_b (Schotz, personal communication). Although the LPL release process from isolated fat cells was not affected by cyclohexamide, all changes in whole tissue LPL activity after insulin therapy were abolished by cyclohexamide. One possible explanation for these apparently conflicting findings might be that there is a rapidly turned over stromal protein required for LPL binding after secretion. The secretion or stromal binding of LPL may be regulatory sites for insulin action.

Borensztajn et al. (1973) examined the possibility that glucagon might be the primary regulator of heart LPLA. They found that the decrease in heart LPLA on refeeding of starved rats could be prevented by glucagon. Glucagon did not alter the rise in adipose tissue LPLA with refeeding. Glucagon administration to fed rats increased heart LPLA but failed to change adipose tissue LPLA. Data for red skeletal muscle have shown that this tissue's activity behaves similarly to cardiac LPLA. The mechanism of the glucagon effect on myocardial LPLA, or its consequences for myocardial energy metabolism, are not defined. Nonetheless, these observations indicate a mechanism by which oppositely directed effects on LPLA might occur. These effects might be teleologically advantageous, since the net effect would be to shift pathways of TGFA utilization away from the adipose organ to tissues with relatively fixed energy requirements.

A second situation in which LPLA is subject to endocrine regulation occurs during pregnancy and lactation. Although the majority of the work in this area has been carried out in animal models, lipemia during the latter portion of human pregnancy and the presence of LPL in human milk suggest that the results of animal studies can be extrapolated to the human. In the pregnant rat, plasma TG concentration increases threefold during the latter portion of pregnancy and, after a brief prepartum dip and rise, falls to low levels throughout lactation. At the same time, adipose tissue LPL declines progressively throughout pregnancy and remains low during lactation. Shortly after parturition, mammary gland LPLA increases from essentially nonexistent levels to high levels during lactation. The maintenance of mammary gland LPLA depends on continued suckling and patency of the lactiferous ducts. During lactation the plasma TG concentration is inversely proportional to mammary gland LPLA (Hamosh et al., 1970; Otway and Robinson, 1968). The expected net effect of these changes would be to shunt TGFA from storage in the mother to secretion in milk.

Zinder et al. (1974) and Garrison and Scow (1975) have studied the effects of prolactin on LPLA in mammary gland and adipose tissue of rats as well as in crop sac and adipose tissue of pigeons. In the lactating rat, hypophysectomy results in decreased LPLA in mammary gland and increased adipose tissue LPLA. Injection of prolactin at the time of hypophysectomy maintained LPLA in mammary gland and suppressed adipose tissue LPLA. Similar findings were reported for pigeon crop sac LPLA.

Since milk LPL is not active at gastric pH, it is unlikely that LPL secreted in milk is of any significance in fat digestion. The mammary gland is able to take up dietary TGFA and to secrete it in milk (Linzell and Peaker, 1971). Mammary LPL may provide fat calories and, perhaps more important, provides a source of essential fatty acids for the newborn.

Estrogenic and progestational hormones are a third example of potentially important endocrine control of LPLA. Several groups have found that the administration of 17β-estradiol lowers LPLA in adipose tissue (Hamosh and Hamosh, 1975; Kim and Kalkhoff, 1975). Ovariectomy increased adipose tissue LPLA, and this effect is reversed by estradiol replacement. Progesterone produces opposite effects (Kim and Kalkhoff, 1975). Kim and Kalkhoff also studied PHLA in estrogen- and progesterone-treated rats. Estrogen treatment decreased PHLA and protamine-resistant hepatic triglyceride lipase (HTGL), whereas progesterone increased both PHLA and protamine-resistant activities. In confirmation of TG kinetic studies in the human, estrogen-induced increases in plasma TG concentration were best correlated with TG entry. In one study in which acetone-ether powders were assayed, heart and lung LPLA were unaffected by either estrogen or progesterone treatment (Hamosh and Hamosh, 1975). In another study in which whole tissue fragments were assayed, adipose tissue LPLA was decreased by estrogen therapy, while heart and skeletal muscle activities were increased (Wilson et al., 1976). These data suggest that tonic effects of estrogen and progesterone on TG entry into and removal from the plasma may regulate the distribution of circulating TGFA among the tissues.

In summary, during starvation, pregnancy, and lactation or with ovarian estrogen secretion, differential effects on LPLA have been found. In each of these instances, differences in the response of LPLA to hormones may provide mechanisms for independent control of TGFA uptake by tissues. Discussion of other possible endocrine modulators of tissue LPLA such as glucocorticoids and catecholamines is beyond the scope of this review (see Krotkiewski et al., 1976).

Reciprocal regulation of LPL and hormone-sensitive lipase. The two enzymes that control TGFA influx and efflux from the adipocyte, LPL and hormone-sensitive lipase (HSL), respectively, appear to be regulated in a reciprocal fashion. Catecholamines stimulate adenyl cyclase, raise intracellular concentrations of cyclic AMP, and stimulate HSL activity. Methyl xanthines inhibit phosphodiesterase, increase cyclic AMP levels, and increase HSL activity. Under these conditions, LPL activity decreases. Several laboratories nearly simultaneously noted that LPL activity was depressed by activators of HSL and increased by antilipolytic agents (Nestel and Austin, 1969; Nikillä and Pykälisto, 1968a, 1968b; Pykälisto, 1970; Wing and Robinson, 1968b). Patten (1970) has studied the relationship between lypolysis and LPL activity in the isolated fat cell. Addition of dibutyryl cyclic AMP produced an immediate rise in glycerol release. Within 20–30 min, LPL activity fell to approximately half of control values. Because of the suspected relationship between protein synthesis and tissue LPL, Patten then measured adipocyte LPL and adipocyte protein synthesis with radiolabeled leucine. Incubation of isolated fat cells with cyclohexamide (10 μg/ml) caused a rapid loss in LPL activity. The addition of dibutyryl cyclic AMP to cyclohexamide-inhibited cells did not further accelerate the loss of LPL activity. These data suggested that the effect of cyclic AMP on LPL activity was mediated through inhibition of protein synthesis. Patten then performed a large number of experiments in which isolated fat cells were incubated with dibutyryl cyclic AMP, cyclohexamide, epinephrine, theophylline, insulin, and glucose. There was a linear relationship ($r = 0.95$) between the rate of protein synthesis from radiolabeled leucine and LPL activity.

The intracellular mediator of the reciprocal control of LPL is not known. In addition to the rise in cyclic AMP, there is intracellular FFA accumulation and depletion of ATP concentrations (Angel et al., 1971). Khoo and Steinberg (1976) offered additional support for an indirect mechanism, since incubation of partially purified LPL with exogenous protein kinase under conditions that markedly affect HSL was without effect on LPL activity. It seems likely, however, that insulin initially exerts its effect on LPL protein synthesis through stimulation of phosphodiesterase and a decrease in intracellular cyclic AMP (Loten and Sneyd, 1970; Desai and Hollenberg, 1975).

Adipose tissue LPL activity in obesity and diabetes. Much of the information about adipose tissue LPLA in obesity and diabetes has appeared only in abstracts. What data are available support the idea that heparin-releasable LPLA in whole adipose tissue is best described as a function of adipocyte volume (Campbell et al., 1974; Guy-Grand and Bigorie, 1975; Pykalisto et al., 1975b; Jaillard et al., 1976). In studies of whole adipose tissue segments from lean and obese humans, LPLA per cell and LPLA per unit surface both increased while LPLA per mass of adipose tissue was relatively constant. With adipocyte enlargement, LPLA per cell increased strikingly (Fig. 6B), (Campbell et al., 1974) but LPLA per mass of adipose tissue did not change or increased slightly (Fig. 6A).

The data for LPLA in isolated adipocytes or for whole adipose tissue (acetone-ether extracts) are not as clear-cut. Bray and Zinder (1974) found a decrease in LPLA per mass of adipose tissue and no change in LPLA per cell in obese volunteers. These experiments would be consistent with the idea that total LPLA was constant regardless of adipocyte size. Other data have shown a positive correlation between adipocyte volume and cellular LPLA in acetone-ether powder or isolated adipocyte preparations (Pykalisto et al.,

1975b; Hartman, 1975). Since stromal LPL may contribute substantially to whole tissue LPLA, it seems reasonable to assume that the effects of increasing cell volume might affect both intracellular and extracellular LPLA (Fig. 4).

Several investigators have shown a positive correlation between fasting immunoreactive insulin and tissue LPLA, which might be predicted if both were the consequence of adipocyte enlargement (Pykalisto et al., 1975b; Guy-Grand and Bigorie, 1973, 1975). The latter investigators found no relationship between immunoreactive insulin levels and LPLA by partial regression analysis if cell size were excluded. This suggests that the effect of cell size on LPLA is not mediated directly by insulin.

Lipoprotein lipase activity in adipose tissue has been decreased in diabetes (Pykalisto et al., 1975a, 1975b; Guy-Grand and Bigorie, 1973, 1975). In such experiments, it is crucial to compare data from adipocyte size-matched samples, particularly since adipocytes from ketosis-prone, insulin-dependent diabetics have been found to be smaller than normal, and so decreased LPLA per cell might be expected (Jaillard et al., 1976) (Fig. 6B).

To summarize then, the method of analysis of LPLA and the manner in which the data are expressed are critical issues in defining the effects of diabetes and obesity on adipose tissue LPLA. Adipose tissue LPLA increases with adipocyte enlargement and can be represented as a function of cell volume. This is, at best, an oversimplification since LPL is found within both adipocytes and stromal elements. In the few published studies in which differences in adipocyte size have been taken into account, adipose tissue LPLA has been depressed in diabetic humans.

Lipoprotein Lipase and Hormone-Sensitive Lipase: Similarities between Triglyceride and Glycogen Storage and Mobilization

Just as the liver and kidney, which store glycogen and contain glucose-6-phosphatase, are storage depots for carbohydrate and provide glucose to other tissues in times of substrate deprivation, the adipose organ is a storage depot for lipid fuels. Both glycogen and triglyceride storage are under endocrine control and both processes shift from storage to release of depot fuels in the fasted state. Glycogen stores in the liver are adequate to provide glucose for less than 24 hr. The release of FFA from adipose tissue during starvation, by contrast, continues for weeks or months. There may be an important intramuscular pool of TGFA as well (Dagenais et al., 1976).

Glycogen storage and breakdown in the liver are regulated by the activities of glycogen synthetase and phosphorylase. In the case of glycogenolysis, the endocrine-stimulated production of cyclic AMP leads to phosphorylation of inactive phosphorylase and to the inactivation of glycogen synthetase (glycogen synthetase D). In the adipocyte, stimulation of the adenyl cyclase mechanism leads to phosphorylation of an inactive hormone-sensitive lipase and stimulation of the hydrolysis of stored TGFA and a rise in plasma FFA concentrations. The regulatory enzyme for the assimilation of lipoprotein TGFA, lipoprotein lipase, is inhibited under these conditions.

The simultaneous stimulation of the catabolic enzyme and inhibition of the anabolic enzyme has the teleological advantage of preventing a "futile cycle." The net result is sparing of TG-rich lipoprotein and production of FFA and ketone bodies for utilization by other tissues.

SUMMARY AND CONCLUSIONS

Diabetes mellitus and hyperlipoproteinemia are prevalent disorders that affect about 1.5% and more than 10% of the population of the United States, respectively. Both have been implicated as important contributors to the atherogenic diathesis and increase mortality and morbidity from coronary heart disease. Independent coronary risk factors are additive, and therefore the coexistence of diabetes mellitus and hyperlipidemia is of special concern.

Within the past decade, our knowledge of and techniques for investigating hyperlipoproteinemia have improved dramatically. New information has been gained from studies of lipoprotein physiology in normal individuals and in patients with primary hyperlipoproteinemias. Our information about the pathogenesis of acquired hyperlipoproteinemias has lagged behind.

Published descriptive clinical studies still leave much to be desired. Increased VLDL and LDL concentrations have been found in diabetes. It is likely that hepatic overproduction of VLDL accounts for much of the hypertriglyceridemia and hypercholesterolemia that have been reported in diabetic populations. Why LDL concentration should also be increased in diabetes is unclear. The importance of decreased plasma HDL in atherogenesis has been rediscovered recently. Older data showed strikingly decreased HDL concentrations in some hyperlipidemic atherosclerotic diabetics. Yet very few data are available for HDL concentrations in unselected diabetic populations. Since HDL concentrations can be altered by drugs (Carlson and Kolmodin-Hedman, 1972; Johansson and Medhus, 1974) this could provide an important avenue of therapeutic attack.

Studies in both experimental animals and humans offer strong circumstantial evidence that LPL activity is abnormal in diabetic-hyperlipoproteinemic states. The role of LPL and abnormal VLDL removal in the pathogenesis of hyperlipoproteinemia in diabetes has not been defined, however. Recent improvements in methodology for measuring LPL activity in postheparin plasma and the realization that PHLA is heterogeneous make it imperative that older studies of PHLA in diabetes be reassessed.

Finally, the genetic relationships between diabetes and hyperlipoproteinemia have not been defined. Some data have suggested that familial hypertriglyceridemia and diabetes mellitus segregate independently. In uncontrolled diabetes and obesity, defective regulation of lipolysis and/or the effects of hyperinsulinism on the liver are the likely causes of mild nongenetic hypertriglyceridemia. However, it seems equally likely that severe hypertriglyceridemia in diabetes has an underlying genetic basis. Answers· to these and many other questions are needed if we are to understand the atherogenic diathesis of diabetes.

REFERENCES

Addison, T. and Gull, W. 1851. On a certain affection of the skin, vitiligoidea a. plana, b. tuberosa. *Guys Hosp. Rep.* 7:265–277.

Ahuja, M. M. S., Kumar, V. and Gossain, W. 1969. Interrelationship of vascular diseases and blood lipids in young Indian diabetics. *Diabetes* 18:670–674.

Alaupovic, P. 1971. Conceptual development of the classification systems of plasma lipoproteins. *Protides Biol. Fluids, Proc. 19th Colloq.* 9–10.

Alaupovic, P., Lee, D. M. and McConathy, W. J. 1972. Studies on the composition and structure of plasma lipoproteins. Distribution of lipoprotein families in major density classes of normal human lipoproteins. *Biochim. Biophys. Acta* 260:689–707.

Albrink, M. J. and Davidson, P. C. 1966. Impaired glucose tolerance in patients with hypertriglyceridemia. *J. Lab. Clin. Med.* 67:573–584.

Albrink, M. J. and Meigs, J. W. 1965. The relationship between serum triglycerides and skinfold thickness in obese subjects. *Ann. N. Y. Acad. Sci.* 131:673.

Albrink, M. J., Lavietes, P. H. and Man, E. B. 1963. Vascular disease and serum lipids in diabetes mellitus. *Ann. Int. Med.* 58:305–323.

Alcindor, L. G., Infante, R., Soler-Argilage Raisonneir, A., Polonovski, J. and Caroli, J. 1970. Induction of the hepatic synthesis of B-lipoproteins by high concentrations of fatty acids. Effect of actinomycin D. *Biochim. Biophys. Acta* 210:483–486.

Anderson, R. F. W., Goldstein, J. L. and Brown, M. S. 1976. Localization of low density lipoprotein receptors on the plasma membrane of normal human fibroblasts and their absence in cells from a familial hypercholesterolemic homozygote. *Proc. Natl. Acad. Sci. U.S.A.* 73:2564–2568.

Angel, A., Desai, K. S. and Halperin, M. L. 1971. Reduction in adipocyte ATP by lipolytic agents: Relation to intracellular free fatty acid accumulation. *J. Lipid Res.* 12:203–213.

Augustin, J., Freeze, H., Boberg, J. and Brown, W. V. 1976. Human postheparin plasma lipolytic activities. In *Lipoprotein metabolism,* ed. H. Greten. Berlin: Springer.

Bagdade, J. D., Porte, D., Jr. and Bierman, E. L. 1967. Diabetic lipemia. A form of fat-induced lipemia. *N. Engl. J. Med.* 276:427–433.

Bagdade, J. D., Porte, D., Jr. and Bierman, E. L. 1968. Acute insulin withdrawal and the regulation of plasma triglyceride removal in diabetic subjects. *Diabetes* 17:127–132.

Baginsky, M. and Brown, W. V. 1977. Differential characteristics of purified hepatic triglyceride lipase and lipoprotein lipase from human plasma. *J. Lipid Res.,* in press.

Ballard, K., Fredholm, B. B., Meng, H. C. and Rosell, S. 1971. Heparin-induced release of lipase activity from perfused canine subcutaneous adipose tissue. *Proc. Soc. Exp. Biol. Med.* 137:1490–1493.

Bar-On, H., Kook, A. I., Stein, O. and Stein, Y. 1973. Assembly and secretion of very low density lipoproteins by rat liver following inhibition of protein synthesis with cyclohexamide. *Biochim. Biophys. Acta* 306:106–114.

Bar-On, H., Roheim, P. S. and Eder, H. A. 1976. Hyperlipoproteinemia in streptozotocin-treated rats. *Diabetes* 25:509–515.

Barr, P. D., Russ, E. M. and Eder, H. A. 1951. Protein-lipid relationships in human plasma. ii. In atherosclerosis and related conditions. *Am. J. Med.* 11:480–493.

Barter, P. J. and Nestel, P. J. 1972. Precursor-product relationship between pools of very low density lipoprotein triglyceride. *J. Clin. Invest.* 51:174–180.

Baxter, J. H. 1966. Origin and characteristics of endogenous lipid in thoracic duct lymph in rat. *J. Lipid Res.* 7:158–166.

Beaumont, J. L., Carlson, L. A., Cooper, G. R., Fejfar, Z., Fredrickson, D. S. and Strasser, T. 1970. Classification of hyperlipidemias and hyperlipoproteinemias. *Bull. WHO* 43:891–915.

Bensadoun, A., Ehnholm, C., Steinberg, D. and Brown, W. V. 1974. Purification and characterization of lipoprotein lipase from pig adipose tissue. *J. Biol. Chem.* 249:2220–2227.

Bergqvist, N. 1970. Serum lipids in an ambulatory diabetic clientele. *Acta Med. Scand.* 187:213–218.

Bernstein, R. S., Grant, N. and Kipnis, D. M. 1975. Hyperinsulinemia and enlarged adipocytes in patients with endogenous hyperlipoproteinemia without obesity or diabetes mellitus. *Diabetes* 24:207–213.

Bezman, A., Felts, J. M. and Havel, R. J. 1962. Relation between incorporation of triglyceride fatty acids and heparin-released lipoprotein lipase from adipose tissue slices. *J. Lipid Res.* 3:427–431.

Bierman, E. L. and Porte, D. Jr. 1968. Carbohydrate intolerance and lipemia. *Ann. Intern. Med.* 68:926–933.

Bierman, E. L., Stein, O. and Stein, Y. 1974. Lipoprotein uptake and metabolism by rat aortic smooth muscle cells in tissue culture. *Circ. Res.* 35:136–150.

Bilheimer, D. W., Eisenberg, S. and Levy, R. I. 1972. The metabolism of very low density lipoprotein proteins. I. Preliminary *in vitro* and *in vivo* observations. *Biochim. Biophys. Acta* 260:212–221.

Birkenhager, J. C. and Tjabbes, T. 1969. Turnover rate of plasma FFA and rate of esterification of plasma FFA to plasma triglycerides in obese humans before and after weight reduction. *Metabolism* 18:18–32.

Björntorp, P. and Östman, J. 1971. Human adipose tissue dynamics and regulation. *Adv. Metab. Disord.* 5:277–329.

Blanchette-Mackie, E. J. and Scow, R. O. 1971. Sites of lipoprotein lipase activity in adipose tissue perfused with chylomicrons. *J. Cell Biol.* 51:1–25.

Blix, G. 1926. Studies on diabetic lipemia I, II, III. *Acta Med. Scand.* 64:142–259.

Borensztajn, J., Sammols, E. R. and Rubenstein, A. H. 1972. Effects of insulin on lipoprotein lipase activity in the rat heart and adipose tissue. *Am. J. Physiol.* 223:1271–1275.

Borensztajn, J., Keig, P. and Rubenstein, A. H. 1973. The role of glucagon in the regulation of myocardial lipoprotein. *Biochem. Biophys. Res. Commun.* 53:603–608.

Borensztajn, J., Rone, M. S. and Sandros, T. 1975. Effects of colchicine and cyclohexamide on the functional and non-functional lipoprotein fractions of rat heart. *Biochim. Biophys. Acta* 398:394–400.

Borut, T. C. and Aladjem, F. 1971. Immunochemical heterogeneity of human high density serum lipoproteins. *Immunochemistry* 8:851–863.

Bray, G. A. and Zinder, O. 1974. Lipoprotein-lipase and lipogenesis in human adipose tissue. *Clin. Res.* 22:188A.

Breslow, J. L., Spaulding, D. R., Lux, S. E., Levy, R. I. and Lees, R. S. 1975. Homozygous familial hypercholesterolemia. A possible biochemical explanation of clinical heterogeneity. *N. Engl. J. Med.* 293:900–903.

Brindley, D. N. and Hubscher, G. 1966. The effect of chain length on the activation and subsequent incorporation of fatty acids into glycerides by the small intestinal mucosa. *Biochim. Biophys. Acta* 125:92–105.

Brockerhoff, H. 1973. A model of pancreatic lipase and the orientation of enzymes at interfaces. *Chem. Phys. Lipids* 10:215–222.

Brown, M. S., Dana, S. E. and Goldstein, J. L. 1975a. Receptor-dependent hydrolysis of cholesteryl esters contained in plasma low density lipoprotein. *Proc. Natl. Acad. Sci. U.S.A.* 72:2925–2929.

Brown, M. S., Faust, J. R., and Goldstein, J. L. 1975b. Role of the low density lipoprotein receptor in regulating the content of free and esterified cholesterol in human fibroblasts. *J. Clin. Invest.* 55:783–793.

Brown, W. V., Baginsky, M., Boberg, J. and Augustin, J. 1975. Lipases and lipoproteins. In *Lipoprotein metabolism*, ed. H. Greten, pp. 2–6. Berlin: Springer-Verlag.

Brunzell, J. D., Hazzard, W. R., Motulsky, A. G. and Bierman, E. L. 1975a. Evidence for diabetes mellitus and genetic forms of hypertriglyceridemia as independent entities. *Metabolism* 24:1115–1121.

Brunzell, J. D., Porte, D., Jr. and Bierman, E. L. 1975b. Reversible abnormalities in postheparin lipolytic activity during the late phase of release in diabetes mellitus (postheparin lipolytic activity in diabetes). *Metabolism* 24:1123–1137.

Campbell, R. G., Faibisoff, B. and Brodows, P. G. 1974. Adipose tissue lipoprotein lipase activity in obesity. *Diabetes* 23(S1):367.

Cardell, R. R., Jr., Badenhausen, S. and Porter, K. P. 1967. Intestinal triglyceride absorption in the rat. An electron microscopical study. *J. Cell Biol.* 34:123–155.

Carlson, L. A. and Kolmodin-Hedman, B. 1972. Hyper-α-lipoproteinemia in men exposed to chlorinated hydrocarbon pesticides. *Acta Med. Scand.* 192:29–32.

Carlson, L. A. and Wahlberg, F. 1966. Serum lipids, intravenous glucose tolerance and their interrelation studied in ischaemic cardiovascular disease. *Acta Med. Scand.* 180:307–315.

Castelli, W. P., Doyle, J. T., Gordon, T., Hames, C., Hulley, S. B., Kagan, A., McGee, D., Vicic, W. J. and Zukel, W. J. 1975. HDL cholesterol levels (HDLC) in coronary heart disease (CHD): A cooperative study. *Circulation* 52(suppl. 11):97a.

Chajek, T., Stein, O. and Stein, J. 1975. Colchicine-induced inhibition of plasma lipoprotein lipase release in the intact rat. *Biochim. Biophys. Acta* 380:127–131.

Chance, G. W., Albutt, E. C. and Edkins, S. M. 1969. Serum lipids and lipoproteins in untreated diabetic children. *Lancet* 2:1126–1128.

Chase, H. P. and Glasgow, A. M. 1976. Juvenile diabetes mellitus and serum lipids and lipoprotein levels. *Am. J. Dis. Child.* 130:1113–1117.

Chen, A. L., Hershgold, E. J. and Wilson, D. E. 1975. One stage assay of heparin. *J. Lab. Clin. Med.* 85:843–854.

Crespin, S. R., Greenough, W. B., III and Steinberg, D. 1972. Effect of sodium linoleate infusion on plasma free fatty acids, glucose, insulin, and ketones in unanesthetized dogs. *Diabetes* 21:1179–1184.

Cryer, A., Davies, P., Williams, E. R. and Robinson, D. S. 1975a. The clearing-factor lipase activity of isolated fat-cells. *Biochem. J.* 146: 481–488.

Cryer, A., McDonald, A., Williams, E. R. and Robinson, D. S. 1975b. Colchicine inhibition of the heparin-stimulated release of clearing-factor lipase from isolated fat cells. *Biochem. J.* 152:717–720.

Cunningham, V. J. and Robinson, D. S. 1969. Clearing-factor lipase in adipose tissue. Distinction of different states of the enzyme and the possible role of the fat cell in the maintenance of tissue activity. *Biochem. J.* 112:203–209.

Dagenais, G. R., Tancredi, R. G. and Zierler, K. L. 1976. Free fatty acid oxidation by forearm muscle at rest, and evidence for an intramuscular lipid pool in the human forearm. *J. Clin. Invest.* 58:421–431.

Desai, K. and Hollenberg, C. H. 1975. Regulation by insulin of lipoprotein lipase and phosphodiesterase activities in rat adipose tissue. *Isr. J. Med. Sci.* 11:540–550.

Eagle, G. R. and Robinson, D. S. 1964. The effect of actinomycin D to increase the clearing-factor lipase activity of rat adipose tissue. *Biochem. J.* 93:10C.

Eder, H. A., Lesser, N. L. and Scholnick, H. R. 1970. Lipid metabolism. In *Diabetes mellitus: Theory and practice,* eds. M. Ellenberg and H. Rifkin, chap. 3. New York: McGraw-Hill.

Egelrud, T. and Olivecrona, T. 1972. The purification of a lipoprotein lipase from bovine skim milk. *J. Biol. Chem.* 274:6212–6217.

Ehnholm, C., Greten, H. and Brown, W. V. 1974a. A comparative study of postheparin lipolytic activity and a purified human plasma triglycerol lipase. *Biochim. Biophys. Acta* 360:68–77.

Ehnholm, C., Shaw, W., Greten, H., Lengfelder, W. and Brown, W. V. 1974b. Characterization of a highly purified human post-heparin lipase. In *Proceedings of the Third International Symposium on Atherosclerosis,* eds. G. Schettler and A. Weizel, pp. 557–560. New York: Springer-Verlag.

Ehnholm, C., Huttunen, J. K., Kinnunen, P. K. J., Miettinen, T. A. and Nikkila, E. A. 1975a. Effect of oxandrolone treatment on the activity of LPL and phospholipase A_1 of human postheparin plasma. *N. Engl. J. Med.* 292:1314–1317.

Ehnholm, C., Kinnunen, P. K. J., Huttunen, J. K., Nikkila, E. A. and Ohta, M. 1975b. Purification and characterization of lipoprotein lipase from pig myocardium. *Biochem. J.* 149:649–655.

Ehnholm, C., Shaw, W., Greten, H. and Brown, W. V. 1975c. Purification from human plasma of heparin-released lipase with activity against triglyceride and phospholipid. *J. Biol. Chem.* 250:6756–6761.

Eisenberg, S. and Levy, R. I. 1975. Lipoprotein metabolism. *Adv. Lipid Res.* 13:1–89.

Eisenberg, S. and Rachmilewitz, D. 1973. Metabolism of rat plasma very low density lipoprotein. II. Fate in circulation of apoprotein subunits. *Biochim. Biophys. Acta* 326:391–405.

Eisenberg, S., Bilheimer, D. W. and Levy, R. I. 1972. The metabolism of very low density lipoproteins. II. Studies on the transfer of apoproteins between plasma lipoproteins. *Biochim. Biophys. Acta* 280:94–104.

Eisenberg, S., Bilheimer, D. W., Levy, R. I. and Lindgren, F. T. 1973. On the metabolic conversion of human plasma very low density lipoprotein to low density lipoprotein. *Biochim. Biophys. Acta* 326:361–377.

Elkeles, R. S. and Williams, E. 1974. Post-heparin lipolytic activity and tissue lipoprotein lipase activity in the alloxan-diabetic rat. *Clin. Sci. Mol. Med.* 46:661–664.

Faergeman, O. and Damgaard-Pedersen, F. 1973. Increase of post-heparin lipase activity by oxandrolone in familial hyperchylomicronemia. *Scand. J. Lab. Invest.* 31:27–31.

Feinstein, A. R. 1963. Boolean algebra and clinical taxonomy. I. Analytic synthesis of the general spectrum of a human disease. *N. Engl. J. Med.* 269:929–938.

Felber, J. P. and Vanotti, A. 1964. Effects of fat infusion on glucose tolerance and insulin plasma levels. *Med. Exp.* 10:153–156.

Felker, T. E., Fainevu, M., Hamilton, R. L. and Havel, R. J. 1976. Secretion of apolipoproteins (AI and ARP) by the isolated perfused rat liver. *Circulation* 53(suppl. 2):92A.

Fielding, C. J. 1970. Human lipoprotein lipase. I. Purification and substrate specificity. *Biochim. Biophys. Acta* 206:109–117.

Fielding, P. E., Shore, V. G. and Fielding, C. J. 1974. Lipoprotein lipase: Properties of the enzyme isolated from post-heparin plasma. *Biochemistry* 13:4318.

Fineberg, S. E. and Merimee, T. J. 1974. Acute metabolic effects of human growth hormone. *Diabetes* 23:499–504.

Fogelman, A. M., Edmond, J., Seager, J. and Popjak, G. 1975. Abnormal induction of 3-hydroxy-3-methylglutaryl coenzyme A reductase in leukocytes from subjects with heterozygous familial hypercholesterolemia. *J. Biol. Chem.* 250:2045–2055.

Ford, S., Jr., Bozian, R. C. and Knowles, H. C., Jr. 1969. Interactions of obesity and glucose and insulin levels in hypertriglyceridemia. *Am. J. Clin. Nutr.* 21:904–910.

Forte, T., Nichols, A., Glomset, J. and Norum, K. 1974. The ultrastructure of plasma lipoproteins in lecithin:cholesterol acyltransferase deficiency. *Scand. J. Lab. Clin. Invest.* 33(suppl. 137):121–132.

Fredrickson, D. S. 1975. It's time to be practical. *Circulation* 51:209–211.

Fredrickson, D. S. and Levy, R. I. 1972. Familial hyperlipoproteinemia. In *The metabolic basis of inherited disease,* eds. J. B. Stanbury, J. B. Wyngaarden and D. S. Fredrickson, 3rd ed., pp. 545–614. New York: McGraw-Hill.

Fredrickson, D. S., Ono, K. and Davis, L. L. 1963. Lipolytic activity of post-heparin plasma in hypertriglyceridemia. *J. Lipid Res.* 4:24–33.

Fredrickson, D. S., Levy, R. I. and Lees, R. S. 1967. Fat transport in lipoproteins—An integrated approach to mechanisms and disorders. *N. Engl. J. Med.* 276:34–44, 94–103, 148–156, 215–225 and 273–281.

Fredrickson, D. S., Gotto, A. M. and Levy, R. I. 1972. Familial lipoprotein deficiency (abetalipoproteinemia, hypobetalipoproteinemia, and Tangier disease). In *The metabolic basis of inherited disease,* eds. J. B. Stanbury, J. B. Wyngaarden and D. S. Fredrickson, 3rd ed., pp. 493–530. New York: McGraw-Hill.

Furman, R. H., Howard, R. P. and Lakshmi, K. 1961. The serum lipids and lipoproteins in normal and hyperlipidemic subjects as determined by preparative ultracentrifugation. *Am. J. Clin. Nutr.* 9:73–102.

Gage, S. H. and Fish, P. A. 1924. Fat digestion, absorption, and assimilation in man and animals as determined by the dark-field microscope, and a fat soluble dye. *Am. J. Anat.* 34:1–85.

Ganesan, D. and Bass, H. B. 1975. Isolation of C-I and C-II activated lipoprotein lipases and protamine insensitive triglyceride lipase by heparin-Sepharose affinity chromatography. *FEBS Lett.* 53:1–4.

Ganesan, D. and Bass, H. B. 1976. The effect of two heparin preparations on the distribution of protamine in sensitive triacylglycerol lipase and C-I and C-II activated lipoprotein lipases in human post-heparin plasma. *Artery* 2:143–152.

Ganesan, D. and Bradford, R. H. 1971. Isolation of apolipoprotein-free lipoprotein lipase from human post-heparin plasma. *Biochem. Biophys. Res. Commun.* 43:544–549.

Gangl, A. and Ockner, R. K. 1975. Intestinal metabolism of lipids and lipoproteins. *Gastroenterology* 68:167–186.

Garcia, M. J., McNamara, P. M., Gordon, T. and Kannel, W. B. 1974. Morbidity and mortality in diabetics in the Framingham population. *Diabetes* 23:105–111.

Garfinkel, A. S. and Schotz, M. C. 1972. Separation of molecular species of lipoprotein lipase from adipose tissue. *J. Lipid Res.* 13:63–68.

Garfinkel, A. S., Baker, N. and Schotz, M. C. 1967. Relationship of lipoprotein lipase activity to triglyceride uptake in adipose tissue. *J. Lipid Res.* 8:274–280.

Garfinkel, A. S., Nilsson-Ehle, P. and Schotz, M. C. 1976. Regulation of lipoprotein lipase: Induction by insulin. *Biochim. Biophys. Acta* 424:264–273.

Garrison, M. M. and Scow, R. O. 1975. Effect of prolactin on lipoprotein lipase in crop sac and adipose tissue of pigeons. *Am. J. Physiol.* 228:1542–1544.

Gibson, T., Fuller, J. H., Grainger, S. L., Jarrett, R. J. and Keen, H. 1974. Intralipid triglyceride and oral glucose tolerance. *Diabetologia* 10:97–100.

Girolamo, M., Howe, M. D., Esposito, J., Thurman, L. and Owens, J. L. 1974. Metabolic pattern and insulin responsiveness of enlarging fat cells. *J. Lipid Res.* 15:332–338.

Glickman, R. M. and Kirsch, K. 1973. Lymph circulation formation during the inhibition of protein synthesis. *J. Clin. Invest.* 52:2910–2920.

Glomset, J. A. 1968. The plasma lecithin:cholesterol acyltransferase reaction. *J. Lipid. Res.* 9:155–167.

Glomset, J. A. and Norum, K. R. 1973. The metabolic role of lecithin:cholesterol acyltransferase: Perspectives from pathology. *Adv. Lipid Res.* 11:1–65.

Glueck, C. J., Levy, R. I. and Fredrickson, D. S. 1969. Immunoreactive insulin, glucose tolerance and carbohydrate inducibility in types II, III, IV and V hyperlipoproteinemia. *Diabetes* 18:739–747.

Glueck, C. J., Fallat, R. W., Millet, F., Gartside, P., Elston, R. C. and Go, R. C. P. 1975. Familial hyper-alpha-lipoproteinemia: Studies in eighteen kindreds. *Metabolism* 24:1243–1265.

Gofman, J. W., deLalla, O., Glazier, F., Freeman, N. K., Lindgren, F. T., Nichols, A. V., Strishower, E. H., and Tamplin, A. R. 1954. The serum lipoprotein transport system in health, metabolic disorders, atherosclerosis and coronary artery disease. *Plasma* 2:413.

Goldstein, J. L. and Brown, M. S. 1974. Binding and degradation of low density lipoproteins by cultured human fibroblasts. Comparison of cells from a normal subject and from a patient with homozygous familial hypercholesterolemia. *J. Biol. Chem.* 249:5133-5162.

Goldstein, J. L. and Brown, M. S. 1975a. Lipoprotein receptors, cholesterol metabolism, and atherosclerosis. *Arch. Pathol.* 99:181-184.

Goldstein, J. L. and Brown, M. S. 1975b. Familial hypercholesterolemia. A genetic regulatory defect in cholesterol metabolism. *Am. J. Med.* 58:147-150.

Goldstein, J. L., Hazzard, W. R. Schrott, H. G., Bierman, E. L. and Motulsky, A. G. 1973a. Hyperlipidemia in coronary heart disease. I. Lipid levels in 500 survivors of myocardial infarction. *J. Clin. Invest.* 52:1533-1543.

Goldstein, J. L., Schrott, H. G., Hazzard, W. R., Bierman, E. L. and Motulsky, A. G. 1973b. Hyperlipidemia in coronary heart disease. II. Genetic analysis of lipid levels of 176 families and delineation of a new inherited disorder, combined hyperlipidemia. *J. Clin. Invest.* 52:1544-1568.

Goldstein, J. L., Dana, S. E., Brunschede, G. Y. and Brown, M. S. 1975. Genetic heterogeneity in familial hypercholesterolemia: Evidence for two different mutations affecting functions of low density lipoprotein receptor. *Proc. Natl. Acad. Sci. U.S.A.* 72:1092-1096.

Gotto, A. M., Levy, R. I., John, K. and Fredrickson, D. S. 1971. On the protein defect in abetalipoproteinemia. *N. Engl. J. Med.* 284:813-818.

Greenberger, N. J., Rodgers, J. B. and Isselbacher, K. J. 1966. Absorption of medium and long chain triglycerides: Factors influencing their hydrolysis and transport. *J. Clin. Invest.* 45:217-227.

Greten, H. and Walter, B. 1973. Purification of rat adipose tissue lipoprotein lipase. *FEBS Lett.* 35:36-40.

Greten, H., Levy, R. I. and Fredrickson, D. S. 1969. Evidence for separate monoglyceride hydrolase and triglyceride lipase in post-heparin human plasma. *J. Lipid Res.* 10:326-330.

Greten, H., Walter, B. and Brown, W. V. 1972. Purification of human postheparin plasma triglyceride lipase. *FEBS Lett.* 27:306-310.

Greten, H., DeGrella, R., Klose, G., Rascher, W., de Gennes, J. L. and Gjone, E. 1976. Measurement of two plasma triglyceride lipases by an immunochemical method: Studies in patients with hypertriglyceridemia. *J. Lipid Res.* 17:203-210.

Guy-Grand, B. and Bigorie, B. 1973. Lipoprotein lipase activity release by human adipose tissue in vitro: Effect of adipose cell size. In *Proceedings of the 4th International Meeting of Endocrinology*, eds. J. Vagne and J. Boyer. International Congress Series No. 315. Amsterdam: Excerpta Medica.

Guy-Grand, B. and Bigorie, B. 1975. Effect of fat cell size, restrictive diet and diabetes on lipoprotein lipase release by human adipose tissue. *Horm. Metab. Res.* 7:471-475.

Hamilton, R. L. 1972. Synthesis and secretion of plasma lipoproteins. *Adv. Exp. Med. Biol.* 26:7-24.

Hamosh, M. and Hamosh, P. 1975. The effect of estrogen on the lipoprotein lipase activity of rat adipose tissue. *J. Clin. Invest.* 55:1132-1135.

Hamosh, M., Clary, T. R., Chernick, S. and Scow, R. O. 1970. Lipoprotein lipase activity of adipose and mammary tissue and plasma triglyceride in pregnant and lactating rats. *Biochim. Biophys. Acta* 210:473-482.

Harlan, W. R., Jr., Winesett, P. S. and Wasserman, A. J. 1967. Tissue lipoprotein lipase in normal individuals and in individuals with exogenous hypertriglyceridemia and the relationship of this enzyme to assimilation of fat. *J. Clin. Invest.* 46:239-247.

Hartman, A. D. 1975. Relationship between adipocyte size and lipoprotein lipase activity in various depots of the rat. *Fed. Proc.* 34:909.

Havel, R. J. 1970. Typing of hyperlipoproteinemias. *Atherosclerosis* 11:3–6.

Havel, R. J. 1971. Mechanisms of hyperlipoproteinemia. *Adv. Exp. Med. Biol.* 26:57–69.

Havel, R. J. 1975. Hyperlipoproteinemia: Problems in diagnosis and challenges posed by the "type III" disorder. *Ann. Intern. Med.* 82:273–274.

Havel, R. J. and Gordon, R. S., Jr. 1960. Idiopathic hyperlipemia: Metabolic studies in an affected family. *J. Clin. Invest.* 39:1777–1790.

Havel, R. J., Kane, J. P., Balasse, E. O., Segel, N. and Basso, L. V. 1970a. Splanchnic metabolism of free fatty acids and production of triglycerides of very low density lipoproteins in normotriglyceridemic and hypertriglyceridemic humans. *J. Clin. Invest.* 49:2017–2035.

Havel, R. J., Shore, V. G., Shore, B. and Bier, D. M. 1970b. Role of specific glycopeptides of human serum lipoproteins in the activation of lipoprotein lipase. *Circ. Res.* 27:595–600.

Havel, R. J., Fielding, C. J., Olivecrona, T., Shore, V. G., Fielding, P. E. and Egelrud, T. 1973a. Cofactor activity of protein components of human very low density lipoproteins in the hydrolysis of triglycerides by lipoprotein lipase from different sources. *Biochemistry* 12:1828–1833.

Havel, R. J., Kane, J. P. and Kashyap, M. L. 1973b. Interchange of lipoproteins between chylomicrons and high density lipoproteins during alimentary lipemia in man. *J. Clin. Invest.* 52:32–38.

Hazzard, W. R., Goldstein, J. L., Schrott, H. G., Motulsky, A. G. and Bierman, E. L. 1973. Hyperlipidemia in coronary heart disease. III. Evaluation of lipoprotein phenotypes of 156 genetically defined survivors of myocardial infarction. *J. Clin. Invest.* 52:1569–1577.

Hedstrand, H. and Vessby, B. 1976. Serum lipoprotein concentration and composition in healthy 50-year-old men. *Upsala J. Med. Sci.* 81:37–48.

Heimberg, M. and Wilcox, H. G. 1972. The effect of palmitic and oleic acids on the properties and composition of the very low density lipoprotein secreted by the liver. *J. Biol. Chem.* 247:875–880.

Ho, Y. K., Brown, M. S., Bilheimer, D. W. and Goldstein, J. L. 1976. Regulation of low density lipoprotein receptor activity in freshly isolated human leukocytes. *J. Clin. Invest.* 58:1465–1474.

Hofmann, A. F. and Borgstrom, B. 1964. The intralumenal phase of fat digestion in man: The lipid content of the micellar and oil phases of intestinal content during fat digestion and absorption. *J. Clin. Invest.* 43:247–257.

Hofmann, A. F. and Mekhjian, H. S. 1973. Bile acids and the intestinal absorption of fat and electrolytes in health and disease. In *The bile acids*, vol. 2. New York: Plenum.

Howard, C. F., Jr. 1975. Diabetes and lipid metabolism in non-human primates. *Adv. Lipid Res.* 13:91–134.

Huttunen, J. D. and Nikkila, E. A. 1973. Postheparin plasma lipase in human subjects. Studies with chylomicrons, very-low density lipoproteins and a fat emulsion. *Eur. J. Clin. Invest.* 3:483–490.

Huttunen, J. K., Ehnholm, C., Nikkila, E. A. and Ohta, M. 1975. Effect of fasting on two postheparin plasma triglyceride lipases and triglyceride removal in obese subjects. *Eur. J. Clin. Invest.* 5:425–445.

Huttunen, J. K., Ehnholm, C., Kekki, M. and Nikkila, E. A. 1976. Postheparin plasma lipoprotein lipase and hepatic lipase in normal subjects and in patients with hypertriglyceridemia. *Clin. Sci. Mol. Med.* 50:249–260.

Jackson, R. L., Morrisett, J. D. and Gotto, A. M., Jr. 1976. Lipoprotein structure and metabolism. *Physiol. Rev.* 56:259–316.

Jaillard, J., Sezille, G., Fruchart, J. C., Dewailly, P. and Romon, M. 1976. Etude de l'activité de la lipoproteine-lipase et de la cellularité au niveau du tissu apideux humain: Influence de l'obésité et du diabète. *Diabete Metab.* 2:5–9.

Jansen, H. and Hülsman, W. C. 1974. Liver and extrahepatic contributions to postheparin serum lipase activity of the rat. *Biochim. Biophys. Acta* 369:387–396.

Jensen, J. 1967. The story of xanthomatosis in England prior to the first World War. *Clio Med.* 2:289–305.

Johansson, B. G. and Medhus, A. 1974. Increase in plasma α-lipoproteins in chronic alcoholics after acute abuse. *Acta Med. Scand.* 195:273–277.

Jones, A. L., Ruderman, N. and Herrera, G. 1967. An electron microscopic and biochemical study of lipoprotein synthesis in the isolated perfused rat liver. *J. Lipid Res.* 8:429–446.

Jones, D. P., Plotkin, G. R. and Arky, R. A. 1966. Lipoprotein lipase activity in patients with diabetes mellitus, with and without hyperlipemia. *Diabetes* 15:565–570.

Kaufmann, R. L., Assal, J. P. H., Soeldner, J. S., Wilmhurst, E. G., Lemaire, J. R., Gleason, R. E. and White, P. 1975. Plasma lipid levels in diabetic children. *Diabetes* 24:672–679.

Khoo, J. C., Steinberg, D., Huang, J. J. and Vagelos, P. R. 1976. Triglyceride, diglyceride, monoglyceride and cholesterol ester hydrolases in chicken adipose tissue activated by adenosine 3':5'-monophosphate-dependent protein kinase. *J. Biol. Chem.* 251:2882–2890.

Kim, H.-J. and Kalkhoff, R. K. 1975. Sex steroid influence on triglyceride metabolism. *J. Clin. Invest.* 56:888–896.

Kompiang, P. I., Bensadoun, A. and Yang, M.-W. W. 1976. Effect of an anti-lipoprotein lipase serum on plasma triglyceride removal. *J. Lipid Res.* 17:498–505.

Korn, E. D. 1955a. Clearing factor, a heparin-activated lipoprotein lipase. I. Isolation and characterization of the enzyme from normal rat heart. *J. Biol. Chem.* 215:1–15.

Korn, E. D. 1955b. Clearing factor, a heparin-activated lipoprotein lipase. II. Substrate specificity and activation of coconut oil. *J. Biol. Chem.* 215:15–26.

Köstner, G. M. 1974. Studies of the composition and structure of human serum lipoproteins. Isolation and partial characterization of apolipoprotein AIII. *Biochim. Biophys. Acta* 336:383–395.

Köstner, G. M., Patsch, J. R., Sailer, S., Braunsteiner, H. and Holasek, A. 1974. Polypeptide distribution of the main lipoprotein density classes separated from human plasma by rate zonal ultracentrifugation. *Eur. J. Biochem.* 45:611–621.

Krauss, R. M., Levy, R. I. and Fredrickson, D. S. 1974. Selective measurement of two lipase activities from normal subjects and patients with hyperlipoproteinemia. *J. Clin. Invest.* 54:1107–1124.

Krotkiewski, M., Bjorntorp, P. and Smith, U. 1976. The effect of long-term dexamethasone treatment on lipoprotein lipase activity in rat fat cells. *Horm. Metab. Res.* 8:245–246.

Kumar, V., Berenson, G. S., Guiz, H., Dalferes, E. R., Jr. and Strong, J. P. 1967. Acid mucopolysaccharides of human aorta. *J. Atheroscler. Res.* 7:573–581.

Kuo, P. T. and Feng, L. Y. 1970. Study of insulin in atherosclerotic patients with endogenous hypertriglyceridemia (types III and IV hyperlipoproteinemia). *Metabolism* 19:372–380.

Kuo, P. T., Feng, L., Cohen, N. N., Fitts, W. T. and Miller, L. D. 1966. Lipogenesis in hepatic tissue; lipogenesis and lipolysis in the adipose tissue of hypertriglyceridemic and atherosclerotic patients. *Trans. Assoc. Amer. Physicians* 79:187–200.

Kyner, J. L., Levy, R. I., Soeldner, J. S., Gleason, R. E. and Fredrickson, D. S. 1976. Lipid, glucose, and insulin interrelationships in normal, prediabetic, and chemical diabetic subjects. *J. Lab. Clin. Med.* 88:345–358.

Langer, T., Strober, W. and Levy, R. I. 1972. The metabolism of low density lipoprotein in familial type II hyperlipoproteinemia. *J. Clin. Invest.* 51:1528–1536.

LaRosa, J. C., Levy, R. I., Herbert, R., Lux, S. E. and Fredrickson, D. S. 1970. A specific apoprotein activator for lipoprotein lipase. *Biochem. Biophys. Res. Commun.* 41:57–62.

LaRosa, J. C., Levy, R. I., Windmueller, H. G. and Fredrickson, D. S. 1972. Comparison of the triglyceride lipase of liver, adipose tissue and postheparin plasma. *J. Lipid Res.* 13:356–363.

Lees, R. S. and Hatch, F. T. 1963. Sharper separation of lipoprotein species by paper electrophoresis in albumin-containing buffer. *J. Lab. Clin. Med.* 61:518–528.

LeMarchand, Y., Singh, A., Assimacopoulos, J., Orci, L., Rouiller, C. and Jeanrenaud, B. 1973. A role for the microtubular system in the release of very low density lipoproteins by perfused mouse livers. *J. Biol. Chem.* 248:6862–6870.

Leren, P. and Haabrekke, O. 1971. Blood lipids in normals. *Acta Med. Scand.* 189:501–504.

Linzell, J. L. and Peaker, M. 1971. Mechanism of milk secretion. *Physiol. Rev.* 51:564–597.

Loten, E. G. and Sneyd, J. G. T. 1970. An effect of insulin on adipose-tissue adenosine-3',5'-cyclic monophosphate phosphodiesterase. *Biochem. J.* 120:187–193.

Luft, R. and Guillemin, R. 1974. Growth hormone and diabetes in man. *Diabetes* 23:783–787.

Man, E. B. and Peters, J. P. 1934. Lipoids of serum in diabetic acidosis. *J. Clin. Invest.* 13:237–261.

Man, E. B. and Peters, J. P. 1935. Serum lipoids in diabetes. *J. Clin. Invest.* 14:579–594.

Marsh, J. B. 1974. Lipoproteins in a noncirculating perfusate of rat liver. *J. Lipid Res.* 15:544–550.

Martin, F. I. R. and Warne, G. L. 1975. Factors influencing the prognosis of vascular disease in insulin-deficient diabetes of long duration: A seven year follow-up. *Metabolism* 24:1–9.

McConathy, W. J. and Alaupovic, P. 1973. Isolation and partial characterization of apolipoprotein D: A new protein moiety of the human plasma lipoprotein system. *FEBS Lett.* 37:178–182.

McGarry, J. C. and Foster, D. W. 1972. Regulation of ketogenesis and clinical aspects of the ketotic state. *Metabolism* 21:471–489.

Meikle, A. W., Klain, G. F. and Hannon, J. P. 1973. Inhibition of glucose oxidation and fatty acid synthesis in liver slices from fed, fasted and fasted-refed rats by glucagon, epinephrine and adenosine-3',5'-monophosphate. *Proc. Soc. Exp. Biol. Med.* 143:379–381.

Miller, H. I., Bortz, W. M. and Durham, B. C. 1968. The rate of appearance of FFA in plasma triglyceride of normal and obese subjects. *Metabolism* 17:515–521.

Mjos, O. D., Faergeman, O., Hamilton, R. L. and Havel, R. J. 1975. Characterization of remnants produced during the metabolism of triglyceride-rich lipoproteins of blood plasma and intestinal lymph in the rat. *J. Clin. Invest.* 56:603–615.

Morley, N. H., Kuksis, A., Buchnea, D. and Myher, J. J. 1975. Hydrolysis of diacylglycerols by lipoprotein lipase. *J. Biol. Chem.* 250:3414–3418.

Moskowitz, M. and Moskowitz, S. 1965. Lipase: Localization in adipose tissue. *Science* 149:72–73.

Motulsky, A. G. 1976. Current concepts in genetics: The genetic hyperlipidemias. *N. Engl. J. Med.* 294:823–827.

Nestel, P. J. 1964. Relationship between plasma triglycerides and the removal of chylomicrons. *J. Clin. Invest.* 43:943–949.

Nestel, P. J. 1967. Relationship between FFA flux and TGFA influx in plasma before and during the infusion of insulin. *Metabolism* 16:1123–1132.

Nestel, P. J. and Austin, W. 1969. Relationship between adipose lipoprotein lipase activity and compounds which affect intracellular lipolysis. *Life Sci.* 8:157–164.

Nestel, P. J. and Whyte, H. M. 1968. Plasma free fatty acid and triglyceride turnover in obesity. *Metabolism* 17:1122–1128.

Nikkila, E. A. 1969. Control of plasma and liver triglyceride kinetics by carbohydrate metabolism and insulin. *Adv. Lipid Res.* 4:63–134.

Nikkila, E. A. 1973. Triglyceride metabolism in diabetes mellitus. *Prog. Biochem. Pharmacol.* 8:271–299.

Nikkila, E. A. and Kekki, M. 1971. Measurement of plasma triglyceride turnover in the study of hyperglyceridemia. *Scand. J. Lab. Invest.* 27:97–104.

Nikkila, E. A. and Kekki, M. 1973. Plasma triglyceride transport kinetics in diabetes mellitus. *Metabolism* 22:1–22.

Nikkila, E. A. and Pelkonen, R. 1975. Serum lipids in acromegaly. *Metabolism* 24:829–838.

Nikkilä, E. A. and Pykälistö, O. 1968a. Induction of adipose tissue lipoprotein lipase by nicotinic acid. *Biochim. Biophys. Acta* 152:421–425.

Nikkilä, E. A. and Pykälistö, O. 1968b. Regulation of adipose tissue lipoprotein lipase synthesis by intracellular free fatty acid. *Life Sci.* 7:1303–1309.

Nilsson-Ehle, P. and Belfrage, P. 1972. A monoglyceride hydrolyzing enzyme in human postheparin plasma. *Biochim. Biophys. Acta* 270:60–64.

Nilsson-Ehle, P., Egelrud, T., Belfrage, P., Olivecrona, T. and Borgstrom, B. 1973. Positional specificity of purified milk lipoprotein lipase. *J. Biol. Chem.* 248:6734–6737.

Noel, S. P. and Rubinstein, D. 1974. Secretion of apolipoproteins in very low density and high density lipoproteins by perfused rat liver. *J. Lipid Res.* 15:301–308.

Noel, S. P., Dolphin, P. J. and Rubinstein, D. 1975. An in vitro model for the catabolism of rat chylomicrons. *Biochem. Biophys. Res. Commun.* 63:764–772.

Ockner, R. K. and Jones, A. L. 1970. An electron microscopic and functional study of very low density lipoproteins in intestinal lymph. *J. Lipid Res.* 11:284–292.

Ockner, R. K., Manning, J. M., Poppenhausen, R. B. and Ho, W. K. L. 1972. A binding protein for fatty acids in cytosol of intestinal mucosa, liver, myocardium, and other tissues. *Science* 177:56–58.

O'Connor, T. P. and Schnatz, J. D. 1968. Lipoprotein lipase activity and hypertriglyceridemia in alloxan diabetic rabbits. *Metabolism* 17:838–844.

Olivecrona, T., Bengtsson, G., Höök, M. and Lindahl, U. 1976. Physiologic implications of the interaction between lipoprotein lipase and some sulfated glycosaminoglycans. In *Lipoprotein metabolism*, ed. H. Greten, pp. 13–19. New York: Springer-Verlag.

Ostrander, L. D., Lamphiear, D. E., Block, W. D., Johnson, B. C. and Epstein, F. H. 1974. Biochemical precursors of atherosclerosis. Studies in apparently healthy men in a general population, Tecumseh, Mich. *Arch. Intern. Med.* 134:224–230.

Otway, S. and Robinson, D. S. 1968. The significance of changes in tissue clearing-factor lipase activity in relation to the lipaemia of pregnancy. *Biochem. J.* 106:677–682.

Patten, R. L. 1970. The reciprocal regulation of lipoprotein lipase activity and hormone-sensitive lipase activity in rat adipocytes. *J. Biol. Chem.* 245:5577–5584.

Persson, B. 1972. Lipoprotein lipase in human adipose tissue. Thesis, Goteborg.

Persson, B. 1973. Lipoprotein lipase activity of human adipose tissue in health and in some diseases with hyperlipidemia as a common feature. *Acta Med. Scand.* 193:457–462.

Phair, R. D., Hammond, M. G., Bowden, J. A., Fried, M., Berman, M. and Fisher, W. R. 1972. Kinetic studies of human lipoprotein metabolism in type IV hyperlipoproteinemia. *Fed. Proc.* 31:421.

Pottenger, L. A., Frazier, L. E., DuBien, L. H., Getz, G. A. and Wissler, R. W. 1973. Carbohydrate composition on lipoprotein apoproteins isolated from rat plasma and from the livers of rats fed orotic acid. *Biochim. Biophys. Res. Commun.* 54:770–776.

Pozza, G., Pappalettera, A., Melogli, O., Viberti, G. and Ghidoni, A. 1971. Lipolytic effects of intraarterial injection of glucagon in man. *Horm. Metab. Res.* 3:291–292.

Pykälistö, O. 1970. Regulation of the adipose tissue lipoprotein lipase by free fatty acids. Dissertation, University of Helsinki.

Pykälistö, O. J., Smith, P. H., Bierman, E. L. and Brunzell, J. H. 1975a. Decreased adipose tissue lipoprotein lipase in untreated diabetic man. *Diabetes* 23:348.

Pykälistö, O. J., Smith, P. H. and Brunzell, J. D. 1975b. Determinants of human adipose tissue lipoprotein lipase. Effect of diabetes and obesity on basal- and diet-induced activity. *J. Clin. Invest.* 56:1108–1117.

Pykälistö, O. J., Smith, P. H. and Brunzell, J. D. 1975c. Human adipose tissue lipoprotein lipase: Comparison of assay methods and expressions of activity. *Proc. Soc. Exp. Biol. Med.* 148:297–300.

Pykälistö, O., Goldberg, A. P. and Brunzell, J. D. 1976. Reversal of decreased human adipose tissue lipoprotein lipase and hypertriglyceridemia after treatment of hypothyroidism. *J. Clin. Endocrinol. Metab.* 43:591–600.

Quarfordt, S. H., Frank, A., Shames, D. M., Berman, M. and Steinberg, D. 1970. Very low density lipoprotein transport in type IV hyperlipoproteinemia and the effects of carbohydrate-rich diets. *J. Clin. Invest.* 49:2281–2297.

Rachmilewitz, D., Stein, O., Roheim, P. S. and Stein, Y. 1972. Metabolism of iodinated high density lipoproteins in the rat. II. Autoradiographic localization in the liver. *Biochim. Biophys. Acta* 270:414–425.

Rachmilewitz, D., Albers, J. J. and Saunders, D. R. 1976. Apoprotein B in fasting and postprandial human jejunal mucosa. *J. Clin. Invest.* 57:530–533.

Randle, P. J. 1966. Carbohydrate metabolism and lipid storage and breakdown in diabetes. *Diabetologia* 2:237–247.

Rao, G. A. and Johnston, J. M. 1966. Purification and properties of triglyceride synthetase from the intestinal mucosa. *Biochim. Biophys. Acta* 125:465–473.

Reaven, G. M., Lerner, R. L., Stern, M. P. and Farquhar, J. W. 1967. Role of insulin in endogenous hypertriglyceridemia. *J. Clin. Invest.* 46:1756–1767.

Rhoads, G. G., Gulbrandsen, C. L. and Kagan, A. 1976. Serum lipoproteins and coronary heart disease. *N. Engl. J. Med.* 294:293–305.

Robinson, D. S. 1970. The function of the plasma triglycerides in fatty acid transport. *Compr. Biochem.* 18:51–116.

Rodger, N. W. and Du, E. L. 1973. Some factors indicative of hypertriglyceridemia in patients investigated for diabetes mellitus. *Can. Med. Assoc. J.* 109:363–368.

Roheim. P. S., Rachmilewitz, D., Stein, O. and Stein, Y. 1971. Metabolism of iodinated high density lipoproteins in the rat. I. Half-life in the circulation and uptake by organs. *Biochim. Biophys. Acta* 248:315–329.

Sabesin, S. M. and Isselbacher, K. J. 1965. Protein synthesis inhibition: Mechanism for the production of impaired fat absorption. *Science* 147:1149–1151.

Santen, R. J., Willis, P. W. and Fajans, S. S. 1972. Atherosclerosis in diabetes mellitus. Correlations with serum lipid levels, adiposity and serum insulin level. *Arch. Intern. Med.* 130:833–843.

Schade, D. S. and Eaton, R. P. 1975. Modulation of fatty acid metabolism by glucagon in man. *Diabetes* 24:502–509.

Schnatz, J. D. and O'Connor, T. P. 1967. Studies on lipemia of diabetic acidosis. *Diabetes* 16:534A.

Schonfeld, G., Birge, E., Miller, J. P., Kessler, G. and Santiago, J. 1974. Apolipoprotein B levels and altered lipoprotein composition in diabetes. *Diabetes* 23:825–834.

Schotz, M. C. and Garfinkel, A. S. 1965. The effect of puromycin and actinomycin on carbohydrate-induced lipase activity in rat adipose tissue. *Biochim. Biophys. Acta* 106:202–205.

Schotz, M. C. and Garfinkel, A. S. 1972. Effect of nutrition on species of lipoprotein lipase. *Biochim. Biophys. Acta* 270:472–478.

Schotz, M. C., Stewart, J. E., Garfinkel, A. S., Whelan, C. F. and Baker, N. 1969. Isolated fat cells: Morphology and possible role of released lipoprotein lipase in disposition of lipoprotein fatty acid. In *Drugs affecting lipid metabolism*, ed. W. L. Holmes, pp. 161–183. New York: Plenum.

Schreibman, P. H., Arons, D. L., Saudek, C. D. and Arky, R. A. 1973. Abnormal lipoprotein lipase in familial exogenous hypertriglyceridemia. *J. Clin. Invest.* 52:2075–2082.

Scow, R. O., Blanchette-Mackie, E. J. and Smith, L. C. 1976. Role of capillary endothelium in the clearance of chylomicrons. A model for lipid transport from blood by lateral diffusion in cell membranes. *Circ. Res.* 39:149–162.

Shafrir, E. and Biale, Y. 1970. Effect of experimental hypertriglyceridemia on tissue and serum lipoprotein lipase activity. *Eur. J. Clin. Invest.* 1:19–24.

Sherrill, B. C. and Dietschy, J. M. 1976. Uptake of lipoproteins of intestinal origin in the isolated perfused liver. *Circulation* 53(suppl. 2):91a.

Shoemaker, W. C., Carruthers, P. J., Elwyn, D. H. and Ashmore, J. 1962. Effect of insulin on fatty acid transport and regional metabolism. *Am. J. Physiol.* 203:919–925.

Siperstein, M. D. 1975. The glucose tolerance test: A pitfall in the diagnosis of diabetes mellitus. *Adv. Intern. Med.* 20:297–323.

Spitzer, J. J. 1953. Influence of protamine on alimentary lipemia. *Am. J. Physiol.* 174:43–45.

Stein, O. and Stein, Y. 1967. Lipid synthesis, intracellular transport, storage, and secretion. I. Electron microscopic radioautographic study of liver after injection of tritiated palmitate or glycerol in fasted and ethanol-treated rats. *J. Cell. Biol.* 33:319–339.

Stein, O. and Stein, Y. 1973. Colchicine-induced inhibition of very low density lopoprotein release by rat liver *in vivo*. *Biochim. Biophys. Acta* 306:142–147.

Stein, O., Scow, R. O. and Stein, Y. 1970. FFA-³H uptake by perfused adipose tissue: Electron microscopic autoradiographic study. *Am. J. Physiol.* 219:510–518.

Steinberg, D. 1966. Catecholamine stimulation of fat mobilization and its metabolic consequences. *Pharmacol. Rev.* 18:217–235.

Steiner, G. 1968. Lipoprotein lipase in fat-induced hyperlipemia. *N. Engl. J. Med.* 279:70–74.

Stern, M. P., Olefsky, J., Farquhar, J. W. and Reaven, G. M. 1973. Relationship between fasting plasma lipid levels and adipose tissue morphology. *Metabolism* 22:1311–1317.

Stewart, J. E. and Schotz, M. C. 1971. Studies on release of lipoprotein lipase activity from fat cells. *J. Biol. Chem.* 246:5749–5753.

Stewart, J. E. and Schotz, M. C. 1974. Release of lipoprotein lipase from isolated fat cells. II. Effect of heparin. *J. Biol. Chem.* 249:904–907.

Stewart, J. E., Whelan, C. F. and Schotz, M. C. 1969. Release of lipoprotein lipase from fat cells. *Biochem. Biophys. Res. Commun.* 34:376–381.

Thannhauser, S. J. 1947. Serum lipids and their value in diagnosis. *N. Engl. J. Med.* 237:515–521, 546–551.

Thannhauser, S. J. 1950. *Lipoidosis.* New York: Oxford.

Thannhauser, S. J. 1958. *Lipoidoses: Disease of the intracellular lipid metabolism,* 3rd ed. New York: Grune & Stratton.

Thannhauser, S. J. and Magendantz, H. 1938. The different clinical groups of xanthomatous diseases: A clinical physiological study of 22 cases. *Ann. Intern. Med.* 11:1662–1746.

Topping, D. L. and Mayes, P. A. 1972. The immediate effects of insulin and fructose on the metabolism of the perfused liver. Changes in lipoprotein secretion, fatty acid oxidation and esterification, lipogenesis and carbohydrate metabolism. *Biochem. J.* 126:295–311.

Twu, J.-S., Garfinkel, A. S. and Schotz, M. C. 1976. Purification and characterization of lipoprotein lipase from human heart. *Atherosclerosis* 24:119–128.

Vaughan, M. and Steinberg, D. 1963. Effect of hormones on lipolysis and esterification of free fatty acids during incubation of adipose tissue in vitro. *J. Lipid Res.* 4:193–199.

Volpe, J. J. and Vagelos, P. R. 1974. Regulation of mammalian fatty-acid synthetase. The role of carbohydrate and insulin. *Proc. Natl. Acad. Sci. U.S.A.* 71:889–893.

Wille, L. E. and Aarseth, S. 1973. Demonstration of hyper-α-lipoproteinemia in three diabetic patients. *Clin. Genet.* 4:281–285.

Wilson, D. E., Schreibman, P. H. and Arky, R. A. 1969. Post-heparin lipolytic activity in diabetic patients with a history of mixed hyperlipemia. *Diabetes* 18:562–566.

Wilson, D. E., Schreibman, P. H., Day, V. C. and Arky, R. A. 1970. Hyperlipidemia in an adult diabetic population. *J. Chronic Dis.* 23:501–506.

Wilson, D. E., Flowers, C. M., Carlile, S. I. and Udall, K. S. 1976. Estrogen treatment and gonadal function in the regulation of lipoprotein lipase. *Atherosclerosis* 24:491–499.

Wilson, F. A. and Dietschy, J. M. 1972. Characterization of bile acid absorption across the unstirred water layer and brush border of the rat jejunum. *J. Clin. Invest.* 51:3015–3025.

Windmueller, H. G. and Spaeth, A. E. 1972. Fat transport and lymph and plasma lipoprotein biosynthesis by isolated intestine. *J. Lipid Res.* 13:92–105.

Windmueller, H. G., Herbert, P. N. and Levy, R. I. 1973. Biosynthesis of lymph and plasma lipoprotein apoproteins by isolated perfused rat liver and intestine. *J. Lipid Res.* 14:215–223.

Wing, D. R. and Robinson, D. S. 1968a. Clearing-factor lipase in adipose tissue. Studies with puromycin and actinomycin. *Biochem. J.* 106:667–676.

Wing, D. R. and Robinson, D. S. 1968b. Clearing-factor lipase in adipose tissue. A possible role of adenosine 3′,5′-(cyclic)-monophosphate in the regulation of its activity. *Biochem. J.* 109:841–849.

Wing, D. R., Fielding, C. J. and Robinson, D. S. 1967. The effect of cyclohexamide on tissue clearing-factor lipase acitivity. *Biochem. J.* 104:45C.

Wood, P. S., Stern, M. P., Silvers, A., Reaven, G. M. and von der Groben, J. 1972. Prevalence of plasma lipoprotein abnormalities in a free-living population at Central Valley, California. *Circulation* 45:114–126.

Zinder, O., Hamosh, M., Fleck, T. R. C. and Scow, R. O. 1974. Effect of prolactin on lipoprotein lipase in mammary gland and adipose tissue of rats. *Am. J. Physiol.* 226:744–748.

Chapter 5

INTERRELATION OF ATHEROSCLEROSIS, ABNORMAL LIPID METABOLISM, AND DIABETES MELLITUS

Edwin L. Bierman and John D. Brunzell

Department of Medicine
Division of Metabolism, Endocrinology, and Gerontology
University of Washington School of Medicine
Seattle, Washington

INTRODUCTION

Atherosclerosis is the leading cause of death in diabetes; coronary artery disease alone accounts for more than half of all diabetic mortality. This represents a remarkable change in the half-century since insulin became available for treatment (Marks and Krall, 1971) (Fig. 1). Although the average life span of diabetics has been greatly increased, they still have a shorter life expectancy (Marks and Krall, 1971) (Fig. 2) and an increased risk of death from coronary artery disease, particularly at younger ages (Garcia et al., 1974; H. H. Marks, unpublished data), when compared to the general population (Fig. 3).

Although accelerated atherosclerosis in diabetes does not differ in either distribution among the large vessels or morphological appearance (Strandness et al., 1964), postmortem studies indicate that diabetics have a greater extent of coronary and aortic atherosclerotic lesions than sex- and age-matched nondiabetics in every country surveyed, whether affected by very high or very low prevalence of coronary artery disease (Robertson and Strong, 1968) (Fig. 4). Clinical studies have also indicated a marked predisposition to atherosclerosis of the coronary and lower extremity arteries (Garcia et al., 1974; Strandness et al., 1964).

Research studies by the authors reported in this chapter were supported by grants AM 06670, HL 18257, AG 00299, and FR-37 from the National Institutes of Health, U.S. Public Health Service. The authors are indebted to Ms. Sharon Kemp for her skillful assistance in the preparation of this manuscript.

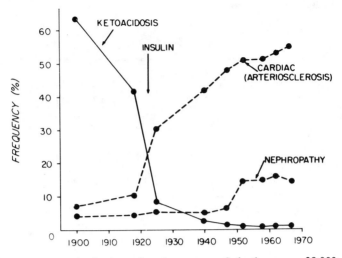

FIGURE 1 Distribution of major causes of death among 28,000 deceased diabetics between 1897 and 1968. Experience of the Joslin Clinic (adapted from Marks and Krall, 1971).

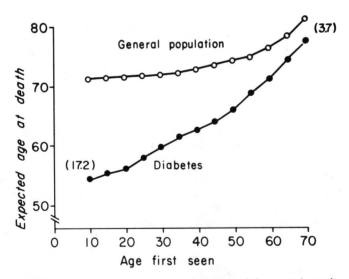

FIGURE 2 Life expectancy among diabetics and the general population (whites) at different ages. Analysis of Joslin Clinic experience (1947–1951 for diabetic patients first observed during 1930–1951) and of the general population of the United States (1949–1951) (adapted from Marks and Krall, 1971).

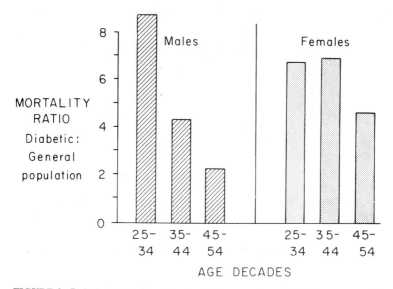

FIGURE 3 Relative mortality from heart disease among diabetics compared to the general population. Experience of the Joslin Clinic with patients of 1950-1958 traced to 1961, attained ages 25-54. The comparison is on the basis of mortality among whites in New England, 1949-1951 (H. H. Marks, unpublished data).

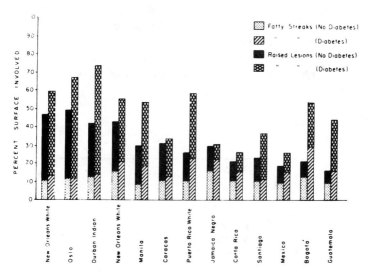

FIGURE 4 Mean extent of atherosclerotic lesions of coronary arteries in men, aged 45-54, by presence (right bar) or absence (left bar) of diabetes mellitus and by location and race group. From a report of the results of the International Atherosclerosis Project (Robertson and Strong, 1968).

189

Why should atherosclerosis be accelerated and more severe in diabetes? If one examines the known risk factors identified for atherosclerosis in large population studies, it can be seen that virtually all of them are intensified in diabetes (Table 1).

RISK FACTORS FOR ATHEROSCLEROSIS IN DIABETICS

Hyperglycemia

Hyperglycemia appears to be an independent risk factor for atherosclerosis. In population surveys, such as the Tecumseh study (Ostrander et al., 1965, 1973), the prevalence of elevated blood glucose levels (1 hr after oral glucose) was significantly higher for subjects with vascular disease than for those without it (Table 2). Preliminary results for the incidence of ischemic heart disease in a subset of hyperglycemic subjects in Tecumseh (Epstein, 1967a) confirm the conclusions drawn from the prevalence study. In the Bedford study (Keen et al., 1965; Keen and Jarrett, 1973), both the prevalence and the incidence of vascular disease were also related to the initial blood glucose levels. In unselected 3 month survivors of myocardial infarction in a total community (Seattle), a high prevalence of diabetes was found (Goldstein et al., 1973b). These studies in a variety of populations confirm an association of hyperglycemia with clinically evident atherosclerotic disease.

Diabetics, by definition, have higher blood glucose levels than those in the general population. However, the risk for atherosclerotic disease does not appear to be grossly related to the severity of hyperglycemia (Stearns et al., 1947; Liebow et al., 1955; Downie and Martin, 1959). Conversely, results in the UGDP study have suggested that reduction of blood glucose does not appear to influence mortality from atherosclerosis, once established (University Group Diabetes Program, 1970). Thus hyperglycemia and atherosclerosis

TABLE 1   Risk Factors for Atherosclerosis
in Diabetes

Risk factor	General population	Diabetics
Hyperglycemia	+	+++
Hypertriglyceridemia	++	+++
Hypercholesterolemia	++	+++
Hypertension	++	+++
Hyperinsulinemia	+	++
Obesity	+	+++
Dietary fat and cholesterol	+	++
"Diabetes"	——	+++
Cigarette smoking	+++	+++

TABLE 2   Prevalence of Hyperglycemia
among Persons with Vascular Disease
in Tecumseh, Michigan

	Observed/expected	
	Male	Female
Coronary heart disease	1.67	1.82
Peripheral and cerebral vascular disease	1.49	1.90
T-wave changes	1.77	1.92

are associated: there is an increased prevalence and incidence of large vessel disease in known diabetics and, conversely, there is an increased prevalence of hyperglycemia in association with clinically apparent atherosclerosis.

Hyperlipidemia

Diabetes mellitus is often associated with an excessive accumulation of one or more major lipids transported in plasma. For clinical purposes, this hyperlipidemia manifests as hypertriglyceridemia, hypercholesterolemia, or both. Thus, levels of lipid-carrying molecular aggregates, the lipoproteins, are elevated (hyperlipoproteinemia). Although the lipoproteins are a continuum of size and composition, they have been divided into triglyceride-rich, very low density (pre-beta) lipoproteins and cholesterol-rich, low-density (beta) lipoproteins. In addition, chylomicrons, the largest and most triglyceride-rich of the lipoproteins, enter the circulation from the gut and may accumulate in plasma in some diabetics, causing turbidity or lactescence of the plasma.

Elevations of triglyceride and cholesterol levels are independently related to atherosclerotic vascular disease in the population as a whole (Keen and Jarrett, 1973; Carlson and Bottiger, 1972). However, high plasma triglycerides appear to be more common than hypercholesterolemia in middle-aged diabetics with vascular disease (New et al., 1963). In a recent study, it was confirmed that hypertriglyceridemia was much commoner than hypercholesterolemia in diabetics with atherosclerosis; diabetics without atherosclerosis had triglyceride levels that were indistinguishable from those in nondiabetic subjects (Santen et al., 1972) (Fig. 5). In the Framingham study (Garcia et al., 1974) serum cholesterol levels were no higher in diabetic men but were slightly higher in diabetic women than in the total study group. The high incidence of cardiovascular disease in diabetics could not be explained by changes in cholesterol levels. In Tecumseh (Ostrander et al., 1967), a group of subjects who had both cardiovascular disease and hyperglycemia initially had significantly higher triglyceride levels than subjects with only one, or neither, of these abnormalities, while serum cholesterol was similar in all groups.

Thus abnormalities in serum lipids appear to be related to athero-

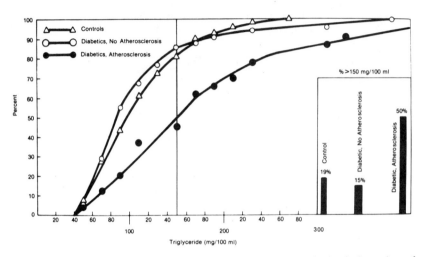

FIGURE 5 Frequency distribution curves of plasma triglyceride levels in male and female diabetics with and without atherosclerosis and in control subjects, all aged 30–59. The insert depicts the proportion of subjects with triglyceride levels above 150 mg/dl (Santen et al., 1972).

sclerotic vascular complications in diabetics in a fashion analogous to their relationship in nondiabetics, but abnormalities in neither triglyceride nor cholesterol regulation alone can adequately explain the increased frequency of atherosclerosis in diabetes (see Fig. 3).

Hypercholesterolemia. Increased plasma cholesterol levels occur in some diabetic patients. This increase either reflects an elevation of low-density lipoproteins (LDL) with normal levels of very low density lipoproteins (VLDL), or, more commonly, is associated with marked elevations in levels of triglyceride-rich very low density lipoproteins, which also contain cholesterol. Familial hypercholesterolemia, as either the monogenic or the polygenic disorder, does not appear to be more frequent in diabetics than in the general population (Fredrickson and Levy, 1972). Hypercholesterolemia, possibly due to secondary abnormalities, has been reported in certain groups of diabetic patients.

Young patients with diabetes have been found to have elevated plasma cholesterol without concomitant hypertriglyceridemia (New et al., 1963), such that hypercholesterolemia has been found to occur more commonly in insulin-treated patients than in those treated by oral sulfonylureas (Pell and D'Alonzo, 1970; Schonfeld et al., 1974). Recently, Kaufmann et al. (1975) suggested that the hypercholesterolemia in the young, insulin-dependent diabetic may be related in part to the diabetic diet used in the past (carbohydrate restriction and a reciprocal increase in fat content). They were able to decrease cholesterol levels in insulin-dependent diabetic children to or below levels found in normal children of the same age by increasing the carbohydrate content and lowering the increased cholesterol and saturated fat content of the diet. These insulin-treated groups of subjects are the ones most likely to live long enough with diabetes to develop renal disease with the nephrotic syndrome. The role of the hypercholesterolemia of the nephrotic syndrome in the increased prevalence of hypercholesterolemia in insulin-treated diabetics has yet to be determined.

Hypertriglyceridemia. The reported prevalence of hypertriglyceridemia in diabetic populations is variable. About 30% of patients followed in diabetes clinics have elevated plasma triglyceride levels (Albrink et al., 1963; Belknap et al., 1967; Wilson et al., 1970; Bergqvist, 1970). Untreated fasting hyperglycemia is frequently associated with hypertriglyceridemia, and plasma triglyceride levels are restored to or toward normal with therapy aimed at reduction of the elevated glucose levels (Thannhauser, 1958; Bagdade et al., 1967b; Brunzell et al., 1975b). Glucose intolerance with normal fasting glucose levels is also a frequent concomitant of hypertriglyceridemia (Glueck et al., 1969). It has been suggested that obesity plays a part both in the increase triglyceride levels and in the glucose intolerance seen in obese, adult-onset mildly diabetic patients (Bierman and Porte, 1968), since weight reduction leads to reversal of both glucose intolerance and hypertriglyceridemia (Olefsky et al., 1974; Bierman and Porte, 1968).

The mechanism of hypertriglyceridemia in untreated overt diabetics could be either a defect in the removal of the VLDL and chylomicrons or an increase in splanchnic production of triglyceride-rich VLDL. The pathogenic mechanism appears to depend on the severity of the insulin deficiency and the presence and type of associated diabetic complications.

Untreated Moderate Fasting Hyperglycemia. Patients with moderate uncontrolled fasting hyperglycemia have a deficiency in adipose tissue lipoprotein lipase (Pykalisto et al., 1975) (Fig. 6), the enzyme responsible for the major portion of plasma triglyceride removal as a result of lipolysis of triglyceride contained in triglyceride-rich lipoproteins (Robinson, 1970). This defect can also be demonstrated as an abnormality in postheparin lipolytic activity (PHLA) during a high-dose heparin infusion (Brunzell et al., 1975) (Fig. 7). During the early phase of the heparin infusion, total PHLA as well as the subcomponents of PHLA (extrahepatic lipoprotein lipase and hepatic triglyceride lipase (Nikkila et al., 1975)) are normal in patients with moderate fasting hyperglycemia. During the later phase of the heparin infusion a defect in total PHLA is found which is an inverse function of the degree of hyperglycemia. Whether this decrease in the later phase of PHLA is specifically due to a decrease in postheparin plasma lipoprotein lipase or hepatic lipase is not known. However, the level of PHLA in this phase of the heparin infusion is an index of the activity of lipoprotein lipase in the adipose tissue (Fig. 8). Support for a functional role for this defect in lipoprotein lipase is obtained from observations that lipoprotein lipase-related plasma triglyceride removal is reduced concomitantly (Brunzell et al., 1972). Diabetics of this

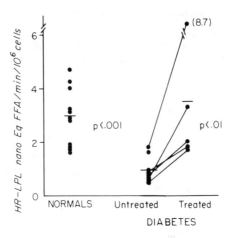

FIGURE 6 Adipose tissue lipoprotein lipase activity (heparin releasable fraction; HR-LPL) in normal subjects and diabetics before and after treatment for uncontrolled symptomatic hyperglycemia (data from Pykalisto et al., 1975).

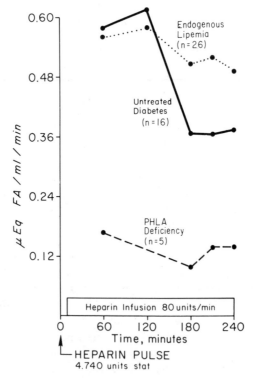

FIGURE 7 Postheparin lipolytic activity during high-dose heparin infusion in subjects with hypertriglyceridemia associated with primary endogenous lipemia, untreated diabetes, and PHLA deficiency.

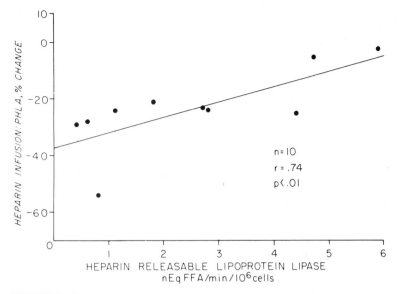

FIGURE 8 Correlation between the decrease in late-phase release of PHLA during high-dose heparin infusion and adipose tissue lipoprotein lipase (heparin-releasable fraction) (unpublished data).

type show impaired plasma triglyceride removal estimated by other methods as well (Lewis et al., 1972; Kissebah et al., 1974).

With several months of insulin or oral sulfonylurea therapy, the defect in plasma PHLA and adipose tissue lipoprotein lipase corrects to normal with a concomitant decrease in plasma triglyceride levels to or toward normal. The reason for the 2-month delay in complete correction of this abnormality is unknown.

Untreated Severe Hyperglycemia. With more severe degrees of hyperglycemia (Bagdade et al., 1967b), with or without ketoacidosis, and after insulin withdrawal in insulin-dependent diabetics (Bagdade et al., 1968), a defect in the early release of plasma PHLA is also found. The low level of PHLA released during a heparin infusion in insulin-deprived diabetics is similar to that seen in patients with genetically determined absence of adipose tissue lipoprotein lipase (Brunzell et al., 1975b) (Fig. 9). The abnormality in these diabetics appears to specifically affect plasma postheparin lipoprotein lipase, while postheparin hepatic triglyceride lipase is normal (Nikkila et al., 1975).

With insulin treatment there is a rapid increase in the early phase of PHLA but no increase in the late phase of PHLA, so that soon after treatment these patients will have a defect similar to that seen in the moderately hyperglycemic diabetic patients described above (Brunzell et al., 1975b) (Fig. 9). Again, this late-phase defect in PHLA will correct after several months of insulin therapy.

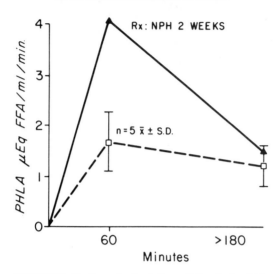

FIGURE 9 Postheparin lipolytic activity during high-dose heparin infusion in subjects with severe hyperglycemia before (dashed line) and after treatment with NPH insulin for 2 wk (unpublished data).

Degree of Hypertriglyceridemia. Plasma triglycerides in patients with untreated fasting hyperglycemia range from high normal to markedly increased levels associated with milky (lipemic) plasma. Several months of insulin or oral sulfonylurea therapy result in a decrease in plasma triglyceride levels. Diabetics who have mild to moderate hypertriglyceridemia (less than 1,000 mg/dl) almost always have normal triglyceride levels following treatment (Brunzell et al., 1975a). Those who have lipemic plasma (triglyceride over 2,000 mg/dl) almost always remain moderately hypertriglyceridemic after antihyperglycemic therapy. This group of subjects includes diabetics with severe chylomicronemia during the untreated hyperglycemic state (and shortly after insulin therapy) who are predisposed to develop eruptive xanthomata (xanthomata diabeticorum) (Parker et al., 1970), lipemia retinalis, and abdominal pain or pancreatitis (Brunzell and Schrott, 1973) (the "diabetic lipemia" syndrome) (Bagdade et al., 1967b).

When the families of untreated diabetic patients who exhibit the wide variation in magnitude of hypertriglyceridemia are examined, diabetics with severe hypertriglyceridemia are found to have nondiabetic hypertriglyceridemic relatives, while diabetics with mild hypertriglyceridemia that corrects to normal with insulin therapy come from families with normal triglyceride levels (Brunzell et al., 1975a) (Fig. 10). Thus, the marked hypertriglyceridemia seen in some diabetics appears to be due to the simultaneous occurrence of (1) a decrease in adipose tissue lipoprotein lipase due to insulin deficiency and (2) a familial form of hypertriglyceridemia. It has been suggested that the familial

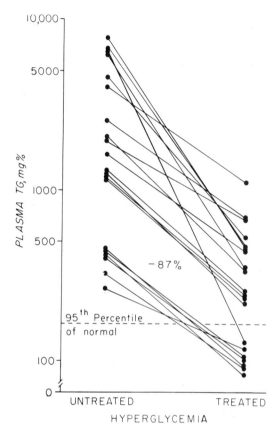

FIGURE 10 Fasting plasma triglyceride (TG) levels in untreated diabetics with hypertriglyceridemia before and after treatment (unpublished data).

forms of hypertriglyceridemia and overt diabetes are inherited together (Glueck et al., 1969; Fredrickson and Levy, 1972). However, recent studies have demonstrated that these two diseases segregate, or are inherited independently (Brunzell et al., 1975a), and suggest that their simultaneous occurrence is by chance only, but leads to preferential selection for study.

Hypertriglyceridemia in the Treated Diabetic. If plasma triglyceride levels are measured in a patient shortly after insulin therapy is begun or shortly after a bout of ketoacidosis, hypertriglyceridemia may be found, resulting from the abnormality in lipoprotein lipase not yet completely corrected.

If the prevalence of the familial forms of hypertriglyceridemia is about 3% in the general population (Goldstein et al., 1973a), one would expect to see about the same prevalence of this independent disorder in the diabetic population. It has been suggested that some of the hypertriglyceridemic individuals in a population of subjects selected for hypertriglyceridemia who also have diabetes show increased splanchnic triglyceride-rich VLDL production (Nikkila and Kekki, 1973). However, neither the presence of an independent familial form of hypertriglyceridemia nor short duration of antihyperglycemic therapy in these studies was excluded. In animals made acutely diabetic, a transient increase in splanchnic triglyceride production occurs (Balasse et al., 1972; Reaven and Reaven, 1974; Woodside and Heimberg, 1976), presumably due to increased free fatty acid mobilization and conversion to triglyceride by an insulinized liver (Topping and Mayes, 1972). This increased free fatty acid esterification disappears within a short period of time (Basso and Havel, 1970; Reaven and Reaven, 1974; Woodside and Heimberg, 1976), while there is continuing hypertriglyceridemia, which suggests a removal defect.

Finally, diabetic patients, including those with normal fasting glucose levels and glucose intolerance after an oral glucose load, have an increased prevalence of obesity, chronic renal failure, and nephrotic syndrome, each associated with hypertriglyceridemia. Obesity and other forms of insulin resistance associated with glucose intolerance could, through compensatory hyperinsulinism, mediate increased triglyceride-rich VLDL production by the liver (Topping and Mayes, 1972; Woodside and Heimberg, 1976). Chronic renal failure, associated with abnormalities in lipoprotein lipase and triglyceride removal (Goldberg et al., 1975), accounts for some of the hypertrigly-ceridemia seen in treated diabetics. And the nephrotic syndrome, common in diabetes, is associated with an increase in plasma triglyceride, as well as in plasma cholesterol levels, independent of the presence or absence of renal failure.

Hypertension

Hypertension has been shown to be an important risk factor for death from atherosclerotic cardiovascular disease (National Heart and Lung Institute, 1971). The risk progressively increases with increasing blood pressure, and mortality is diminished by therapeutic reduction of blood pressure (Veterans Administration Co-operative Study Group, 1967, 1970).

There is a widespread clinical impression that arterial pressure tends to be higher in diabetics than nondiabetics. Apart from the diabetics with renal disease, there is indeed evidence linking diabetes with hypertension. A large autopsy study (Goldenberg et al., 1958) showed that hypertension, diagnosed as cardiac enlargement without valvular disease, was twice as common in diabetics than nondiabetics, and a survey of nonhospitalized subjects (Pell and D'Alonzo, 1967) found that hypertension was 54% more common in diabetics than nondiabetics matched for age, sex, and social class. In the large population study in Tecumseh (Ostrander et al., 1965), it was found that hypertension was more common than expected in diabetic women, but had a

TABLE 3   Prevalence of Hypertension
among Diabetics (Tecumseh Study)

| Age | Diastolic hypertension, observed/expected | |
	Male	Female
20–39	1.7	3.3
40–59	0.7	2.5
60+	1.2	1.2
Total	1.0	1.8

variably increased frequency in diabetic men (Table 3). Conversely, hypergly-cemia was more common in subjects with hypertension than in the population as a whole (Ostrander et al., 1965). Of interest in this regard, the risk of hyperglycemia for cardiovascular disease was independent of its association with hypertension and was at least as important as hypertension (Epstein, 1967b). Similar conclusions were drawn from the population study in Bedford, England (Keen et al., 1965). In the Framingham study (Garcia et al., 1974), blood pressure was significantly higher in diabetics than in the study population as a whole, but the high incidence of cardiovascular disease in diabetics could not be entirely explained by this one risk factor.

Thus hypertension appears to be slightly more common in diabetics than in the general population. Age, sex, obesity, renal disease, and duration of diabetes may influence the association of diabetes and hypertension. The coexisting presence of hypertension will increase the risk of atherosclerosis, but since many atherosclerotic diabetics are normotensive, excess hypertension alone cannot account for the increased atherosclerosis in diabetics.

Obesity

In general, morbidity and mortality from atherosclerotic heart disease are higher in direct relation to the degree of overweight (Kannel et al., 1967b) (Fig. 11). Despite this some of the major epidemiological studies of coronary heart disease have not demonstrated an *independent* relationship between this condition and anything less than gross obesity (Keys et al., 1972). However, obesity is a disorder closely associated with other potent risk factors such as hypertriglyceridemia (Bagdade et al., 1971), hypercholesterolemia (Montoye et al., 1966), and hypertension (Kannel et al., 1967a). The relationship between obesity and atherosclerosis is thus multifaceted, and since in practice obesity does not occur "independently," it must be considered a risk factor.

Obesity is considerably more common in diabetics than in the popula-tion as a whole (Pyke and Please, 1957) and vascular disease is more common in diabetics who have gained weight than in those who have not (Reinheimer et al., 1967). Diabetics who gained weight but lost it again had a lower

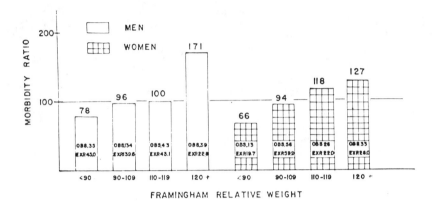

FIGURE 11   Risk of developing coronary heart disease (CHD) in 12 yr according to relative weight in the Framingham population, age 30–59 at entry to the study (Kannel et al., 1967b, by permission of the American Heart Association, Inc.).

frequency of vascular disease, and those who lost more weight had a lower frequency than those who lost little weight (Reinheimer et al., 1967). Although another study of large numbers of diabetics revealed no relationship between atherosclerosis and obesity (Stearns et al., 1947), Santen et al. (1972) found more obese subjects among their diabetics with atherosclerotic disease than among those without diabetic complications.

Obesity is closely related to circulating triglyceride levels in both diabetics (Santen et al., 1972) and nondiabetics (Bagdade et al., 1971), but triglyceride levels and obesity may be independently related to atherosclerosis in diabetics (Santen et al., 1972). The relationship between obesity and triglyceride levels could be mediated through the elevated insulin levels associated with obesity (Bagdade et al., 1971). There is a relationship between body weight and cholesterol levels (Montoye et al., 1966), and obesity is associated with increased total body cholesterol synthesis (Nestel et al., 1969; Miettinen, 1971), presumably splanchnic very low density lipoprotein cholesterol. Hypertension is also related to body weight (Kannel et al., 1967a; Chiang et al., 1969) and blood pressure is reduced by weight reduction (Chiang et al., 1969).

Thus, the role of obesity in the atherosclerotic disease of diabetes may be indirect. While weight reduction results in improved glucose tolerance, lower triglyceride levels, and often lower blood pressure, it is not known whether the development of atherosclerosis is slowed or reversed by this measure.

Hyperinsulinemia

It has been postulated that insulin may directly affect arterial wall metabolism, predisposing to atherosclerosis (Stout and Vallance-Owen, 1969).

Obesity is associated with higher circulating levels of insulin, both in the basal state and after stimulation (Bagdade et al., 1967a). Since obesity is related to atherosclerosis (both directly and through hypertension, hypertriglyceridemia, and hypercholesterolemia), it is not surprising that many studies have shown a relationship between serum insulin levels, particularly after oral glucose, and atherosclerotic disease of the coronary and peripheral arteries (Peters and Hales, 1965; Nikkila et al., 1965; Tzagournis et al., 1968; Sloan et al., 1971). A few studies, however, have suggested that this association is independent of obesity (Christiansen et al., 1968; Malherbee et al., 1970).

In diabetics, a clear distinction must be made between the reduction in the insulin secretory response to glucose stimulation (the hallmark of glucose intolerance and fasting hyperglycemia [Brunzell et al., 1976]) and the actual levels of insulin in the circulation. Thus obese diabetics, in direct relation to their degree of adiposity, have higher basal and stimulated serum insulin levels than thin nondiabetics, even though their insulin response to the glucose stimulus is relatively impaired (Bagdade et al., 1967a). Since obesity is so common in adult-onset diabetes, many diabetics have higher circulating insulin levels throughout the day than most nondiabetics.

Diabetics requiring treatment with exogenous insulin also have abnormally high circulating insulin levels at various times during the day (Heding, 1972; Rasmussen et al., 1975). Not only are the injected amounts usually excessive in terms of endogenous secretion, but exogenous insulin reaches peripheral tissues before the liver, instead of the more physiological portal route from the pancreas. Thus the quantity of insulin perfusing the large arteries in diabetics may be inordinately high. If a direct effect of insulin on the arterial wall can be shown to be involved in the pathogenesis of atherosclerosis (see below), the diabetic is again in greater jeopardy.

A few clinical studies of the relationship between circulating insulin levels and atherosclerosis in diabetics suggest that otherwise matched diabetics with clinical evidence of atherosclerosis have higher basal and stimulated serum insulin levels than diabetics without manifest atherosclerosis (Kashyap et al., 1970; Santen et al., 1972).

Dietary Fat and Cholesterol

Epidemiological studies among various population groups have supported an association between an increased intake of dietary fat and cholesterol and the prevalence of atherosclerosis (McGandy et al., 1967), perhaps mediated by increased serum cholesterol levels.

Traditionally, diabetics were frequently advised to adhere to a restricted carbohydrate diet which, if total calories were not reduced, had an excessively high saturated fat and cholesterol content. The role of the typical diabetic high-fat, low-carbohydrate diet in the genesis of hypercholesterolemia in diabetes, particularly among younger diabetics, has not been resolved. However, a recent study (Kaufmann et al., 1975) carried out in a diet-managed diabetic summer camp suggests that diet plays a significant role; juvenile diabetics had lower cholesterol levels on lower-fat, higher-carbohydrate diets than on their usual diabetic diet. As shown by the study of Stone and Connor (1963), insulin-requiring diabetics maintained on a low-fat, low-cholesterol, high-carbohydrate diet had lower cholesterol levels than matched diabetics taking a more usual diabetic diet, while their triglyceride levels and insulin requirements were not different. Whether such a dietary regimen reduces or prevents atherosclerosis in diabetes remains unknown. However, diabetics in countries such as Japan, Yemen, and Sri Lanka, who receive a diet on the average much higher in carbohydrate and lower in fat than that of their Western counterparts, have very little coronary or peripheral atherosclerosis (Rudnick and Anderson, 1962; Brunner et al., 1964; de Zoysa, 1951).

On the other hand, it has been suggested by retrospective analysis that an increase in the proportion of carbohydrates in the diabetic diet is associated with an increase in the frequency of atherosclerotic complications (Albrink et al., 1962), perhaps mediated by carbohydrate-induced increases in serum triglyceride levels. However, there is little evidence to support the idea that a higher-carbohydrate, lower-fat diet is harmful to diabetics. Although increasing the proportion of carbohydrate in the diet induces short-term elevation of circulating fasting triglyceride levels (Ahrens et al., 1961), this phenomenon appears to be transient in both diabetic (Bierman and Hamlin, 1961; Stone and Connor, 1963) and nondiabetic subjects (Antonis and Bersohn, 1961) and is restricted to the basal (overnight fasted) state, since triglyceride levels over a 24 hr period are actually lower in subjects consuming high-carbohydrate diets (Schlierf et al., 1971). Increasing dietary carbohydrate tends to improve glucose tolerance in mild diabetics (Brunzell et al., 1971) and lowers fasting glucose levels with no increase in glycosuria or the insulin requirements of severe diabetics (Brunzell et al., 1974).

Thus it seems likely that the fundamental role of dietary fat and cholesterol in atherosclerosis is the same in diabetics as in nondiabetics. Since diabetics have been exposed to higher-fat diets, perhaps their risk for atherosclerosis has been enhanced to some unknown extent.

Cigarette Smoking

Cigarette smoking is not only one of the more potent risk factors for atherosclerosis in humans (National Heart and Lung Institute, 1971; Dawber, 1975), it is also the factor that, if reduced or eliminated clearly results in a reduction of risk. There is no evidence that diabetics smoke more or with greater frequency than nondiabetics. However, preliminary results in hemodialysis patients, another atherosclerosis-prone population, indicate an impressive interaction of cigarette smoking with other risk factors, resulting in a marked enhancement of mortality from atherosclerosis (H. Haire et al., unpublished data). Since such interaction is likely but has not been proved for diabetics, special attention needs to be focused on this potentially reversible problem.

"Diabetes Mellitus" Gene Effect

The fundamental genetic abnormality in human diabetes mellitus remains unknown. In addition to all of the risk factors mentioned above that are either the same or amplified in diabetics compared to the rest of the population, diabetes could provide a unique contribution to atherogenesis, depending on the nature of the inherited abnormality.

It has been suggested that genetic diabetes mellitus in humans represents a cellular abnormality intrinsic to all cells (Goldstein, 1971; Vracko and Benditt, 1974), resulting in decreased life span and increased cell turnover. If arterial endothelial and smooth muscle cells are intrinsically defective in diabetes, then accelerated atherogenesis can be readily postulated on the basis of current concepts of pathogenesis.

PATHOGENESIS OF ATHEROSCLEROSIS—GENERAL

A working hypothesis consistent with a wide variety of experimental evidence is that the sequence of events in atheroma formation begins with "injury" to the endothelium and exposure of the subendothelial tissue to increased concentrations of plasma constituents (Ross and Glomset, 1976). Platelets adhere, form microthrombi, and release their granular contents which, in conjunction with other plasma constituents including cholesterol-rich lipoproteins (Ross and Glomset, 1973) and insulin (Stout et al., 1975), stimulate migration and focal proliferation of smooth muscle cells. The multipotential arterial smooth muscle cell is the predominant cell type in the intima and media of large arteries and appears to play a fundamental role in the pathogenesis of atherosclerosis in both humans and experimental animals (Ross and Glomset, 1973). These cells not only migrate into the intima and proliferate early in atheroma formation, perhaps as a monoclonal response (Benditt and Benditt, 1973), but they accumulate intracellular lipid in the presence of increased concentrations of extracellular lipoprotein to become the characteristic "foam cells," and they deposit extracellular connective tissue proteins. As the lesion progresses, it is characterized by increased numbers of lipid-laden smooth muscle cells, increased connective tissue matrix, and accumulation of extracellular lipid. A fibrous plaque is formed that encroaches on the lumen of the artery, which ultimately can calcify and rupture, leading to thrombosis and complete occlusion.

In addition to a potent proliferation-stimulating factor released from platelets (Ross et al., 1974), there are several key plasma constituents that appear to be involved in the process, which may relate to their role as risk factors. Cholesterol-rich LDL have been shown to stimulate the proliferation of cultured arterial smooth muscle cells (Ross and Glomset, 1974). Despite their large size, both LDL and the triglyceride-rich VLDL are avidly and specifically bound and internalized by human arterial smooth muscle cells in tissue culture (Bierman and Albers, 1975), and the LDL apoprotein can be readily demonstrated by immunological techniques in human atheroma (Smith and Slater, 1973). A close relationship exists between plasma cholesterol and arterial lipoprotein cholesterol concentration (Smith and Slater, 1972). Thus, these and other lines of evidence suggest that the cholesterol ester that characteristically accumulates in the lesion appears to be mainly derived from plasma lipoproteins (Stein and Stein, 1973), predominantly LDL and VLDL.

Another important plasma constituent that may be involved in atheroma formation is insulin. In physiological concentrations as low as 10 μU/ml, insulin has been shown to stimulate proliferation of cultured arterial smooth muscle cells, and the effect was directly related to insulin concentration (Stout et al., 1975). Insulin also appears to enhance endogenous lipid synthesis in the arterial wall (Stout, 1968, 1969); however, little is known of its effect on the handling of lipoprotein by these cells.

The role of glucose in atheroma formation, if any, is poorly understood. Hyperglycemia is known to affect aortic wall metabolism. Sorbitol, a production of the insulin-independent aldose reductose pathway of glucose metabolism (the polyol pathway), accumulates in the arterial wall in the presence of high glucose concentrations, which results in osmotic effects, including increased cell water content and decreased oxygenation (Morrison et al., 1972). Preliminary results suggest that increased glucose also stimulates proliferation of cultured smooth muscle cells (Turner and Bierman, 1976).

PATHOGENESIS OF ATHEROSCLEROSIS IN DIABETES

Risk Factor Interaction in Diabetes and Role in the Pathogenesis of Atherosclerosis

Not only are the individual risk factors for atherosclerosis intensified in diabetes, but they also interact to produce a marked enhancement of atherogenesis. A scheme summarizing the interaction of risk factors in the pathogenesis of atherosclerosis related to diabetes is represented in Fig. 12. As already indicated, obesity is closely associated with the development of hypertension, hypertriglyceridemia, and hypercholesterolemia, as well as hyperglycemia. The insulin resistance in adipose tissue and muscle in obesity results in impaired glucose utilization and compensatory hyperinsulinism. Elevated insulin levels associated with obesity, with or without concomitant hyperglycemia, can influence atherogenesis in several ways. First, insulin enhances the production of triglyceride-rich lipoproteins by the liver (Topping and Mayes, 1972), resulting in elevations in both plasma triglyceride and cholesterol levels. Higher circulating levels, in turn, result in increased lipoprotein accumulation in the arterial wall smooth muscle cells (Smith and

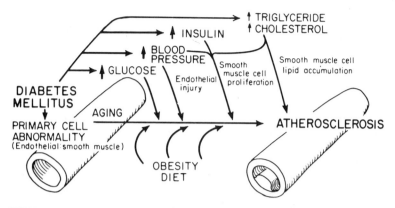

FIGURE 12 Interaction of risk factors in the pathogenesis of atherosclerosis related to diabetes.

Slater, 1972). Insulin may also directly affect arterial wall lipid metabolism, leading to lipid accumulation (Stout, 1968, 1969). Finally, insulin in physiological concentrations has been shown to accelerate the proliferation of smooth muscle cells in tissue culture (Stout et al., 1975).

Hypertension can interact in producing the same effects. Experimental hypertension accelerates smooth muscle cell proliferation, resulting in increased thickness of the intimal smooth muscle layer in the arterial wall and increased connective tissue elements (Ross and Harker, 1976). In addition, hypertension could result in additional lipid accumulation in arterial smooth muscle cells by altering the permeability of intact endothelial lining cells, allowing more lipoproteins to be transported through them, or by directly producing endothelial injury through mechanical stress on endothelial cells at specific high-pressure sites in the arterial tree. Hypercholesterolemia in experimental animals has also been shown to result in endothelial damage and smooth muscle cell proliferation (Ross and Glomset, 1976; Ross and Harker, 1976).

Hyperglycemia can also conceivably lead to changes in endothelial cells (injury or altered permeability); accelerate smooth muscle cell proliferation, as shown in tissue culture studies (Turner and Bierman, 1976); and enhance lipid accumulation in arterial wall smooth muscle cells.

Finally, the postulated primary cellular abnormality in diabetes could result in decreased life span of endothelial and smooth muscle cells in the artery. These effects would resemble the growth properties of aging cells and thus genetic diabetes mellitus could represent premature aging. Aging itself has been associated with lessened endothelial integrity, focal intimal thickening (smooth muscle cell proliferation), and increased intimal lipid accumulation (Bierman and Ross, 1977). Any of the risk factors that increase cell death would accelerate this process. In this regard, clonal senescence of arterial wall cells (the ultimate failure of a clone of cells to continue dividing) has been implicated in the pathogenesis of atherosclerosis (Martin et al., 1975).

Atherosclerosis in Experimental Diabetes

Attempts to produce atherosclerotic lesions in animals with experimental "diabetes" (pancreatic beta cell ablation) have been remarkably unsuccessful (Stout et al., 1975). Experimental animal models of diabetes are those in which insulin deficiency is produced, either surgically by removing most or all of the pancreas or chemically by use of alloxan or streptozotocin, which, among other effects, destroy pancreatic islet beta cells. In addition, strains of spontaneously diabetic animals have been developed that are almost always characterized by obesity and/or hyperphagia coupled with hyperinsulinism. The comparability of any of these animal models to the full syndrome of genetic diabetes in humans is open to serious question.

However, when insulin-deficient animals are fed high-cholesterol diets, atherosclerosis develops just as in cholesterol-fed normal animals. However, cholesterol-fed diabetic animals appear to have less extensive atherosclerosis than do nondiabetic animals (Duff and McMillan, 1949; McGill and Holman, 1949), and insulin replacement reverses this protective effect (Duff et al., 1954). While insulin-deficient animals do develop hyperlipidemia, the artery of the experimentally diabetic animal does not appear to be more susceptible than that of the nondiabetic animal for any level of serum lipid (Wilson et al., 1967). Thus, it does not seem that insulin deficiency *per se* in association with hyperglycemia will experimentally produce atherosclerotic lesions or increase atherogenesis produced by other experimental manipulations.

In contrast, insulin infusion into the artery of diabetic animals will produce arterial thickening and lipid deposition (Cruz et al., 1961). The level of circulating insulin appears to modulate lipid accumulation in the artery and the development of arterial lesions in experimental animals (Stout, 1970). Thus elevated insulin levels, characteristic of both adult obese diabetics and insulin-treated diabetics, would promote endogenous lipid synthesis, reduce lipid mobilization, and perhaps enhance uptake.

Therefore, if insulin is involved in atherogenesis, it does not appear to be related to hyperglycemia and insulin deficiency alone. Genetic diabetes in humans then must provide additional pathogenic factors for the development of atherosclerosis. These are likely to include the risk factors discussed above, unique to the human syndrome and not reproduced in any of the experimental animal models to date.

CONCLUSION

Atherosclerosis is the leading cause of death in diabetes and occurs more frequently and prematurely than in normal populations. Many of the risk factors for atherosclerosis, such as hyperglycemia, hypertriglyceridemia, hyper-cholesterolemia, hypertension, obesity, hyperinsulinemia, and increased dietary fat and cholesterol, are more prevalent in diabetes. Smoking may interact with these risk factors and with the basic predisposition for atherosclerosis in diabetes in more than an additive fashion.

A recent model for atherogenesis has been adapted and modified in an attempt to explain the increased atherogenesis seen in diabetes.

REFERENCES

Ahrens, E. H., Hirsch, J., Oette, K., Farquhar, J. W. and Stein, Y. 1961. *Trans. Assoc. Am. Physicians* 74:134.

Albrink, M. J., Lavietes, P. H. and Man, E. B. 1963. *Ann. Intern. Med.* 58:305.

Antonis, A. and Bersohn, I. 1961. *Lancet* 1:3.

Bagdade, J. D., Bierman, E. L. and Porte, D., Jr. 1967a. *J. Clin. Invest.* 46:1549.

Bagdade, J. D., Porte, D., Jr. and Bierman, E. L. 1967b. *N. Engl. J. Med.* 276:427.

Bagdade, J. D., Porte, D., Jr. and Bierman, E. L. 1968. *Diabetes* 17:127.

Bagdade, J. D., Bierman, E. L. and Porte, D., Jr. 1971. *Diabetes* 20:664.

Balasse, E. O., Bier, D. M. and Havel, R. J. 1972. *Diabetes* 21:280.

Basso, L. V. and Havel, R. J. 1970. *J. Clin. Invest.* 49:537.

Belknap, B. H., Bagdade, J. D., Amaral, J. A. P. and Bierman, E. L. 1967. In *Tolbutamide after ten years,* eds. W. J. H. Butterfield and W. Van Westering, p. 171. Amsterdam: Excerpta Medica.

Benditt, E. P. and Benditt, J. M. 1973. *Proc. Natl. Acad. Sci. U.S.A.* 70:1753.

Bergqvist, N. 1970. *Acta Med. Scand.* 187:213.

Bierman, E. L. and Albers, J. J. 1975. *Biochim. Biophys. Acta* 388:198.

Bierman, E. L. and Hamlin, J. T. 1961. *Diabetes* 10:432.

Bierman, E. L. and Porte, D., Jr. 1968. *Ann. Intern. Med.* 68:926.

Bierman, E. L. and Ross, R. 1977. In *Atherosclerosis reviews II,* eds. R. Paoletti and A. M. Gotto. New York: Raven. In press.

Brunner, D., Altman, S., Nelken, L. and Reider, J. 1964. *Diabetes* 13:268.

Brunzell, J. D. and Schrott, H. G. 1973. *Trans. Assoc. Am. Physicians* 86:245.

Brunzell, J. D., Lerner, R. L., Hazzard, W. R., Porte, D., Jr. and Bierman, E. L. 1971 *N. Engl. J. Med.* 284:521.

Brunzell, J. D., Porte, D., Jr. and Bierman, E. L. 1972. *Diabetes* 21 (Suppl. 1):342.

Brunzell, J. D., Lerner, R. L., Porte, D., Jr. and Bierman, E. L. 1974. *Diabetes* 23:138.

Brunzell, J. D., Hazzard, W. R., Motulsky, A. G. and Bierman, E. L. 1975a. *Metab. Clin. Exp.* 24:1115.

Brunzell, J. D., Porte, D., Jr. and Bierman, E. L. 1975b. *Metab. Clin. Exp.* 24:1123.

Brunzell, J. D., Robertson, R. P., Lerner, R. L., Hazzard, W. R., Ensinck, J. W., Bierman, E. L. and Porte, D., Jr. 1976. *J. Clin. Endocrinol. Metab.* 42:222.

Carlson, L. A. and Bottiger, L. E. 1972. *Lancet* 1:865.

Chiang, B. N., Perlman, L. V. and Epstein, F. H. 1969. *Circulation* 39:403.

Christiansen, I., Deckert, T., Kjerulf, K., Midtgaard, K. and Worning, H. 1968. *Acta Med. Scand.* 184:283.

Cruz, A. B., Amatuzio, D. S., Grande, F. and Hay, L. J. 1961. *Circ. Res.* 9:39.

Dawber, T. R. 1975. Risk factors for atherosclerotic disease. Current concepts, prepared by the Upjohn Company, Kalamazoo, Michigan 49001.

de Zoysa, V. P. 1951. *Arch. Intern. Med.* 88:812.

Downie, E. and Martin, F. I. R. 1959. *Diabetes* 8:383.

Duff, G. L. and McMillan, G. C. 1949. *J. Exp. Med.* 89:611.

Duff, G. L., Brechin, J. H. and Finkelstein, W. E. 1954. *J. Exp. Med.* 100:371.

Epstein, F. H. 1967a. *Proc. R. Soc. Med.* 60:56.

Epstein, F. H. 1967b. *Circulation* 36:609.

Fredrickson, D. S. and Levy, R. I. 1972. In *Metabolic basis of inherited disease,* 3rd ed., eds. J. B. Stanbury, J. B. Wyngaarden and D. S. Fredrickson, pp. 545–614. New York: McGraw-Hill.

Garcia, M. J., McNamara, P. M., Gordon, T. and Kannel, W. B. 1974. *Diabetes* 23:105.

Glueck, C. J., Levy, R. I. and Fredrickson, D. S. 1969. *Diabetes* 18:239.

Goldberg, A., Sherrard, D. and Brunzell, J. 1975. *Clin. Res.* 24:361A.

Goldenberg, S., Alex, M. and Blumenthal, H. T. 1958. *Diabetes* 7:98.

Goldstein, J. L., Hazzard, W. R., Schrott, H. G., Bierman, E. L. and Motulsky, A. G. 1973a. *J. Clin. Invest.* 52:1544.

Goldstein, J. L., Hazzard, W. R., Schrott, H. G., Bierman, E. L. and Motulsky, A. G. 1973b. *J. Clin. Invest.* 18:1533.

Goldstein, S. 1971. *Humangenetik* 12:83.

Heding, L. G. 1972. *Diabetologia* 8:260.

Kannel, W. B., Brand, N., Skinner, J. J., Dawber, T. R. and McNamara, P. M. 1967a. *Ann. Intern. Med.* 67:48.

Kannel, W. B., LeBauer, E. J., Dawber, T. R. and McNamara, P. M. 1967b. *Circulation* 35:734.

Kashyap, L., Magill, F., Rojes, L. and Hoffman, M. M. 1970. *Can. Med. Assoc. J.* 102:1165.

Kaufman, R. L., Assal, J. P., Soeldner, J. S., Wilmhurst, E. G., Lemaire, J. R., Gleason, R. E. and White, P. 1975. *Diabetes* 24:672.

Keen, H. and Jarrett, R. J. 1973. *Adv. Metab. Disord.* (Suppl. 2):3.

Keen, H., Rose, G., Pyke, D. A., Boyns, D., Chlouverakis, C. and Mistry, S. 1965. *Lancet* 2:505.

Keys, A., Aravanis, C., Blackburn, H., Van Buchem, F. S. P., Buzino, R., Djordjevic, B. S., Fidanza, F., Karvonen, M. J., Menotli, A., Puddo, V. and Taylor, H. L. 1972. *Ann. Intern. Med.* 77:15.

Kissebah, A. H., Adams, P. Q. and Wynn, V. 1974. *Diabetologia* 10:119.

Lewis, B., Mancini, M., Mattock, M., Chait, A. and Fraser, T. R. 1972. *Eur. J. Clin. Invest.* 2:445.

Liebow, I. M., Hellerstein, H. K. and Miller, M. 1955. *Am. J. Med.* 18:438.

Malherbee, C., de Gasparo, M., Berthet, P., de Hertogh, R. and Hoet, J. J. 1970. *Eur. J. Clin. Invest.* 1:265.

Marks, H. H. and Krall, L. F. 1971. In *Joslin's diabetes mellitus,* eds. A. Marble, P. White, R. F. Bradley and L. P. Krall, chap. 9, pp. 209–254. Philadelphia: Lea & Febiger.

Martin, G., Ogburn, C. and Sprague, C. 1975. In *Explorations in aging,* eds. V. J. Cristofalo, J. Roberts and R. C. Adelman, p. 163. New York: Plenum.

McGandy, R. B., Hegsted, D. M. and Stare, F. J. 1967. *N. Engl. J. Med.* 277:186.

McGill, H. G. and Holman, R. L. 1949. *Proc. Soc. Exp. Biol. Med.* 72:72.

Miettinen, T. A. 1971. *Circulation* 44:842.

Montoye, H. J., Epstein, F. H. and Kjelsberg, M. O. 1966. *Am. J. Clin. Nutr.* 18:397.

Morrison, A. D., Clements, R. S. and Winegrad, A. I. 1972. *J. Clin. Invest.* 51:3114.

National Heart and Lung Institute. 1971. *Arteriosclerosis—A report by the NHLI Task Force on Arteriosclerosis.* Bethesda, Md.: National Institutes of Health.

Nestel, P. J., Whyte, H. M. and Goodman, D. S. 1969. *J. Clin. Invest.* 48:982.

New, M. I., Roberts, T. N., Bierman, E. L. and Reader, G. G. 1963. *Diabetes* 12:208.

Nikkila, E. A. and Kekki, M. 1973. *Metabolism* 22:1.

Nikkila, E. A., Miettinen, T. A., Vesenne, M. R. and Pelkonen, R. 1965. *Lancet* 2:508.

Nikkila, E. A., Huttunen, J. K., Ehnholm, C. and Kekki, M. 1975. *Eur. Assoc. Study Diabetes Abstr. 201.*

Olefsky, J., Reaven, G. M. and Farquhar, J. W. 1974. *J. Clin. Invest* 53:64.

Ostrander, L. D., Francis, T., Hayner, N. S., Kjelsberg, M. O. and Epstein, F. H. 1965. *Ann. Intern. Med.* 62:1188.

Ostrander, L. D., Neff, B. J., Block, W. D., Francis, T. and Epstein, F. H. 1967. *Ann. Intern. Med.* 67:34.

Ostrander, L. D., Block, W. D., Lamphiear, D. E. and Epstein, F. H. 1973. *Adv. Metab. Disord.* (Suppl. 2):73.

Parker, F., Bagdade, J. D., Odland, G. F. and Bierman, E. L. 1970. *J. Clin. Invest.* 49:2172.

Pell, S. and D'Alonzo, C. A. 1967. *J. Am. Med. Assoc.* 202:10.

Pell, S. and D'Alonzo, C. A. 1970. *J. Am. Med. Assoc.* 214:1833.

Peters, N. and Hales, C. N. 1965. *Lancet* 1:1144.

Pykalisto, O. J., Smith, P. H. and Brunzell, J. D. 1975. *J. Clin. Invest.* 56:1108.

Pyke, D. A. and Please, N. W. 1957. *J. Endocrinol.* 15:xxvi.

Rasmussen, S. M., Heding, L. G. and Parbst, E. 1975. *Diabetologia* 11:151.

Reaven, E. P. and Reaven, G. M. 1974. *J. Clin. Invest.* 54:1167.

Reinheimer, W., Bliffen, G., McCoy, J., Wallace, D. and Albrink, M. J. 1967. *Am. J. Clin. Nutr.* 20:986.

Robertson, W. B. and Strong, J. P. 1968. *Lab. Invest.* 18:538.

Robinson, D. S. 1970. *Compr. Biochem.* 18:51.

Ross, R. and Glomset, J. 1973. *Science* 180:1332.

Ross, R. and Glomset, J. 1976. *N. Engl. J. Med.* 295:420.

Ross, R. and Harker, L. 1976. *Science,* in press.

Ross, R., Glomset, J., Kariya, B. and Harker, L. 1974. *Proc. Natl. Acad. Sci. U.S.A.* 71:1207.

Rudnick, P. A. and Anderson, P. S. 1962. *Diabetes* 11:533.

Santen, R. J., Willis, P. W. and Fajans, S. S. 1972. *Arch. Intern. Med.* 130:833.

Schlierf, G., Reinheimer, W. and Stossberg, V. 1971. *Nutr. Metab.* 13:80.

Schonfeld, G., Birge, C., Miller, J. P., Kessler, G. and Santiago, J. 1974. *Diabetes* 23:827.

Sloan, J. M., Mackay, J. S. and Sheridan, B. 1971. *Diabetologia* 7:431.

Smith, E. B. and Slater, R. S. 1972. *Lancet* 1:463.

Smith, E. B. and Slater, R. S. 1973. In *Atherogenesis: Initiating factors. Ciba Found. Symp.* 12:39.

Stearns, S., Schlesinger, M. J. and Rudy, A. 1947. *Arch. Intern. Med.* 80:463.
Stein, Y. and Stein, O. 1973. In *Atherogenesis: Initiating factors. Ciba Found. Symp.* 12:165.
Stone, D. B. and Connor, W. E. 1963. *Diabetes* 12:127.
Stout, R. W. 1968. *Lancet* 2:702.
Stout, R. W. 1969. *Lancet* 2:467.
Stout, R. W. 1970. *Br. Med. J.* 3:685.
Stout, R. W. and Vallance-Owen, J. 1969. *Lancet* 1:1078.
Stout, R. W., Bierman, E. L. and Brunzell, J. D. 1975a. In *Diabetes, its physiological and biochemical basis,* ed. by J. Vallance-Owen, p. 125. Lancaster: MTP Press.
Stout, R. W., Bierman, E. L. and Ross, R. 1975b. *Circ. Res.* 36:319.
Strandness, D. E., Jr., Priest, R. E. and Gibbons, G. E. 1964. *Diabetes* 13:366.
Thannhauser, S. J. 1958. In *Lipidoses: Diseases of the intracellular lipid metabolism,* 3rd ed. p. 296. New York: Grune & Stratton.
Topping, D. L. and Mayes, P. A. 1972. *Biochem. J.* 126:295.
Turner, J. L. and Bierman, E. L. 1976. *Diabetes* 25 (Suppl. 1):336.
Tzagournis, M., Chiles, R., Ryan, J. M. and Skillman, T. G. 1968. *Circulation* 38:1156.
University Group Diabetes Program. 1970. *Diabetes* 19 (Supple 2).
Veterans Administration Co-operative Study Group on Antihypertensive Agents. 1967. *J. Am. Med. Assoc.* 202:1028.
Veterans Administration Co-operative Study Group on Antihypertensive Agents. 1970. *J. Am. Med. Assoc.* 213:1143.
Vracko, R. and Benditt, E. P. 1974. *Am. J. Pathol.* 75:204.
Wilson, D. E., Schreibman, P. H., Day, V. C. and Arky, R. A. 1970. *J. Chron. Dis.* 23:501.
Wilson, R. B., Martin, J. M. and Hartroft, W. S. 1967. *Diabetes* 16:71.
Woodside, W. F. and Heimberg, M. 1976. *J. Biol. Chem.* 251:13.

Chapter 6

RELATIONSHIP OF OBESITY TO DIABETES: SOME FACTS, MANY QUESTIONS

M. Berger, W. A. Muller, and A. E. Renold
Institut de Biochimie Clinique
University of Geneva
Geneva, Switzerland

INTRODUCTION

A convincing association between diabetes and obesity was observed by physicians as early as 100 or more years ago (Bouchardat, 1875; Lanceraux, 1880). However, at that time it was not clear whether, in humans, obesity is a consequence ("diabetogenic obesity") or a cause ("lipogenic diabetes") of carbohydrate intolerance. To be sure, Allen reported in 1917 that in partially pancreatectomized dogs overt diabetes could be induced when the animals were made obese by overfeeding, but that pioneering experimental observation was not sufficient in itself to guide further clinical thinking.

Later, on the basis of extensive clinical records, Joslin et al. (1936) convincingly suggested that diabetes more often develops secondary to the onset of obesity, and that overweight (or overnutrition) might indeed precipitate the manifestation and worsen the prognosis of diabetes. The early reports have since been substantiated by a multitude of clinical and epidemiological observations, overnutrition and obesity being presently regarded as probably the main environmental determinant in the clinical manifestation of diabetes mellitus, especially the adult-onset form of the disease.

Despite the generally accepted evidence for a strong association between glucose intolerance and obesity, the nature of the association is not a simple one; many of its details remain obscure, as discussed so well by Keen (1975) in more recent times.

This work was supported by grant 3.774.076 SR from the Swiss National Scientific Foundation, Berne; by a grant from the Juvenile Diabetes Research Foundation, Miami, Florida; and by a grant-in-aid from Hoechst Pharmaceuticals, Frankfurt-Hoechst, Germany.

EPIDEMIOLOGICAL EVIDENCE

Population Screening Studies

Although textbooks of medicine often refer to "ample epidemiological evidence" linking the incidence rates of diabetes and obesity, critical evaluation reveals that adequately controlled quantitative data are available to a limited extent only, some difficulties inherent in the epidemiological approach having been insufficiently considered. The main problem, of course, is that inherent in the arbitrary aspects of the diagnostic definition of either obesity or diabetes. Both definitions are subject to controversy and may vary widely from one study to another.

Obesity. In very few studies was the degree of adiposity—that is, the relationship of adipose tissue mass to total body weight—measured directly. Weight-over-height indices are most often used to describe relative weight (body weight in relation to body height); alternatively, body weight is quantified in relation to life insurance ideal-weight tables, the validity of which is presently under dispute (Keys and Grande, 1973; Dyer et al., 1975; Weinsier et al., 1976). Even more generally, "obesity" is a cultural concept and its definition must vary with climate, food availability, need for physical exercise, and the socioeconomic system. Hence, direct comparison and evaluation of data obtained in different studies will be necessarily difficult.

In addition, much evidence suggests that, even when adiposity as a whole is the same, its distribution over different areas of the body (Albrink and Meigs, 1964; Vague, 1950, 1956; Vague et al., 1971; Feldman et al., 1969) or the mean fat cell size achieved (Björntorp et al., 1971) might influence carbohydrate tolerance in a manner independent of overall adiposity alone. Most epidemiological studies have insufficiently differentiated between such probable subtypes of obesity, or not even considered their existence.

Diabetes mellitus. Here also, no consensus exists as to the criteria needed for the diagnosis of diabetes mellitus. A variety of methods have been employed, but it is only recently that understanding of pathogenetic differences between the maturity-onset type of diabetes (MOD) and the primarily insulin-dependent juvenile-onset type (JOD) has made real progress; whereas JOD bears little or no relation to overweight (Pyke and Please, 1957; Joslin et al., 1936; Tattersall and Pyke, 1973), the association is clear-cut in MOD. It is also noteworthy that MOD is not necessarily confined to older age groups, since adolescents with the characteristic syndrome of a primarily insulin-independent diabetes (MODY) have also been described (Tattersall and Fajans, 1975; Martin and Martin, 1973). As for other differences between the two types (JOD and MOD) of diabetes—for example, the association with certain HLA antigens, the occurrence of anti-islet autoantibodies, or the relative predominance of the role of genetics (*Lancet,* 1977)—the association with obesity similarly separates quite clearly between JOD and MOD.

Differences in the relative time course of the two associated disorders also need to be appreciated: the overweight maturity-onset diabetic may, of course, lose weight, either through deterioration of the metabolic state or as a consequence of proper treatment. Hence, in some studies (Grönberg et al., 1967; Reid et al., 1974) there was at first glance little difference in the prevalence of obesity among the general population and treated diabetics. However, when newly diagnosed diabetics were evaluated (Reid et al., 1974; Pyke and Please, 1957) or when the highest remembered or fully documented weight of treated diabetics was taken into account (Keen, 1975; Joslin et al., 1936), the prevalence of obesity was again remarkably higher among the diabetic than the appropriately selected control groups. In Pima Indians, on the other hand, a significant association between obesity and carbohydrate intolerance was demonstrable only below the age of 35, not above the age of 45 (Bennett et al., 1976).

Of course, additional environmental and/or genetic factors that are known to influence the prevalence rates of diabetes as well as of obesity (e.g., age, sex, parity, physical activity, and racial and nutritional determinants), as well as others as yet unknown, also should be or will have to be taken into account when estimating and comparing the coincidence rate of the two diseases in different populations.

Because of the reservations summarized in this section, a valid *quantitative* assessment of the prevalence of combined and/or isolated obesity and diabetes, as compared to an appropriate control population, cannot be definitively established on the basis of presently available epidemiological screening studies. Such a *general* association of obesity and diabetes is nevertheless well documented by mortality figures from life insurance companies (Dublin and Marks, 1952), standardized multinational comparative studies (West, 1974), and studies on selected population samples (Eriksen et al., 1970; Claussen et al., 1970; Eschwege et al., 1974).

For the prevalence of obesity *at some time* in the life history of diabetics, the values reported may be as high as 80% (Joslin et al., 1936), but are more often in the range 30–50%, varying greatly between different diabetic cohorts and in different countries or socioeconomic environments. On the other hand, the prevalence of carbohydrate intolerance in grossly obese patients has been repeatedly found to be around 50%, varying somewhat with age, sex, race, and so on (Paullin and Sauls, 1922; John, 1929; Knowles, 1968; Duncan et al., 1968; Grott et al., 1962; Berchtold et al., 1977). Why only every second grossly obese individual develops glucose intolerance—and therefore why every second grossly obese individual retains entirely normal glucose tolerance—remains both obscure and of considerable interest. Furthermore, the prevalence of carbohydrate intolerance in obese populations may be only weakly correlated to the *degree* of obesity (Berchtold et al., 1977), whereas in some studies the association with the *duration* of obesity may be somewhat stronger (Allison, 1927; Ogilvie, 1935; Newburgh and Conn, 1939;

Martin and Martin 1973; Bierman et al., 1968). It remains nevertheless true that neither differences in degree nor differences in duration of obesity suffice to discriminate clearly between overweight patients with and those without glucose intolerance.

Certain subtypes of obesity may be more markedly associated with diabetes than others (Vague, 1956; Feldman et al., 1969); also, the otherwise seemingly unrelated genetic background most likely influences the rate of onset of glucose intolerance in obese subjects (Tyner, 1933; Medley, 1965; Keen, 1975; Paulsen et al., 1968; Chiumello et al., 1969). However, since precisely controlled quantitative data are lacking, neither statement should be taken more seriously than the collective affirmation of observers with considerable experience.

Additional studies comparing prevalence figures in highly selected populations have occasionally revealed major and unexpected exceptions to these more general rules. For example, when comparing glucose tolerance among several racial groups in South Africa, Jackson (1972) observed the lowest prevalence of diabetes in Bantu women, even though they were the most obese. Likewise, Eskimos seem to exhibit a relatively high prevalence of obesity without any of the expected associated glucose intolerance (Mouratoff et al., 1967). Finally, the extreme and well-documented prevalence of diabetes in Pima Indians cannot be related easily to their also prevalent obesity (Bennett et al., 1976).

In comparative studies, West (1972, 1974) and Baird (1972) were unable to identify one or several nutritional factors and/or specific components of the diet as possible causes of difference prevalent rates of diabetes, independent of the influence of obesity. It is tempting—but still idle—to speculate that apparent exceptions to the general association between obesity and diabetes, in both individual cases and population studies, are due to genetic influences.

Longitudinal Studies in Selected Population Groups

It has been reported repeatedly that in a given population the prevalence of diabetes and also that of obesity—more precisely, of relative over- and underfeeding—responds to socioeconomic situations associated with major alterations of food intake and/or physical exercise. It is not surprising, therefore, that the lowest rates of diabetes, or diabetes-associated morbidity, have been observed with war-associated major decreases of food intake, as first emphasized by Bouchardat (1875) during the widespread starvation associated with the 1870 siege of Paris. In the United Kingdom (Himsworth, 1949), Japan (Goto et al., 1958), and Germany (Schliack, 1954) decreased mortality from diabetes or its decreased prevalence was associated less with the state of war itself than with the times, either during or after the war, when rationing was most severe.

More conclusive (because better controlled) evidence in support of the association between the prevalence of diabetes and altered overall nutrition resulting in obesity has evolved from longitudinal prospective studies in selected cohorts of normal or obese subjects. Thus, obesity was repeatedly shown to enhance the probability of manifestation of diabetes in later life (Paffenbarger and Wing, 1973; Bennett et al., 1976; O'Sullivan, 1969; Medalie et al., 1975; Kannel et al., 1970; Comstock et al., 1966). Also, both prospective and retrospective studies have established that persistence of obesity over years has often been associated with continuing deterioration of glucose tolerance, until clinically manifest diabetes mellitus finally developed (Allison, 1927; Ogilvie, 1935; John, 1950; Berger et al., 1975). On the other hand, beginning with the observations of Newburgh and Conn (1939), it has been unequivocally shown that weight loss may often (but not always: Newburgh, 1942; Berger et al., 1975) result in improved glucose tolerance, often even full normalization of the overt diabetes of overweight subjects (Pfeiffer, 1974; Kalkhoff et al., 1971; Rabinowitz, 1970). Even in subjects of normal weight with normal glucose tolerance, strictly enforced overfeeding resulting in "acute" overweight may produce glucose intolerance and other endocrine-metabolic anomalies characteristic of spontaneous obesity (Sims et al., 1971). In these subjects, discontinuation of the calorically excessive diets similarly resulted in a prompt return to normal weight and normal endocrine-metabolic indices (Sims et al., 1968).

Finally, Berger et al. (1975) reported a long-term study in which acute nutritional influences could be excluded; they observed that when obesity was associated with subclinical (chemical) diabetes, a further gradual weight change in either direction, and over a period of 5 yr, again resulted in a significantly correlated improvement or deterioration of glucose tolerance.

Summary of Epidemiological Observations to Date in Humans

An overall association of obesity (or overnutrition) and diabetes is indeed supported by ample epidemiological evidence, obtained in both studies on populations and longitudinal studies of selected groups of subjects. Nevertheless, the available data do not as yet permit a truly quantitative assessment and quantitative description of the relationship between quantifiable overweight and similarly quantifiable carbohydrate intolerance and/or resistance to insulin. Since only some 50% of grossly obese, middle-aged patients exhibit significant glucose intolerance, additional factors are likely to come into play and must be diligently looked for. It is, of course, most likely that the relationship between obesity and diabetes will prove to be dependent on a number of genetically transmitted factors in the population or the patient under study.

For the time being, however, it must be conceded that the epidemiological evidence does not easily reveal the nature of the possible pathophysiological mechanisms that must, somehow, link obesity with glucose intolerance and even overt diabetes in a great number of instances.

EPIDEMIOLOGY OF SPONTANEOUS HYPERGLYCEMIA
AND OBESITY IN SMALL LABORATORY ANIMALS

It probably came as some surprise to early workers with laboratory rodents that a very similar association of obesity and hyperglycemia is a frequent occurrence in several laboratory animals, especially during inbreeding and in the species most frequently used in mammalian genetics, the laboratory mouse. For almost 100 yr (Lataste, 1883; Cuenot, 1905; Danforth, 1927) mutation-controlled (i.e., genetic) obesity has been known, while other mutations resulting in obesity have been described since in genetically analyzed inbred mouse strains. This was the case, for example, in the Jackson Laboratories, Bar Harbor, Maine (Ingalls et al., 1950) and in the strain observed for many years at the University of Otago, New Zealand, by Bielschowsky and Bielschowsky (1953). In all, about a dozen somatic mutations associated with the development of obesity have so far been described in mice, some of which have since been shown to be identical. At least six syndromes presently remain as undoubtedly separate mutations of separate genes, even though considerable similarity may link two of them. From the point of view of epidemiology and, more particularly, genetics, the main lesson to be drawn from the existence of these animal models of adiposity is clearly related to this genetic multiplicity, including entirely different modes of transmission (dominant, recessive, dominant requiring one or more recessive modifiers, polygenic).

With reference to the topic of this chapter, it is of considerable interest that all of the overweight mice demonstrate at some point during their life more or less severe metabolic anomalies highly suggestive of what, in humans, we would term glucose intolerance and/or diabetes mellitus. Also, several observers have clearly and convincingly established that the detailed clinical (or phenotypic) expression of obesity and glucose intolerance in several of these inbred mice requires more than the mere presence of a single or double dose of the abnormal allele. Whenever such mutant alleles may be transferred to the related but not fully identical genomes of related but not identical inbred strains, the clinical syndrome induced by the mutation in each inbred strain may be profoundly modified.

It is impossible to state today that one or the other "model" of obesity associated with greater or lesser severity of inappropriate hyperglycemia is the best, or even a better or a worse model, for the study of coincidence of obesity and hyperglycemia in humans. It seems evident to us that much has already been learned from all of them together: most likely, overweight and/or carbohydrate intolerance are not genetically simpler in humans than in mice. The real difference is that a meaningful analysis may be attempted in mice but will remain impossible in humans because of the frequency of both phenotypic expressions and the laws governing such matters in most countries.

PATHOGENETIC MECHANISM(S)

General Considerations

That human obesity is likely to be associated with increased activity of the β-cells of the islets of Langerhans was first given solid experimental support by Ogilvie (1933), who demonstrated hyperplasia of these islets in 11 of 19 grossly obese patients having come to autopsy in Edinburgh. Since then, it has been amply confirmed that elevated serum levels of immunoreactive as well as biologically active insulin are characteristic markers of obesity, both in the basal state and following stimulation of the β-cells by various means (Karam et al., 1963; Bagdade et al., 1967; Kreisberg et al., 1967; Perley and Kipnis, 1966; Rabinowitz, 1970; Samaan and Fraser, 1963; Schade and Eaton, 1974; Stern and Hirsch, 1972). Indeed, in nondiabetic obese subjects, fasting insulin levels and/or serum insulin response to glucose are significantly elevated whether the presence of obesity was assessed by relative body weight or by more precise measures of adiposity (El-Khodary et al., 1972; Bagdade et al., 1967; Abrams et al., 1969; Gibson et al., 1975).

The relationship between overweight and serum immunoreactive insulin becomes more complex when obesity and diabetes coincide. Thus, in overweight patients with subclinical (chemical) diabetes, mild to moderate hyperinsulinemia (compared with levels of nonobese controls) is usually seen, even though the temporal profile of insulin secretion may be of the delayed type. Once diabetes is clinically overt, serum concentrations of immunoreactive insulin in excess of values in nonobese persons are no longer seen, even when overweight is still present, and the insulin secretion profile in response to glucose is usually both delayed and markedly decreased. To be sure, the response may still be in excess of what would be expected with the same degree of glucose intolerance or overt diabetes *without* concurrent excess weight (Kipnis, 1970).

The most likely interpretation of these findings is that obesity and diabetes exert opposite overall influences on serum levels of immunoreactive insulin. Accordingly, it is not surprising that a variety of insulin secretion patterns has been reported, whenever the two disorders coincide.

However, it remains difficult to avoid the conclusion that the simultaneous occurrence in obesity of greatly increased basal and/or postprandial serum insulin levels, together with blood glucose concentrations that are either elevated or within the normal range, must mean diminished effectiveness of that serum insulin and, most likely, decreased tissue sensitivity to the circulating hormone. The resistance to endogenous insulin action is a rather general one, concerning the metabolism of glucose, of branched-chain amino acids (Felig et al., 1969), and of free fatty acids (Opie and Walfish, 1963). Decreased sensitivity to exogenous insulin has been confirmed by demonstrating decreased responsiveness to the injection of insulin in obese subjects (Godlowsky, 1946; Rabinowitz, 1970; Mahler, 1974).

The concept now emerging seems attractively simple: as resistance to insulin action augments with increasing severity of obesity and with the passage of time, the functional capacity of the insulin-secreting cells of the islets of Langerhans first increases, as a result of hypertrophy and perhaps also limited hyperplasia. When the total functional capacity of the system is reached, however, decompensation and perhaps true exhaustion of the insulin-producing ability occurs. The timing of the β-cell decompensation might be set either by a genetically controlled overall reserve capacity or by more complex sequences—for example, increased susceptibility to factors detrimental to multiplication or functional growth of β-cells.

This gradual process of increasing resistance to insulin action, followed by first increased and then decreased function of the insulin-producing β-cells, may well serve to explain the clinically amply documented gradual yet continuous deterioration of glucose tolerance in the patients with obesity who are likely to end by developing overt diabetes. Also consistent with this hypothesis is the long-maintained capacity of patients with overweight and as yet modest glucose intolerance to revert to normal glucose tolerance after significant weight loss. It should nevertheless be understood that the detailed mechanisms underlying these still descriptive and empirical sequences are far from clear. Thus, the mechanism of resistance to insulin action is still unknown, and whether the same mechanism is likely to be operative in all insulin-sensitive tissues, or whether different insulin-sensitive tissues vary as to the severity and/or mechanism of obesity-related resistance, is also unknown. Similarly, the nature of the apparent relationship between hyperinsulinism and resistance to insulin action remains to be clarified and, finally, both the nature and the time course of the still largely hypothetical mechanism(s) leading to "exhaustion of β-cell function" are mysterious at best.

These general considerations have served to introduce the subject of what we presently know—or do not know—about the pathogenetic mechanisms of interrelations of obesity and diabetes. We will now analyze in somewhat greater detail the two principal components that must be accounted for before any semblance of understanding of the pathogenesis involved can be reached. These two components are (1) resistance to insulin action and (2) elevation of circulating "insulin" (IRI and/or ILA) levels in serum.

Resistance to Insulin Action

The decreased effectiveness of endogenous as well as exogenous insulin in tissues of obese subjects was described first indirectly (as already discussed) but then promptly and directly at the organ and tissue level in humans. Thus:

1. Localized studies, including the measurement of organ blood flow and of arteriovenous concentration differences across the organ, have established that in forearm tissues of obese individuals insulin is less effective on glucose uptake, potassium uptake, and the release of free fatty acids and branched-chain amino acids (Rabinowitz and Zierler, 1962; Butterfield et al., 1965; Sims et al., 1973);
2. Catheterization studies have also revealed resistance to insulin action in liver of obese subjects (Felig and Wahren, 1975);
3. Adipose cells and slices from biopsies of adipose tissue obtained from obese subjects for incubation *in vitro* demonstrated marked resistance to the action of insulin (Englhardt et al., 1971; Sims et al., 1973; Smith, 1970; Salans et al., 1968);
4. Insulin resistance demonstrated by the direct means described in either forearm tissues (Butterfield and Whichelow, 1968) or isolated adipocytes (Salans et al., 1968; Olefsky et al., 1974) could be improved toward normal or abolished entirely by prior weight reduction.

Although these observations fully confirm, directly on tissues, the general concept of resistance to insulin action concurrent with obesity, two important qualifications must be added. It has so far been impossible to obtain data demonstrating precisely and over a wide range a quantitative relationship between the measured degree of adiposity and the measured severity of tissue resistance to insulin action. Also, evidence for a quantitative relationship between measured insulin resistance and measured decrease in carbohydrate tolerance is similarly variable. The present interpretation of these limitations leads us to conclude that although reversible resistance to insulin action is a part of the endocrine metabolic syndrome of obesity, this resistance cannot by itself serve to explain all anomalies of carbohydrate tolerance observed in different obese individuals.

What, specifically, is the mechanism of insulin resistance in obesity? We shall first dispose of the less likely hypotheses: since decreased responsiveness to insulin may be demonstrated equally well when the variable is endogenous serum insulin activity or when it is administered exogenous insulin, secretion of an abnormal insulin molecule in obesity is unlikely; similarly, the parallel demonstration of resistance to the hormone of tissues normally situated *in vivo* and of tissues incubated *in vitro*, even after dispersion into single cells, speaks strongly against a major role for circulating antagonists to insulin action. Metabolic antagonists, such as fatty acids and ketone bodies, do interfere with glucose oxidation in a variety of tissues (Randle et al., 1966; Cuendet et al., 1975; Berger et al., 1976), but the production or concentrations of these lipid metabolites in obesity (especially in normoglycemic but nonetheless hyperinsulinemic obese subjects) is often in the normal range or, at least, not increased to any major extent. Furthermore, a direct inhibition of glucose uptake by these metabolites is exerted only on a rather limited part of the insulin-sensitive body mass, as recently demonstrated by Berger et al. (1976).

Most available evidence presently favors a cell-based reduction of sensitivity to insulin action; accordingly, the most likely (and most recently fashionable) proposed mechanism involves one or several types of disturbance of the interaction between insulin and its receptor(s) on, or in, the plasma cell membrane. Additional factors may include some of those which have just been ruled out as principal or major factors—for example, intracellular disturbances of the metabolic flow of substrates, with resulting accumulation of normal and possibly abnormal metabolites of glucose and/or other nutrients (Olefsky, 1976). We refer here to the extensive review by Reaven and Olefsky (Chap. 7), especially as related to differences in the genesis of resistance in different tissues.

How does resistance to insulin action relate, directly or indirectly, to hypersecretion of insulin? Although it may seem logical that resistance to the effectiveness of an essential biological messenger should result in hypertrophy of the messenger's production system (as in the case of hypertrophy of muscles that need to overcome greater resistance), the fact remains that a suitable signal must be identified in each instance before this type of response may be seriously considered.

For obesity with insulin resistance, several possible signals that might result in increased secretory activity of β-cells have been suggested; for example, a self-sensed enlargement of individual adipocytes (Stern and Hirsch, 1972), or increased blood levels of substrates or metabolites, especially free fatty acids, glucose, or certain amino acids, including the branched-chain ones (Opie and Walfish, 1963; Felig et al., 1969; Rabinowitz, 1970). These might indeed be suitable signals, but a satisfactory correlation of any one of the indices with increased insulin secretion, or even with increased serum concentrations of the hormone, has not yet been seen. It is conceivable that continuous 24 hr monitoring of blood glucose and insulin levels (Thum et al., 1975) might yield differences in blood glucose sufficiently small, and sufficiently brief but also repetitive, to be effective and yet easy to miss; such small but repetitive elevations may yield the one likely signal for hyperinsulinism in obesity. On the other hand, Streja et al. (1977) measured glucose turnover rates in grossly obese patients and reported that they are within the normal range. For the time being, therefore, we are forced to conclude that the search must continue for a signal able to carry to the pancreatic islets the information that insulin resistance is operative and that insulin production must be increased.

Hyperinsulinism

When considering pathogenetic mechanisms in obesity and diabetes, one of the unanswered questions is what comes first as overweight becomes established—resistance to insulin action or hyperinsulinism. In the preceding section, this relationship has been discussed from the more traditional standpoint that resistance to insulin action probably comes first. It is becoming increasingly clear, however, that there is no definitive evidence to support that view. Indeed, more recent observations suggest that hypersecretion of insulin and elevated concentrations of the circulating hormone induce *decreased* sensitivity of responsive tissues to insulin (Roth et al., 1977); this concept receives support from the probable decrease in the number of insulin-binding sites ("receptor" sites) observed after prolonged hyperinsulinemia. Again, the reader is referred to Chap. 7 for a more complete discussion of the topic. It may also be worth recalling that resistance to insulin action (with carbohydrate intolerance) has been induced by long-term infusion of exogenous insulin to humans (Fineberg and Merimee, 1974) and repeated subcutaneous insulin injections in rats (Sagalnik et al., 1974). Similarly, we will briefly discuss in the next section the observation that the diminished sensitivity to endogenous or exogenous insulin seen in certain genetic obesity syndromes of mice may be restored to normal by inhibiting pancreatic insulin secretion with appropriate (low) doses of β-cytotoxic agents.

If it becomes likely that hyperinsulinemia indeed comes first in obesity, and resistance to insulin action second, it is also evident that emphasis must shift to understanding just what is the primary cause of hyperinsulinemia in the obese. At present there is no convincing evidence for delayed metabolic breakdown of insulin in the obese human or mouse (Genuth, 1970; Coore and Westman, 1970). Persistent hyperinsulinemia must therefore result from increased secretion of the hormone, either because of hypertrophy or because of hyperplasia of the β-cell system. The mechanisms that might be involved are many, and some of them have been reviewed by Mahler (1974). They include increases in the circulating levels of other hormones; increased availability of substrates, probably combined with nutritionally induced hyperresponsiveness; genetically or environmentally induced hyperresponsiveness of the insulinogenic β-cells, with or without overnutrition and with or without participation of the autonomic nervous system; decreased levels of inhibitors of insulin secretion (Patel et al., 1976); and increased production of gastrointestinal hormones (Ebert et al., 1976), at least some of which are, and many more may be β-cytotropic.

Well-controlled experimental studies that result in the imposed production of obesity in human subjects without a spontaneous tendency to obesity are, of course, rare. Accordingly, considerable attention has been focused on the studies by Sims, Horton, and their collaborators (Sims et al., 1968, 1971, 1973, 1974) in which significant overweight was induced by gross overfeeding, accepted over periods of months. Some carbohydrate intolerance was induced, as well as most hormonal and metabolic features usually associated with spontaneous human obesity; also, all of these indices reverted to normal when the forced hypercaloric nutrition ceased, with prompt return (over 2 or 3 wk) to each volunteer's original normal weight. In general terms, therefore, we may presently assume that overnutrition, at least relative overnutrition, is the primary factor concerned with the induction, possibly adaptive, of excess adiposity, hyperinsulinism, and tissue resistance to insulin action. When our understanding progresses, it is likely that the primary pathogenetic event will be associated with overnutrition, perhaps as a result of faulty control of appetite and satiety at the level of the hypothalamus, as presently assumed for at least two of the best studied genetic obesities associated with glucose intolerance in mice.

PATHOGENETIC MECHANISMS IN LABORATORY RODENTS WITH ADIPOSITY AND HYPERGLYCEMIA

Within the scope of this chapter, the pathogenetic mechanisms so far explored in laboratory animals with obesity and hyperglycemia do represent a separate topic since they have been both intensively studied and extensively reviewed (Renold, 1968; Stauffacher et al., 1971; Cameron et al., 1972; Herberg and Coleman, 1977).

A striking feature is that, as in humans, hyperinsulinism (here usually associated with gross hyperplasia of the islets of Langerhans—primarily of their β-cells) and resistance to insulin action are very clearly associated. In the instance studied so far, there is also association of hyperinsulinemia and decreased cell surface density of receptors for insulin. Hyperphagia, at least during the early or active phase of weight gain, is of considerable importance in the mouse disorders, and an especially dynamic area of investigation concerns the possible role of other endocrine cells, either in the intestinal mucosa or in the pancreas.

Finally, Herberg and Coleman (1977) most appropriately ended their recent review as follows:

> Based on the clear association of hyperphagia and obesity in all of these mutants with the subsequent development of diabetes, we suggest that those pathways involved in hormonal influences over feeding behavior may be the most effective areas to probe in ensuring studies with other animal models and human obesity and diabetes. It is hoped that these detailed studies, also covering hypothalamic feeding mechanisms, will stimulate further investigations on other animal species and provide knowledge of the interaction of hyperphagia and obesity on the development and pathogenesis of diabetes in humans.

REFERENCES

Abrams, M. E., Jarrett, R. J., Keen, H., Boyns, D. R. and Crossley, J. N. 1969. Oral glucose tolerance and related factors in a normal population sample. II. Interrelationship of glycerides, cholesterol and other factors with the glucose and insulin response. *Br. Med. J.* 1:599–602.

Albrink, M. J. and Meigs, J. W. 1964. Interrelationship between skinfold thickness, serum lipids and blood sugar in normal men. *Am. J. Clin. Nutr.* 15:255–261.

Allen, F. M. 1917. The role of fat in diabetes. *Am. J. Med. Sci.* 153:360–373.

Allison, R. S. 1927. Carbohydrate tolerance in overweight and obesity. *Lancet* 1:537–540.

Bagdade, J. D., Bierman, E. L. and Porte, D., Jr. 1967. The significance of basal insulin levels in the evaluation of the insulin response to glucose in diabetic and nondiabetic subjects. *J. Clin. Invest.* 46:1549–1557.

Baird, J. D. 1972. Diet and the development of clinical diabetes. *Acta Diabetol. Lat.* 9 (Suppl. 1):621–639.

Bennett, P. H., Rushforth, N. B., Miller, M. and Lacompte, P. M. 1976. *Recent Prog. Horm. Res.* 32:333–376.

Berchtold, P., Berger, M., Greiser, E., Dohse, M., Irmscher, K., Gries, F. A. and Zimmerman, H. 1977. Cardiovascular risk factors in obesity. *Int. J. Obesity* 1:219–229.

Berger, M., Baumhoff, E. and Gries, F. A. 1975. Effect of weight reduction upon glucose tolerance in obesity. A follow up study of five years. In *Recent advances in obesity research,* ed. A. Howard, vol. 1, pp. 128–130. London: Newman.

Berger, M., Hagg, S. A., Goodman, M. N. and Ruderman, N. B. 1976. Glucose metabolism in perfused skeletal muscle. *Biochem. J.* 158:191–202.

Bielschowsky, M. and Bielschowsky, F. 1953. A new strain of mice with hereditary obesity. *Proc. Univ. Otago Med. Sch.* 31:29–31.

Bierman, E. L., Bagdade, J. D. and Porte, D. Jr. 1968. Obesity and diabetes: The odd couple. *Am. J. Clin. Nutr.* 21:1434–1437.

Björntorp, P., Berchtold, P. and Tiblin, G. 1971. Insulin secretion in relation to adipose tissue in man. *Diabetes* 20:65–70.

Bouchardat, A. 1875. De la glycosurie au diabète sucré. Paris: Gerner-Baillière.

Butterfield, W. J. H. and Whichelow, M. J. 1968. Fenfluramine and muscle glucose uptake in man. *Lancet* 2:109 (letter).

Butterfield, W. J. H., Hanley, T. and Whichelow, M. J. 1965. Peripheral metabolism of glucose and free fatty acids during oral glucose tolerance tests. *Metabolism* 14:851–864.

Cameron, D. P., Stauffacher, W. and Renold, A. E. 1972. Spontaneous hyperglycemia and obesity in laboratory rodents. In *Handbook of Physiology,* Sect. 7: *Endocrinology,* Vol. 1: *Endocrine pancreas,* eds. D. F. Steiner, N. Freinkel, and S. R. Geiger, pp. 611–625, American Physiological Society, Washington, D.C.

Chiumello, G., Del Guercio, M. J., Carnelutti, M. and Bidone, G. 1969. Relationship between obesity, chemical diabetes and beta pancreatic function in children. *Diabetes* 18:238–243.

Claussen, F., Jahnke, K., Daweke, H., Liebermeister, H. and Oberdisse, K. 1970. Diabetesmorbidität in einer soziologisch definierten Bevölkerungsgruppe (Bäckermeister einer Grosstadt). *Dtsch. Med. Wochenschr.* 95:431–437.

Comstock, G. W., Kendrick, M. A. and Livesay, V. T. 1966. Subcutaneous fatness and mortality. *Am. J. Epidemiol.* 83:548–563.

Coore, H. G. and Westman, S. 1970. Disappearance of serum insulin in obese hyperglycemic mice. *Acta Physiol. Scand.* 78:274–279.

Cuendet, G. S., Loten, E. G. and Renold, A. E. 1975. Evidence that the glucose fatty acid cycle is operative in isolated skeletal (soleus) muscle. *Diabetologia* 11:336 (abstract)

Cuenot, L. 1905. Les races pures et leurs combinaisons chez les souris. *Arch. Zool. T.* 3:123–132.

Danforth, C. H. 1927. Hereditary adiposity in mice. *J. Hered.* 18:153–162.

Dublin, L. I. and Marks, H. H. 1952. Mortality among insured overweights in recent years. *Trans. Assoc. Life Ins. Med. Dir. Am.* 35:235–266.

Duncan, G. C., Duncan, T. G. and Schatanoff, J. 1968. Refractory obesity and diabetes. *Ann. N.Y. Acad. Sci.* 148:906–913.

Dyer, A. R., Stamler, J., Berkson, D. M. and Lindberg, H. A. 1975. Relationship of relative weight and body mass index to 14-year mortality in the Chicago Peoples Gas Company study. *J. Chronic Dis.* 28:109–123.

Ebert, R., Willms, B., Brown, J. C. and Creutzfeldt, W. 1976. Serum gastric inhibitory polypeptide (GIP) levels in obese subjects and after weight reduction. *Eur. J. Clin. Invest.* 6:327 (abstract)

El-Khodary, A. Z., Ball, M. F., Oweiss, I. M. and Canary, J. J. 1972. Insulin secretion and body composition in obesity. *Metabolism* 21:641–655.

Englhardt, A., Kasperek, R., Liebermeister, H. and Jahnke, K. 1971. Studies on glucose utilization and insulin responsiveness of human subcutaneous adipose tissue in obese and non-obese subjects. *Horm. Metab. Res.* 3:266–272.

Eriksen, M., Deckert, T. and Hansen, P. F. 1970. Glucosetolerans his 70 öarige personer. *Nord. Med.* 83:748–753.

Eschwege, E., Rosselin, G., Lellouch, J., Vallerón, A. J., Claude, J. R., Warnet, J. M. and Richard, J. L. 1974. Epidemiological study of adipose mass in a population of men in their fifties: Relationship to glucose, lipid, insulin, growth hormone and cortisol levels. *Excerpta Med. Int. Congr. Ser.* no. 315, p. 208–214.

Feldman, R., Sender, H. J. and Siegelaub, A. B. 1969. Difference in diabetic and non-diabetic fat distribution patterns by skinfold measurements. *Diabetes* 18:478–486.

Felig, P. and Wahren, J. 1975. The liver as site of insulin and glucagon action in normal, diabetic and obese humans. *Isr. J. Med. Sci.* 11:528–539.

Felig, P., Marliss, E. and Cahill, G. F., Jr. 1969. Plasma amino acid levels and insulin secretion in obesity. *N. Engl. J. Med.* 281:811–816.

Fineberg, S. E. and Merimee, T. J. 1974. The effects of hyperinsulinism upon insulin sensitivity. *Clin. Res.* 22:467A.

Genuth, S. M. 1970. Metabolic clearance and delivery rates of insulin in man. *Diabetes* 19:367–368.

Gibson, T. C., Horton, E. S. and Whorton, E. B. 1975. Interrelationships of insulin, glucose, lipid and anthropometric data in a natural population. *Am. J. Clin. Nutr.* 28:1387–1394.

Godlowsky, Z. 1946. Carbohydrate metabolism in obesity. *Edinburgh Med. J.* 53:574–582.

Goto, Y., Nakayama, Y. and Yagi, T. 1958. Influence of World War II food shortage on the incidence of diabetes mellitus in Japan. *Diabetes* 7:133–135.

Grönberg, A., Larsson, T. and Jung, J. 1967. Diabetes in Sweden. A clinico-statistical, epidemiological and genetic study of hospital patients and death certificates. *Acta Med. Scand. Suppl. 477.*

Grott, J. W., Marzec, L., Grintowt-Dziwill, W., Korzon, J., Pieter, R., Poskuta, W. and Zurkowski, J. W. 1962. La fréquence du diabète et de l'état prédiabétique chez 1000 personnes à 40 ans passés, obèses ou prédisposées à l'obésité. *Diabète* 10:5–13.

Herberg, L. and Coleman, D. L. 1977. Laboratory animals exhibiting obesity and diabetes syndromes. *Metabolism* 26:59–99.

Himsworth, H. P. 1949. Diet in the etiology of human diabetes. *Proc. R. Soc. Med.* 42:323–326.

Ingalls, A. M., Dickie, M. M. and Snell, G. D. 1950. Obese, a new mutation in the house mouse. *J. Hered.* 41:317–318.

Jackson, W. P. V. 1972. Diabetes and related variables among the five main racial groups in South Africa; comparisons from population studies. *Postgrad. Med. J.* 48:391–398.

John, H. J. 1929. A summary of the findings in 1100 glucose tolerance estimations. *Endocrinology* 13:388–392.

John, H. J. 1950. Statistical study of 6000 cases of diabetes. *Ann. Intern. Med.* 33:925–940.

Joslin, E. P., Dublin, L. J. and Marks, H. H. 1936. Studies in diabetes mellitus IV. Etiology. Part II. *Am. J. Med. Sci.* 192:9–23.

Kalkhoff, R. K., Kim, H. J., Cerletty, J. and Ferrou, C. A. 1971. Metabolic effects of weight loss in obese subjects: Changes in plasma substrate levels, insulin and growth hormone responses. *Diabetes* 20:83–91.

Kannel, W. B., Pearson, G. and McNamara, P. M. 1970. Obesity as a force of morbidity and mortality in adolescents. In *Nutrition and growth,* ed. F. P. Heald, p. 51. New York: Appleton-Century-Crofts.

Karam, J. H., Grodsky, G. M. and Forsham, P. H. 1963. Excessive insulin response to glucose in obese subjects as measured by immunochemical assay. *Diabetes* 12:197–204.

Keen, H. 1975. The incomplete story of obesity and diabetes. 1975. In *Recent advances in obesity research,* ed. A. Howard, vol. 1, pp. 116–127. London: Newman.

Keys, A. and Grande, F. 1973. Body weight, body composition and caloric status. In *Modern nutrition in health and disease,* eds. R. S. Goodhart and M. E. Shils, pp. 1–27. Philadelphia: Lea & Febiger.

Kipnis, D. M. 1970. Does diabetes begin with insulin resistance? In *Pathogenesis of diabetes mellitus,* eds. E. Cerasi and R. Luft. *Proceedings of the 13th Nobel Symposium,* pp. 45–46. Stockholm: Almquist and Wiksell.

Knowles, H. C. 1968. Prevalence and development of diabetes. *Fed. Proc.* 27:945–947.

Kreisberg, R. A., Boshell, B. R., Di Placido, J. and Roddam, R. F. 1967. Insulin secretion in obesity. *N. Engl. J. Med.* 276:314–319.

Lanceraux, E. 1880. Etude comparative du diabète maigre et du diabète gras. *Union Med. Paris* 39:161.

Lancet. 1977. The beta cell in diabetes—More sinned against than sinning? *Lancet* 1:177–178 (editorial).

Lataste, F. 1883. Trois questions. Naturaliste. *Bull Sci. Dip Nord* 7–8:364.

Mahler, R. J. 1974. The pathogenesis of pancreatic islet cell hyperplasia and insulin insensitivity in obesity. *Adv. Metab. Disord.* 7:213–241.

Martin, M. M. and Martin, A. L. A. 1973. Obesity, hyperinsulinism, and diabetes mellitus in childhood. *J. Paediatr.* 83:192–201.

Medalie, J. H., Papier, C. M., Goldbourt, N. and Herman, J. D. 1975. Major factors in the development of diabetes mellitus in 10,000 men. *Arch. Intern. Med.* 135:811–817.

Medley, D. R. K. 1965. The relationship between diabetes and obesity: A study of susceptibility to diabetes in obese people. *Q. J. Med.* 34:111–132.

Mouratoff, G. J., Carroll, N. V. and Scott, E. M. 1967. Diabetes mellitus in Eskimos. *J. Am. Med. Assoc.* 199:107–112.

Newburgh, L. H. 1942. Control of the hyperglycemia of the obese "diabetics" by weight reduction. *Ann. Intern. Med.* 17:935–942.

Newburgh, L. H. and Conn, J. W. 1939. New interpretation of hyperglycemia in obese middle aged persons. *J. Am. Med. Assoc.* 112:7–11.

Ogilvie, R. F. 1933. The islands of Langerhans in 19 cases of obesity. *J. Pathol. Bacteriol.* 37:473–481.

Ogilvie, R. F. 1935. Sugar tolerance in obese subjects. A review of 64 cases. *Q. J. Med.* 4:345–358.

Olefsky, J. M. 1976. The insulin receptor: Its role in insulin resistance of obesity and diabetes. *Diabetes* 25:1154–1162.

Olefsky, J. M., Farquhar, J. W. and Reaven, G. M. 1974. The effects of weight reduction on obesity: Studies of carbohydrate and lipid metabolism in normal and hyperlipoproteinaemic subjects. *J. Clin. Invest.* 53:64–76.

Opie, L. H. and Walfish, P. G. 1963. Plasma free fatty acid concentrations in obesity. *N. Engl. J. Med.* 268:757–760.

O'Sullivan, J. B. 1969. Population retested for diabetes after 17 years: New prevalence study in Oxford, Massachusetts. *Diabetologia* 5:211–214.

Paffenbarger, R. S. and Wing, A. L. 1973. Chronic disease in former college students. XII. Early precursors of adult-onset diabetes mellitus. *Am. J. Epidemiol.* 97:314–322.

Patel, Y. C., Orci, L., Bankier, A. and Cameron, D. P. 1976. Decreased pancreatic somatostatin (SRIF) concentration in spontaneously diabetic mice. *Endocrinology* 99:1415–1418.

Paullin, J. E. and Sauls, H. C. 1922. A study of the glucose tolerance test in the obese. *South. Med. J.* 15:249–253.

Paulsen, E. P., Richendorfer, L. and Ginsberg-Fellner, F. 1968. Plasma glucose, free fatty acids, and immunoreactive insulin in sixty-six obese children. *Diabetes* 17:261–269.

Perley, M. J. and Kipnis, D. M. 1966. Plasma insulin responses to glucose and tolbutamide of normal weight and obese diabetic and non-diabetic subjects. *Diabetes* 15:867–874.

Pfeiffer, E. F. 1974. Obesity, islet function and diabetes mellitus. *Horm. Metab. Res. Suppl.* 4:143–152.

Pyke, D. A. and Please, N. W. 1957. Obesity, parity, diabetes. *J. Endocrinol.* 15:26–33.

Rabinowitz, D. 1970. Some endocrine and metabolic aspects of obesity. *Annu. Rev. Med.* 21:241–258.

Rabinowitz, D. and Zierler, K. L. 1962. Forearm metabolism in obesity and its response to intra-arterial insulin. Characterization of insulin resistance, i.e. evidence for adaptive hyperinsulinism. *J. Clin. Invest.* 41:2173–2181.

Randle, P. J., Garland, P. B., Hales, C. N., Newsholme, E. A., Denton, R. M. and Pogson, C. I. 1966. Interactions of metabolism and the physiological role of insulin. *Recent Prog. Horm. Res.* 22:1–43.

Reid, D. D., Brett, G. Z., Hamilton, P. J. S., Jarrett, R. J., Keen, H. and Rose, G. 1974. Cardiorespiratory disease and diabetes among middle-aged civil servants. A study of screening and intervention. *Lancet* 1:469–473.

Renold, A. E. 1968. Spontaneous diabetes and/or obesity in laboratory rodents. *Adv. Metab. Disord.* 3:49–84.

Roth, J., Neville, D. M., Kahn, C. R. and Gorden, P. 1977. Hormone resistance and hormone sensitivity. *N. Engl. J. Med.* 296:277–278.

Sagalnik, R. F., Merrtvetsov, N. P., Gordienko, D. E., Chesuskov, V. N. and Semensva, L. A. 1974. Impairment of induction of glycolytic enzymes and development of insulin resistance in rats as a result of continuous insulin treatment. *Acta Endocrinol. (Kbhn.)* 76:319–337.

Salans, L. B., Knittle, J. L. and Hirsch, J. 1968. The role of adipose cell size and adipose tissue insulin sensitivity in the carbohydrate tolerance of human obesity. *J. Clin. Invest.* 47:153–165.

Samaan, W. and Fraser, R. 1963. "Typical" and "atypical" serum insulin-like activity in untreated diabetes mellitus. *Lancet* 2:311–314.

Schade, D. S. and Eaton, R. P. 1974. Role of insulin and glucagon in obesity. *Diabetes* 23:657–661.

Schliack, V. 1954. Mangelernährung und Diabetesmorbidität. Untersuchungen and 11294 Diabetikern. *Z. Klin. Med.* 151:382–396.

Sims, E. A. H., Goldman, R. F., Gluck, C. M., Horton, E. S., Kelleher, P. C. and Rowe, D. W. 1968. Experimental obesity in man. *Trans. Assoc. Am. Physicians* 81:153–170.

Sims, E. A. H., Horton, E. S. and Salans, L. B. 1971. Inducible metabolic abnormalities during the development of obesity. *Annu. Rev. Med.* 22:235–250.

Sims, E. A. H., Danforth, E., Jr., Horton, E. S., Bray, G. A., Glennon, J. A. and Salans, L. B. 1973. Endocrine and metabolic effects of experimental obesity in man. *Recent Prog. Horm. Res.* 29:457–496.

Sims, E. A. H., Bray, G. A., Danforth, E., Jr., Glennon, J. A., Horton, E. S., Salans, L. B. and O'Connell, M. 1974. Experimental obesity in man. VI: The effect of variations in intake of carbohydrate on carbohydrate, lipid, and cortisol metabolism. *Horm. Metab. Res. Suppl.* 4:70–77.

Smith, U. 1970. Insulin responsiveness and lipid synthesis in human fat cells of different sizes: Effect of the incubation medium. *Biochim. Biophys. Acta* 218:417–423.

Stauffacher, W., Orci, L., Cameron, D. P., Burr, I. M. and Renold, A. E. 1971. Spontaneous hyperglycemia and/or obesity in laboratory rodents. An example of the possible usefulness of animal disease models with both genetic and environmental components. *Recent. Prog. Horm. Res.* 27:41–95.

Stern, J. S. and Hirsch, J. 1972. Obesity and pancreatic function. In *Handbook of physiology*, Sect. 7: *Endocrinology*, vol. 1, pp. 641–651. Washington, D.C.: American Physiological Society.

Streja, D. A., Steiner, G., Marliss, E. B. and Vranic, M. 1977. The turnover and recycling of glucose in man during prolonged fasting. *Metabolism*, in press.

Tattersall, R. B. and Fajans, S. S. 1975. A difference between the inheritance of clinical juvenile-onset and maturity onset type diabetes of young people. *Diabetes* 24:44–53.

Tattersall, R. B. and Pyke, D. A. 1973. Growth in diabetic children: Studies in identical twins. *Lancet* 2:1105–1109.

Thum, Ch., Laube, H., Schröder, K. E., Raptis, S. and Pfeiffer, E. F. 1975. Das kontinuierliche Blutzuckertagesprofil in Korrelation zum Seruminsulin bei idealgewichtigen und normalgewichtigen Stoffwechselgesunden. *Dtsch. Med. Wochensch.* 100:1595–1599.

Tyner, J. D. 1933. The prediabetic state: Its relation to obesity and to diabetic heredity. *Am. J. Med. Sci.* 185:704–710.

Vague, J. 1950. The value of measurement of adipose tissue distribution in pathology. *Bull. Soc. Med. Hop. Paris* 66:1572–1574.

Vague, J. 1956. The degree of masculine differentiation of obesities, a factor determining predisposition to diabetes, atherosclerosis, gout and uric calculous disease. *Am. J. Clin. Nutr.* 4:20–34.

Vague, J., Vague, P., Boyer, J. and Cloix, M. C. 1971. Anthropometry of obesity, diabetes, adrenal and beta-cell functions. *Excerpta Med. Int. Congr. Ser.* 231:517–525.

Weinsier, R. L., Fuchs, R. J., Kay, T. D., Triebwasser, J. H. and Lancaster, M. C. 1976. Body fat: Its relationship to coronary heart disease, blood pressure, lipids and other risk factors measured in a large male population. *Am. J. Med.* 61:815–824.

West, K. M. 1972. Epidemiologic evidence linking nutritional factors to the prevalence and manifestations of diabetes. *Acta Diabetol. Lat.* 9 (Suppl. 1):405–431.

West, K. M. 1974. Epidemiology of adiposity. *Excerpta Med. Int. Congr. Ser.* no. 315, p. 201–207.

Chapter 7

ROLE OF INSULIN RESISTANCE IN THE PATHOGENESIS OF HYPERGLYCEMIA

Gerald M. Reaven and Jerrold M. Olefsky
Department of Medicine
Stanford University
Stanford, California

INTRODUCTION

Under normal conditions the fasting plasma glucose concentration is maintained within a relatively narrow range, and the elevations of plasma glucose that follow eating are relatively transitory. Euglycemia is maintained through an intricate series of relationships between circulating hormones and substrates and complex enzymatic systems in a variety of organs. Failure of this system can result in the appearance of either hypoglycemia or hyperglycemia, and our ability both to detect the presence of these abnormalities and to define the mechanisms responsible for their development is reasonably well advanced. In general, hypoglycemia occurs relatively rarely, possibly because the impact of this phenomenon on the organism is so devastating. On the other hand, an abnormal degree of hyperglycemia, either fasting or postprandial, is not uncommon. Of all the factors responsible for preventing hyperglycemia, insulin is probably the most potent, and it is tempting to always view the development of hyperglycemia as indicative of a failure of insulin secretion. However, it is now apparent that hyperglycemia can occur in a variety of different situations in which the rate of insulin secretion is not diminished. Consequently, one can only continue to maintain that insulin deficiency plays the central role by modifying the above generalization to state that hyperglycemia is always due to insulin deficiency, either absolute *or* relative. Although this formulation is true by definition, we are not sure it is useful. The fact that hyperglycemia can occur in the absence of an absolute deficiency of insulin leads to the obvious conclusion that in these situations the hyperglycemia must be at least partly due to a defect in the effectiveness of the circulating insulin. Continuing to view these conditions as being due to a relative deficiency of insulin simply seems to focus attention away from efforts aimed at defining the mechanism by which hyperglycemia can develop in situations characterized by normal or increased rates of insulin secretion.

In this chapter we review the evidence that resistance to the action of insulin exists in a variety of clinical situations. For this purpose we have chosen to discuss the role of insulin resistance in the glucose intolerance of obesity, nonketotic diabetes mellitus, chronic renal failure, and states of adrenal corticoid excess. We have selected these four conditions because they present common situations in which insulin resistance seems to play a role in the pathogenesis of hyperglycemia. In addition to presenting the evidence that implicates resistance to insulin as the cause of the hyperglycemia in these four conditions, we will attempt to summarize current thinking as to the mechanism(s) responsible for the insulin resistance.

OBESITY

A relationship between obesity and deterioration of glucose tolerance has been known for many years (Smith and Levine, 1964; Berkowitz, 1964). For example, a high incidence of abnormal glucose tolerance is found in obese subjects (Smith and Levine, 1964; Berkowitz, 1964), and the degree of diabetes is exaggerated by weight gain and improved by weight loss (Sims et al., 1968; Farrant et al., 1969; Kalkhoff et al., 1971; Knittle and Ginsberg-Fellner, 1972; Kosaka et al., 1972; Hewing et al., 1973; Olefsky et al., 1974). Although this effect on plasma glucose levels is well known, obesity has a more striking impact on plasma insulin levels. In 1963, Karam et al. first recognized this important association. These workers found excessive plasma insulin levels in ten nondiabetic obese patients following ingestion of oral glucose, and concluded that "obese subjects require increased amounts of insulin to maintain normal glucose levels." Bagdade et al. (1967) also found that obese subjects were hyperinsulinemic, but in addition focused attention on the relationship between the degree of obesity and the degree of elevation of the basal insulin level. Extensive evidence has accrued since these studies to document the fact that obesity in humans and animals is associated with increased insulin secretion (Kreisberg et al., 1967; Sims et al., 1968; Farrant et al., 1969; Kalkhoff et al., 1971; Frohman et al., 1972; Kosaka et al., 1972; York et al., 1972; Olefsky et al., 1974).

The dual observations of hyperglycemia and hyperinsulinemia indicate an insulin-resistant state. Insulin resistance has been widely described in obesity, in both animals and humans, and the first direct studies on this subject were carried out by Rabinowitz and Zierler (1962). Using the forearm perfusion technique to study insulin sensitivity in various groups of patients, these workers found that the administration of intra-arterial insulin had a decreased ability to promote glucose uptake by forearm muscle and adipose tissue in obese patients. Others have confirmed this observation in the overall organism by finding attenuated hypoglycemic responses to exogenous insulin in both humans (Kreisberg et al., 1967; Olefsky et al., 1974) and animals (York et al., 1972).

Mechanisms of Insulin Resistance

In obesity, insulin resistance could theoretically be due to an abnormal β-cell secretory product, circulating insulin antagonists, or tissue insensitivity to insulin's effect. Since resistance to exogenous insulin is seen in obesity, it seems unlikely that the insulin resistance of obesity is related to secretion of abnormal endogenous insulin molecules. The case for a circulating insulin antagonist in obesity has recently been reviewed (Rabinowitz, 1970; Bray et al., 1972). Although slight differences in cortisol (Schteingart et al., 1963) and growth hormone (Roth et al., 1963; Yalow et al., 1965) secretion have been described in obesity, the evidence indicates that this is not responsible for the insulin resistance of this state. Therefore, available information suggests that tissue insulin insensitivity is responsible for the insulin resistance, and this will be the focus of the remainder of this section.

Insulin Receptors

It is well established that the initial step in insulin's cellular action involves binding to specific protein receptors located on the plasma membranes of target tissues (Roth, 1973; Birnbaumer et al., 1974; Cuatrecasas, 1974). Thus, it seems appropriate to begin evaluating the cellular basis for insulin resistance in obesity by focusing on this aspect of insulin's action. In this regard, Kahn et al. (1973a) were the first to study the insulin receptor in obesity. These workers found a striking decrease in insulin binding to liver plasma membranes from the genetically obese (ob/ob) mouse. This decrease in binding was entirely accounted for by a decreased number of insulin receptor sites, and this was true whether plasma membranes or isolated hepatocytes were used. A variety of control studies were performed to further clarify this phenomenon. For example, since these obese animals were hyperinsulinemic, it was possible that *in vivo* occupancy of receptors led to "masking" of binding sites during the *in vitro* assay. However, this proved not to be the case since liver membranes prepared from lean mice who had been injected with pharmacologic amounts of insulin 60 min prior to sacrifice showed normal insulin binding. Subsequent work from the same group (Soll et al., 1975b) has demonstrated that although fewer in number the insulin receptors of the ob/ob mouse are functionally normal. Decreased insulin receptors have also been found in fat (Freychet et al., 1972), cardiac muscle (Freychet and Forgue, 1975), and lymphoid (Soll et al., 1974) tissue from the ob/ob mouse.

Decreased insulin receptors have also been found in a wide variety of other obese states in both animals and humans. Thus, decreased insulin receptors have been found in liver membranes from mice made obese by hypothalamic injection of gold thioglucose (Soll et al., 1975a); in adipocytes (Olefsky and Reaven, 1975; Olefsky, 1976a; L. Lesko et al., submitted), adipocyte membranes (Robinson et al., 1972), liver membranes (Freeman et al., 1973), and skeletal muscle (Olefsky et al., 1976) from old, spontaneously obese rats; and in circulating monocytes (Archer et al., 1973, 1975; Olefsky, 1976b; Bar et al., 1977) and isolated adipocytes (Marinetti et al., 1972; Olefsky, 1976b; Harrison et al., 1976) from obese humans. Thus, decreased insulin binding has been widely described in a variety of obese states.

However, somewhat contrary results have been reported by Amatruda et al. (1975) and Livingston et al. (1972). These workers found that adipocytes from spontaneously obese rats (Livingston et al., 1972) and obese humans (Amatruda et al., 1975) have the same number of insulin receptors as those from lean controls. Although these results seem to be in conflict with all the studies discussed above, it is possible that these differences are more apparent than real. Thus, insulin binding is a membrane phenomenon, and it might be appropriate to express the data in terms of plasma membrane surface area. Following this line of reasoning, adipocytes in obesity become larger and have a greater surface area. Therefore, the data of Livingston et al. and Amatruda et al. show that while adipocytes from obese humans and rats have normal numbers of insulin receptors per cell, they have fewer receptors per unit surface area, and in this sense would be consistent with the concept of decreased insulin binding in obesity.

On the other hand, it has been shown that only hyperinsulinemic insulin-resistant obese patients have decreased insulin receptors (Olefsky, 1976b; Harrison et al., 1976), and that young adult obese patients, with the onset of obesity in childhood, do not demonstrate decreased insulin binding (Olefsky, 1976b). The patients studied by Amatruda et al. (1975) were relatively young (mean age 33 yr), and it is also possible that patient selection contributes to these differences in results. In summary, taking all of the available data from a variety of different species and tissues into account, it seems most probable that in obesity the number of insulin receptors per cell (and certainly per unit of surface area) is decreased. (For another viewpoint on this subject, see Chap. 8.)

Mechanism of Regulation of Receptors

The cause of this decrease in cellular insulin receptors has received considerable attention. The notion that in obesity chronic hyperinsulinemia somehow leads to "adaptive" insulin resistance has been repeatedly suggested in recent years (Rabinowitz, 1970; Grey and Kipnis, 1971; Olefsky et al., 1975a). However, Gavin et al. (1974) were the first investigators to report positive evidence to support this hypothesis. These workers found that high media insulin concentrations led to decreased insulin receptors on cultured human lymphocytes. They further suggested that *in vivo* the plasma insulin concentration inversely regulates the number of cellular insulin receptors, and that in obesity the hyperinsulinemia causes the decreased insulin binding. Results consistent with this hypothesis have been reported by Bar et al. (1977), Olefsky (1976b), and Harrison et al. (1976), who found a highly significant inverse relationship between the plasma insulin concentration and insulin receptors in obesity.

On the other hand, this inverse association does not prove causality, and the alternative hypothesis cannot be excluded—that is, that a primary decrease in insulin receptors leads to insulin resistance and subsequent hyperinsulinemia. Nevertheless, there is considerable information in support of the hypothesis that insulin regulates its own receptors (Gavin et al., 1974; Soll et al., 1975a; Olefsky, 1976b; Bar et al., 1977; Harrison et al., 1976), and Kosmakos and Roth (1976) have shown that this "down regulation" requires intact intracellular metabolic machinery. On the other hand, situations do exist in which hyperinsulinemia occurs without a reduction in receptors [e.g., acromegaly (Archer et al., 1973)]. It has also been shown that receptors change in the absence of a corresponding inverse change in plasma insulin levels [hyperthyroidism (Kobayashi and Meek, 1976)]. These studies indicate that factors in addition to the plasma insulin level participate in receptor regulation. Thus, it seems probable that insulin (or more likely a cellular metabolic effect of insulin) is an important regulator of cellular insulin receptors and that additional factors also modulate this process. Clearly much work remains to be done to delineate the exact mechanisms responsible for receptor regulation.

Relationship between Decreased Receptors and Insulin Resistance

Regardless of the mechanism of the decreased insulin binding in obesity, it seems reasonable to suggest that the decreased binding is responsible for the insulin resistance. However, this potential relationship is not as clear as it would seem, since the relationship between insulin receptors and ultimate insulin action is not at all straightforward. Therefore, let us examine the functional consequences, at the cellular level, of a decrease in insulin receptors.

Much of our information on this subject has come from studies on isolated adipocytes. These cells provide a good model for insulin action because they are easy to obtain in a metabolically active state and they readily respond to insulin. For example, it is known that maximal insulin stimulation of glucose metabolism occurs when only a small fraction (about 10%) of adipocyte insulin receptors are occupied (Fig. 1). This was first noted by Kono and Barham (1971) and has subsequently been corroborated by other workers (Gammeltoft and Gliemann, 1973; Olefsky, 1975, 1976b). This "spare receptor" theory holds that cells have more receptors than necessary to elicit maximal responses, but that all of the receptors are potentially fully functional. Thus, it is merely a random statistical event that determines which particular 10% of receptors are occupied at any point in time, and any group of occupied receptors would lead to the same metabolic response.

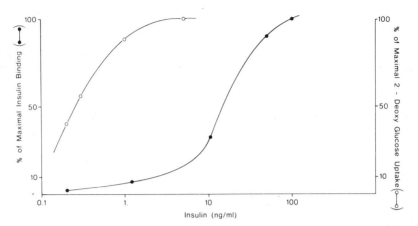

FIGURE 1 Relationship between dose-response curves of insulin binding (●—●) and 2-deoxyglucose uptake (○—○). Open circles represent the percentage of maximal insulin-mediated sugar uptake at the indicated insulin concentrations. Closed circles represent the percentage of maximal specific insulin binding for both groups of cells. For this analysis, maximal insulin binding is taken as the amount of insulin specifically bound at a total insulin concentration of 100 ng/ml (or 2,400 μU/ml) (reprinted from Olefsky, 1975).

Direct experimental evidence in support of this hypothesis has been provided by Gliemann et al. (1975), who found that at an insulin concentration of 0.28 n*M*, adipocytes demonstrated a maximal rate of conversion of glucose to cell lipids, while at 1.4 n*M* insulin the fractional receptor saturation was greater and lipogenesis was the same. On the other hand, when the cells were allowed to equilibrate with these two insulin concentrations and then were placed into insulin-free media, the maximal insulin effect lasted much longer in the cells incubated at the higher insulin concentration, and did not decrease until enough insulin had dissociated from the cells to give a receptor occupancy less than that needed to elicit a maximal insulin response. Further support for the idea that all "spare" receptors are potentially fully functional has been reported by others (Kono and Barham, 1971; Olefsky, 1975, 1976a).

Given this relationship between insulin binding and insulin action, the functional consequence of a decreased number of receptors would be a diminished insulin response only at insulin levels that saturate less than the number of receptors required for a maximal effect, with normal responses to maximally effective insulin levels. Therefore, the result of decreased insulin binding should be simply a shift in the insulin dose-response curve to the right; that is, decreased insulin action at submaximal insulin levels and normal insulin action at maximally effective insulin levels. Such an effect can be seen when a relatively early step of insulin action is measured. Thus, when uptake of the nonmetabolizable sugar 2-deoxyglucose is used to assess glucose transport, a rightward shift in the insulin-glucose transport dose-response curve is found in large adipocytes from older obese rats (Olefsky, 1976a) (Fig. 2). Analogous findings were reported by Czech (1976), who used 3-*O*-methylglucose to assess glucose transport, and by Di Girolamo and Rudman (1968), who found that higher concentrations of insulin were necessary to achieve maximal rates of glucose oxidation in large compared to small adipocytes.

Although higher insulin levels are necessary to reach maximal rates of glucose transport in large adipocytes, the absolute rates of glucose oxidation are always greatly decreased in these cells (Di Girolamo and Rudman, 1968; Salans and Dougherty, 1971; Livingston and Lockwood, 1974; Czech, 1976; Olefsky, 1976a). Therefore, if the activity of the glucose transport system is normal in these cells but the rate of glucose oxidation is greatly decreased, it follows that an intracellular defect in glucose metabolism exists in the large adipocyte. Indeed, several laboratories have reported such results (Livingston and Lockwood, 1974; Olefsky, 1976a; Czech, 1976), and all of these workers have concluded that the most significant metabolic abnormality of the large adipocyte involves intracellular metabolism.

The nature of this intracellular lesion(s) has been partially identified. Using glucose labeled in either the 1 or 6 position, it has been found that the defect in glucose oxidation resides in the hexose monophosphate shunt, and that glycolytic and Krebs cycle oxidative activity are relatively normal in large adipocytes (Olefsky, 1977). Furthermore, glucose conversion to fatty acids is also greatly inhibited in these cells (Di Girolamo and Rudman, 1968; Czech,

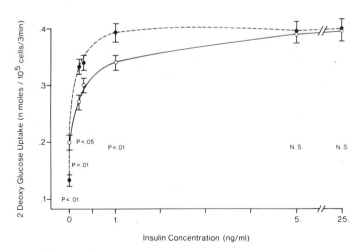

FIGURE 2 Ability of small (●) and large (○) adipocytes to take up 2-deoxyglucose. Cells were preincubated with or without insulin (at the indicated concentrations) for 45 min at 24°C. Uptake was then measured at the end of a 3 min incubation with [2-^{14}C]deoxyglucose (0.125 mM). Data represent the mean (± SE) of 11 experiments for each group, and p values were obtained by use of the nonpaired t-test. (reprinted from Olefsky, 1976a).

1976; Olefsky, 1977), and it seems possible that this is linked to the decreased pentose pathway activity. In other words, decreased fatty acid synthesis leads to accumulation of NADPH with an increased NADPH/NADP ratio. This increased ratio could then inhibit the pentose pathway, and this would make the decrease in glucose oxidation secondary to the block in fatty acid synthesis. Evidence for this hypothesis has recently been described (Czech and Richardson, 1976).

In summary, several mechanisms for cellular insulin resistance can exist, and "insulin-resistant" large adipocytes can be compared to normal cells at several steps. First, insulin binding is decreased in the large adipocyte, and the functional consequence of this decrease in insulin receptors—a rightward shift in the insulin dose-response curve—can be demonstrated provided early steps of insulin action are assessed (glucose transport). On the other hand, maximal insulin-stimulated rates of glucose consumption and oxidation are greatly decreased in the large adipocyte, indicating that the major metabolic abnormality of these cells is an intracellular defect in glucose metabolism. This defect can be further characterized as a linked inhibition of fatty acid synthesis and hexose monophosphate shunt glucose oxidation.

Finally, although the mechanisms of the insulin resistance of the large adipocyte have been reasonably well described, it does not necessarily follow that similar mechanisms will exist in other tissues. Thus, while the intracellular defect in glucose metabolism rather than the decrease in insulin receptors is the major abnormality in the large adipocyte, it is possible that decreased insulin binding may assume a more important role in causing the insulin resistance in muscle and liver tissues in obesity. If this were the case, then one would expect that very high insulin concentrations would overcome the insulin resistance of these tissues—that is, a rightward shift in the response curve. Precise *in vitro* evidence bearing on this issue is not currently available, but in an important *in vivo* study Felig et al. (1974) have found that at low plasma insulin concentrations hepatic glucose output is not suppressed normally in obese patients, whereas at high insulin levels suppression is normal. Although much work remains to be done, it seems reasonable to suggest at this stage that in obesity different causes for insulin resistance may exist in different tissues; in adipocytes an intracellular abnormality predominates, whereas in liver and muscle tissue it is possible that decreased insulin receptors may be paramount.

NONKETOTIC DIABETES MELLITUS

Evidence for the Existence of Insulin Resistance

The notion that insulin resistance might exist in patients with diabetes mellitus was first suggested by Himsworth (1936), who indicated that patients with diabetes could be differentiated into "insulin sensitive" and "insulin insensitive" types on the basis of their blood glucose response to insulin administered with a glucose load. This notion received support from early attempts to estimate circulating insulin levels by the use of various bioassays. The results of several such studies indicated that many patients with non-ketotic diabetes appeared to have normal or increased plasma insulin levels (Bornstein and Trewhella, 1950; Bornstein and Lawrence, 1951; Vallance-Owen et al., 1955; Davidson and Haist, 1958; Samaan and Fraser, 1963; Steinke et al., 1961).

However, these methods were not totally satisfactory, and the realization that hyperglycemia could occur in patients with diabetes mellitus in the absence of a decrease in circulating insulin levels became completely appreciated only with the publication by Yalow and Berson (1960) of their epochal study of the immunoassay of endogenous plasma insulin in humans. In that publication they first described their immunological method for measuring insulin, which combined specificity with the degree of sensitivity needed to measure the minute concentrations of insulin present in the circulation. They used this new method to compare plasma immunoreactive insulin levels in normal subjects to those of patients with nonketotic diabetes and found that the insulin levels were, on the average, higher in the diabetic patients. On the basis of these results they concluded "that the tissues of the maturity-onset diabetic do not respond to his insulin as well as the tissues of the non-diabetic subject respond to his insulin." Or, to use Himsworth's terminology, patients with diabetes were insulin insensitive.

Thus, the idea that hyperglycemia in nonketotic diabetes might be secondary to insulin resistance is the result of reports which indicated that exogenous insulin was not as effective in patients with diabetes and that hyperglycemia could exist in the presence of normal and/or elevated levels of endogenous insulin. Considerable evidence has been gathered in support of both of these general observations, and in the following section we will review this information.

Plasma insulin levels in patients with nonketotic diabetes mellitus. The original observation by Yalow and Berson (1960) of normal to elevated levels of plasma insulin in response to oral glucose in patients with nonketotic diabetes raised the possibility that diabetes may be entirely due to a decrease of insulin sensitivity. However, it soon became apparent that patients with either ketotic diabetes or nonketotic diabetes with significant fasting hyper-glycemia had very low insulin concentrations (Berson and Yalow, 1962; Hales and Randle, 1963; Ehrlich and Bambers, 1964). Unfortunately, insulin responses to oral glucose cannot be simply divided into two categories. Thus, as oral glucose tolerance begins to deteriorate, absolute plasma insulin response to oral glucose is equal to or greater than normal in the nonketotic diabetics (Berson and Yalow, 1962, 1965; Hales and Randle, 1963; Buchanan and McKiddie, 1967; Reaven and Miller, 1968; Chiles and Tzagournis, 1970; Savage et al., 1975). However, with increasing degrees of glucose intolerance and the appearance of significant fasting hyperglycemia, the plasma insulin response becomes attenuated, and with severe fasting hyperglycemia the insulin response is much less than in normal control subjects (Berson and Yalow, 1962; Hales and Randle, 1963; Ehrlich and Bambers, 1964; Buchanan and McKiddie, 1967; Reaven and Miller, 1968; Chiles and Tzagournis, 1970; Savage et al., 1975). Although it is difficult to define any sharp cutoff point, it is clear that substantial numbers of patients currently diagnosed as having diabetes are not insulin-deficient. For example, one-third of the patients studied by the University Group Diabetes Program (1970) did not have fasting hyperglycemia, and almost certainly had plasma insulin responses to oral glucose that were comparable to those of normal subjects.

At about the same time that it became clear that not all diabetics were insulin-deficient, proinsulin was found in the plasma (Roth et al., 1968; Rubenstein et al., 1968). Since proinsulin has much less biological activity than insulin (Shaw and Chance, 1968; Steiner et al., 1968), the possibility arose that the increased plasma insulin levels seen in some diabetics might be due to excessive secretion of proinsulin. This would account for the apparent insulin resistance of patients with diabetes by attributing the combination of hyperglycemia and hyperinsulinemia to pancreatic secretion of the relatively ineffective proinsulin molecule. However, several studies have indicated that the high levels of immunoreactive insulin (IRI) in patients with diabetes are not due to an increase in the relative secretion of proinsulin by these patients (Gorden and Roth, 1970; Melani et al., 1970; Duckworth and Kitabachi, 1972). Thus, many patients with diabetes are hyperglycemic in spite of having plasma insulin levels which in absolute terms are equal to or greater than normal.

Although there is general agreement that many patients with mild diabetes do not have an absolute deficiency of insulin, the conclusion that hyperglycemia in these subjects is due to insulin resistance is not equally well accepted. Thus, Karam et al. (1965) indicated that the plasma insulin response of nonketotic diabetics to oral glucose was less than normal in the thin subjects and greater than normal in the obese ones. They then concluded that the plasma insulin response to glucose was lower in patients with diabetes than in normal subjects matched for weight, and that the increased levels of plasma insulin that had been reported in these diabetics were secondary to the presence of obesity. Unfortunately, although they matched diabetics with controls on the basis of weight, they did not match them on the basis of degree of hyperglycemia. Since the thin diabetic patients were significantly more hyperglycemic than the obese diabetics, their diminished insulin response could simply reflect the fact that patients with severe diabetes, thin or obese, secrete less insulin. Indeed, most studies indicate that when normal subjects and diabetic patients are matched for weight, patients with mild diabetes, as a group, have insulin levels equal to or greater than those of normal subjects. On the other hand, hypoinsulinemia is seen when significant fasting hyperglycemia supervenes (Berson and Yalow, 1965; Buchanan and McKiddie, 1967; Reaven and Miller, 1968; Chiles and Tzagournis, 1970; Savage et al., 1975). Furthermore, although the obese subjects tend to have a greater insulin response to oral glucose than do the nonobese individuals, there is a marked overlap of the insulin responses of obese and nonobese subjects with similar glucose tolerance to an oral glucose challenge (Berson and Yalow, 1965; Buchanan and McKiddie, 1967; Reaven and Miller, 1968). Finally, although loss of weight may lead to a marked decrease in the insulin response to glucose of obese subjects (Sims et al., 1968; Farrant et al., 1969; Kosaka et al., 1972), a similar degree of reduction can also be seen when the patient remains obese even after weight loss (Yalow et al., 1965; Olefsky et al., 1974). Thus, although obesity modulates the insulin response to oral glucose, its impact should not be overestimated, and for any given degree of obesity patients with mild nonketotic diabetes mellitus have greater plasma insulin levels than normal subjects. Therefore, one cannot simply attribute the increased insulin levels that are seen in many nonketotic diabetics to the coexistence of obesity.

Another basis for disagreement with the conclusion that insulin resistance may be causally related to hyperglycemia in patients with mild diabetes is based on a difference in the interpretation of the fact that insulin levels are not always absolutely low in such patients. Thus, it has been argued that the hyperglycemia in patients with mild diabetes should elicit even greater insulin levels than it does, and the absence of this "appropriate" response indicates that the diabetic state is associated with a reduction, albeit a relative one, in insulin secretory capacity. The manner of calculating the appropriateness of the insulin response to glucose varied from such simple manipulations as determining the insulin/glucose ratio (Perley and Kipnis, 1966b) or the ratio between the incremental changes in plasma glucose and insulin levels (Seltzer et al., 1967) to a much more complicated analysis using an analog computer model (Cerasi, 1967). These approaches have two features in common. They focus on what the plasma insulin response "should be," rather than what it actually is, and they are based on the assumption that the plasma insulin response to an oral glucose load in normal subjects is a linear function of the coexisting plasma glucose level. Unfortunately, there seems to be little experimental data in support of the latter assumption and considerable evidence to the contrary (Hales and Randle, 1963; Castro et al., 1970; Peterson and Reaven, 1971; Reaven and Olefsky, 1974).

Another attempt to define the appropriateness of the pancreatic response in diabetics has been based on determining the plasma insulin response under conditions in which the glycemic stimulus was supposedly equalized in normal and diabetic subjects. This condition was attained by producing "normal" and "diabetic" blood glucose profiles by infusing glucose to stimulate the mean response to a 100 g oral glucose load (Perley and Kipnis, 1967). When this was done, the insulin response was lower in the diabetic subjects, and it was concluded that pancreatic insufficiency was present in these patients. As before, this argument assumes that the plasma insulin response is a linear function of coexisting glucose concentration, and that both groups were responding to an equivalent glycemic stimulus. However, to achieve similar glucose levels in the two groups of patients it was necessary to infuse more than twice as much glucose into the normal subjects. There is no reason to assume that the amount of glucose infused may not also modify the insulin response, and for this reason the two groups of subjects were not necessarily responding to identical "glycemic stimuli." Indeed, recent experimental data strongly suggest this notion, and demonstrate that plasma insulin levels are more closely correlated to the amount of glucose infused than to glucose concentration and rise throughout a prolonged glucose infusion, even when the plasma glucose levels are falling during the latter part of the infusion (Olefsky et al., 1973b). Somewhat similar results have been reported by Hoshi and Shreeve (1973), who indicated that insulin release by perfused rat pancreatic islets increased when glucose solutions of the *same* concentration were delivered at a more rapid flow rate.

Thus, there appears to be considerable difficulty in proving that the plasma insulin response to glucose of the patient with mild diabetes is inappropriate to the degree of hyperglycemia. Indeed, it seems to us that the crucial point that remains is that although similar loads of glucose elicit normal or increased insulin levels in patients with mild diabetes, the removal of these loads is attenuated in these patients. In this regard it seems at least as reasonable to ask why the insulin is ineffective in these patients as to speculate on what constitutes an appropriate insulin response to glucose.

Still another objection to the notion that insulin resistance is responsible for hyperglycemia in patients with mild diabetes is based on consideration of the rate of appearance of insulin following a glucose challenge. Indeed, it has been suggested that the inability of patients with mild diabetes to respond promptly to a glucose load is the basic lesion in this disease (Cerasi and Luft, 1967; Seltzer et al., 1967). This suggestion derives from the first observations of Yalow and Berson (1960), in which they indicated that mean plasma insulin levels in patients with diabetes were lower than the normal mean 30 min after the glucose load. However, the patients they studied were heterogeneous in their degree of glucose intolerance: several of the subjects had fasting hyperglycemia and the mean fasting glucose level was 127 mg%. Since the insulin response to glucose decreases as the severity of glucose intolerance increases (Berson and Yalow, 1962; Hales and Randle, 1963; Ehrlich and Bambers, 1964; Buchanan and McKiddie, 1967; Reaven and Miller, 1968; Chiles and Tzagournis, 1970; Savage et al., 1975), it is likely that the lower mean insulin level at 30 min in these diabetic patients was due to the patients with fasting hyperglycemia. Indeed, if the insulin levels following oral glucose are compared in normal subjects and patients with chemical diabetes, the absolute plasma insulin level in the diabetic patients is equal to or greater than normal at every time interval during the tolerance test (Berson and Yalow, 1965; Reaven and Miller, 1968; Chiles and Tzagournis, 1970; Reaven et al., 1971; Danowski et al., 1973; Savage et al., 1975; Tchobroutsky et al., 1973).

Furthermore, it has been shown that glucose tolerance does not deteriorate when two oral glucose tests are performed 3 hr apart (Yalow et al., 1969), in spite of the fact that a delayed insulin response is seen during the second test. Finally, the fact that dogs with alloxan-induced diabetes develop a delay in the rate of appearance of insulin in response to a glucose load (Pupo et al., 1976) suggests that this can occur secondary to the diabetic state itself. Thus, the absolute levels of insulin in patients with mild diabetes are, in general, equal to or greater than normal at all times after an oral glucose load. A delayed insulin response to glucose can be produced experimentally and not lead to hyperglycemia in normal humans, and a delayed insulin response can occur as a secondary phenomenon in experimental diabetics.

In view of this evidence, it seems reasonable to conclude that hyperglycemia in patients with mild diabetes cannot simply be ascribed to a delay in the rate of insulin release. Furthermore, the prolongation of the insulin response (i.e., the delay in reaching peak insulin levels) in patients with mild diabetes seems most reasonably attributed to the continued hyperglycemia in such patients, and the persistence of hyperglycemia in the presence of hyperinsulinemia serves as evidence for the presence of insulin resistance in these patients. It should be emphasized that the delay in reaching peak insulin levels that occurs in patients with significant fasting hyperglycemia is also associated with an absolute decrease in the magnitude of the insulin levels throughout the tolerance test. Under these conditions, insulin deficiency seems to serve as a reasonable explanation for the hyperglycemia, and there is no reason to invoke the presence of a primary abnormality of impaired insulin sensitivity in such patients.

Effectiveness of insulin in patients with nonketotic diabetes mellitus. In order to assess directly insulin sensitivity in patients with nonketotic diabetes, a number of studies have been performed in which the ability of exogenous insulin to increase glucose disposal has been determined (Bearn et al., 1951; Heller et al., 1958; Kalant et al., 1963; Zierler and Rabinowitz, 1963; Stocks and Martin, 1969; Alford et al., 1971). These approaches have involved administration of insulin to normal and diabetic patients, followed by measurement of some aspect of glucose removal. The results of these studies are all consistent with the notion that patients with nonketotic diabetes are insulin-resistant. For example, Zierler and Rabinowitz (1963), using the forearm perfusion technique, found that forearm muscle of diabetic patients demonstrated decreased insulin sensitivity as compared to controls, and the magnitude of the defect increased with the severity of the diabetics. Using a different approach, Alford et al. (1971) administered an intravenous glucose load followed by insulin (0.1 U/kg) to normal subjects, patients with chemical diabetes, and nonketotic patients with fasting hyperglycemia. By measuring the rate of fall in glucose concentration following the administration of insulin they found that the effectiveness of insulin decreased as diabetes progressed; that is, patients with fasting hyperglycemia were the least insulin-sensitive, the group with chemical diabetes had an intermediate response to insulin, and the normals were the most insulin-sensitive.

Stocks and Martin (1969) also measured the glucose concentration following administration of insulin (0.1 U/kg) in normal and nonketotic diabetic subjects with fasting hyperglycemia. They calculated a glucose assimilation index from their data as a measure of insulin sensitivity, and indicated that the diabetic subjects were insulin-resistant; that is, their glucose assimilation index was less than that of normal subjects. Kalant et al. (1963) administered insulin to normal and nonketotic diabetic patients and measured subsequent plasma glucose concentrations and glucose outflow using an isotopic technique. Diabetic subjects had an attenuated hypoglycemic response to the administered insulin, and this was shown to be due to the diminished rate of glucose outflow in response to insulin.

All of the studies discussed above were conducted when the plasma glucose and insulin concentrations were in non-steady-state conditions. It is difficult to quantify this phenomenon while the rates of plasma insulin entry and removal and glucose entry and removal are rapidly changing. To circumvent this problem we designed an experimental approach in which we directly measure the ability of different groups of patients to dispose of comparable glucose loads under the influence of identical insulin stimuli during steady-state conditions (Shen et al., 1970). This is done by giving each patient a constant infusion of insulin, glucose, epinephrine, and propranolol for 150 min. Steady-state plasma concentrations of insulin and glucose are achieved within 90 min of the start of the infusion and are measured every 10 min during the final 60 min of the study. This approach is based on the known ability of epinephrine and propranolol to suppress endogenous insulin secretion, resulting in comparable steady-state plasma levels of exogenous insulin in all subjects [102 μU/ml; coefficent of variation, 10% (Olefsky et al., 1974)]. In these studies the height of the steady-state plasma glucose (SSPG) concentration is a direct reflection of a subject's overall efficiency of insulin-mediated glucose disposal. In this fashion, we can quantify the ability of similar circulating levels of exogenous insulin to promote disposal of comparable glucose loads in a variety of subjects.

Using this technique, we have found that steady-state plasma glucose concentrations are elevated in patients with chemical diabetes as compared to normals (220 $\pm$ 20 mg% compared to 120 $\pm$ 10 mg%) (Ginsberg et al., 1974). Diabetic patients with fasting hyperglycemia have even greater elevations of SSPG levels during these infusions (Ginsberg et al., 1975b). These results provide direct evidence for a graded increase in the degree of insulin resistance as the severity of hyperglycemia increases in nonketotic diabetic subjects.

However, many patients with nonketotic diabetes are overweight, and the relationship between obesity and insulin resistance has already been discussed. Therefore, it is theoretically possible that the insulin resistance in patients with nonketotic diabetes is due to the coexisting obesity in these subjects. However, in several of the studies described above the control and diabetic groups were matched for weight (Zierler and Rabinowitz, 1963; Stocks and Martin, 1969; Alford et al., 1971). Furthermore, in our own studies (Ginsberg et al., 1974, 1975b), we included only subjects who were nonobese. Finally, within the range of percentage adiposity of our nonobese subjects, no relationship is seen between insulin resistance and percentage of adiposity (Olefsky et al., 1973a). This latter finding suggests that significant levels of obesity must be reached before adiposity has an appreciable influence on insulin resistance. Thus, while obesity will accentuate insulin resistance, the insulin resistance described in patients with nonketotic diabetes seems to be independent of this factor.

These results indicate resistance to the action of insulin in patients with nonketotic diabetes mellitus. This generalization based on investigation of diabetic patients receives a certain degree of support from *in vitro* studies of tissue obtained from patients with diabetes. Thus, Kahlenberg and Kalant (1964) studied glucose uptake by adipose tissue from normal and nonketotic diabetic subjects. Their results indicated that adipose tissue from diabetic patients exhibits decreased glucose uptake in both the basal and insulin-stimulated states. This decreased insulin responsiveness was apparent if the data were expressed in either absolute terms or as percentage stimulation above basal. In similar studies, Bjorntorp (1966) measured the ability of insulin to promote glucose oxidation in adipose tissue isolated from normal and nonketotic diabetic subjects (fasting blood sugar > 150 mg per 100 ml). He also indicated that adipose tissue from diabetic subjects has decreased insulin responsiveness compared to that from normal subjects. Finally, Galton et al. (1971) studied glucose metabolism in adipose tissue fragments from 30 diabetic subjects (only two of whom required insulin therapy). They found that when diabetic and normal subjects were matched for weight, basal glucose utilization by adipose tissue from diabetic subjects was decreased at all glucose concentrations in the media. Insulin responsiveness was not determined. These results are all consistent with the hypothesis that glucose uptake is decreased in diabetic subjects, and that the tissues of these patients are relatively insensitive to the action of insulin.

Significance of Insulin Resistance in the Pathogenesis of Nonketotic Diabetes

The evidence presented to this point strongly suggests that patients with nonketotic diabetes are more resistant than normal subjects to the action of insulin, and that the degree of insulin resistance increases with the severity of glucose intolerance. It now seems reasonable to ask what role, if any, the insulin resistance plays in the pathogenesis of the glucose intolerance. The situation is perhaps clearest in the case of patients classified as having chemical diabetes. These individuals are not insulin-deficient—their plasma insulin response to an oral glucose load is in absolute terms at least equal to that of normal individuals. Furthermore, insulin is not as effective in promoting glucose uptake in these patients as in normal subjects. Thus, in these patients it seems possible to attribute carbohydrate intolerance entirely to insulin resistance. There seems to be no reason to postulate the concomitant presence of insulin deficiency.

Unfortunately, the situation is more complex in the case of patients who have nonketotic diabetes with significant fasting hyperglycemia. These patients appear to be both insulin-deficient and insulin-resistant. Thus, as we have described earlier, they respond to an oral glucose load with insulin levels that are less than normal *and* they are resistant to the *in vivo* and *in vitro* action of insulin.

There appear to be two explanations for the hyperglycemia of these individuals. Although both abnormalities may exist, and both may be primary lesions, it would be simpler if one could be shown to be secondary to the other. For example, it could be postulated that the basic lesion in patients with significant fasting hyperglycemia is an absolute deficiency of insulin, resulting in a fall in glucose uptake rate, increased hepatic glucose production, and hyperglycemia. The hyperglycemia stimulates the pancreas, resulting in fasting insulin levels, which are now equal to or greater than normal, and the combination of adequate insulin levels and fasting hyperglycemia restores glucose uptake and hepatic glucose production rates to normal and inhibits ketone body formation.

However, for reasons as yet unclear, the adaptation of the organism to the insulin-deficient state results in a decrease in normal cellular responsiveness to insulin; that is, insulin resistance. Although we do not understand the mechanism involved in the development of the insulin resistance, we do know that resistance to the action of insulin to promote efficiency of glucose uptake and inhibit hepatic glucose production exists in patients with fasting hyperglycemia (Kimmerling et al., 1976). If this formulation is correct, patients with insulin deficiency should be more resistant to the action of insulin than normal subjects. Whether this is the case remains to be clarified. For example, although it is often stated that patients or animals with diabetes secondary to loss of pancreatic function are markedly insulin-sensitive, data in this regard are difficult to come by. However, we have used our infusion technique to compare the insulin resistance of patients with fasting hyperglycemia (> 110 mg%, < 190 mg%) secondary to either chronic pancreatitis or chemical diabetes (Ginsberg et al., 1975b). The results of this study indicated that subjects with chronic pancreatitis were more insulin-sensitive than patients with chemical diabetes. In contrast, Pupo and associates (1976) have indicated that dogs with mild insulin deficiency and fasting hyperglycemia secondary to alloxan are more insulin-resistant than normal dogs. Unpublished observations from our own laboratory indicate that insulin resistance does not develop in dogs following the induction (by alloxan) of mild insulin deficiency, but does occur in dogs who are severely insulin-deficient. Obviously, this question requires further study, and the development of insulin resistance secondary to insulin deficiency may vary with many factors, including the severity of the insulin-deficient state, the cause of the insulin-deficient state, the secretory status of other hormones, and so on. Therefore, we must emphasize that our suggestion that the insulin resistance of patients with significant fasting hyperglycemia is secondary to the insulin deficiency is only a suggestion. However, given this constraint, our current belief is that insulin deficiency, not insulin resistance, is the fundamental defect responsible for the glucose intolerance in nonketotic patients with significant fasting hyperglycemia. Therefore, as a result of these views we believe that insulin resistance plays a different role in the glucose intolerance of different kinds of patients with nonketotic diabetes. This distinction will receive further emphasis in the next section.

Mechanism(s) of Insulin Resistance
in Nonketotic Diabetes

The evidence presented to this point makes it clear that insulin resistance exists in patients with nonketotic diabetes, and that hyperglycemia in these patients can no longer be considered as solely due to lack of insulin. The insulin resistance of patients with nonketotic diabetes theoretically could be due to the secretion of abnormal forms of insulin, the presence of circulating insulin antagonists, or cellular unresponsiveness to the action of insulin. There is essentially no evidence that patients with nonketotic diabetes secrete an abnormal form of insulin, and we have reviewed the evidence indicating that these patients do not respond normally to exogenous insulin. Thus, there is little reason to believe that the first alternative is responsible for the insulin resistance of patients with nonketotic diabetes. However, the two other possible mechanisms still provide viable explanations, and we will separately review the evidence for each below.

Circulating antagonists to insulin. Many suggestions have been made over the years as to the role that various circulating insulin antagonists might play in the pathogenesis of diabetes. This subject was extensively reviewed several years ago (Berson and Yalow, 1965; Katzen and Glitzer, 1968). At that time it appeared that there was little evidence that any known circulating insulin antagonist is responsible for the glucose intolerance of diabetes. However, in the intervening period considerable new evidence has accumulated concerning the possible role of growth hormone and glucagon in this regard, and it seems important to once again consider the possibility that circulating insulin antagonists are involved in ths insulin resistance of nonketotic diabetes.

Growth Hormone. The diabetogenic effect of growth hormone has been appreciated for some time (Houssay and Anderson, 1949), but our ability to measure endogenous hormone levels is more recent. Since the availability of a sensitive radioimmunoassay, several reports have appeared which indicate that abnormal elevations of growth hormone levels are seen under a variety of conditions in patients with insulin-deficient diabetes (Johansen and Hansen, 1969, 1971; Yde, 1969, 1970; Hansen and Johansen, 1970; Hansen, 1970, 1973a; Molnar et al., 1972; Vigneri et al., 1976). Abnormal elevations of growth hormone have also been reported in patients with maturity-onset diabetes (Yde, 1970; Hansen, 1973b; Kjeldsen et al., 1975; Vigneri et al., 1976). However, in the latter instance the differences between diabetic and normal are less striking and often do not reach statistical significance, particularly if obese patients with maturity-onset diabetes are compared with obese normals (Molnar et al., 1972; Hansen, 1973b; Kjeldsen et al., 1975; Vigneri et al., 1976). The latter observations suggest that the elevations in plasma growth hormone levels seen in diabetics are secondary to the insulin-deficient state. This is supported by several observations that indicate the return toward a normal growth hormone response can occur with improvement in degree of diabetic control (Johansen and Hansen, 1971; Hansen, 1971; Molnar et al., 1972; Vigneri et al., 1976). Indeed, there is evidence from the studies cited above that normalization of hyperglycemia can lead to total return to normal growth hormone responsiveness. However, it appears that the abnormal growth hormone response can be normalized in juvenile diabetes only with the most rigid control of the hyperglycemia.

Thus, it would seem likely that most insulin-deficient patients are exposed to abnormal elevations of growth hormone in their daily existence, and these increased growth hormone levels may be of clinical significance. It is possible that this could account for at least part of the resistance to the acute effects of insulin that characterizes nonketotic diabetic patients with significant fasting hyperglycemia, and increased levels of growth hormone might be one of the causes of the secondary insulin resistance that we feel develops as a result of insulin deficiency in these patients. On the other hand, based on this evidence there is little reason to suspect that an abnormality in growth hormone response is responsible for the insulin resistance seen in the patients with chemical diabetes who have normal to increased plasma insulin levels. We believe that primary insulin resistance exists in these patients, and elevated growth hormone levels do not appear to play a role.

Glucagon. The potential role of glucagon as a factor in the pathogenesis of diabetes has received considerable recent interest, and a series of reports have been published indicating that hyperglucagonemia, either absolute or relative, is seen in human diabetes of both juvenile- and adult-onset types (Aguilar-Parada et al., 1969; Unger et al., 1970; Muller et al., 1970; Buchanan and McCarroll, 1972). Hyperglucagonemia has also been described in a variety of forms of spontaneous and experimentally induced diabetes in animals (Katsilambros et al., 1970; Samols et al., 1971; Muller et al., 1970; Meir et al.,

1972; Buchanan and Mawhinney, 1973; Laube et al., 1973; Frankel et al., 1974; Weir et al., 1976). Obviously, as in the case of elevated growth hormone levels, these abnormalities could be either primary or secondary to the insulin-deficient state. Earlier reports indicated that the hyperglucagonemia of alloxan-induced insulin deficiency was promptly corrected by administration of small amounts of insulin (Muller et al., 1970; Braaten et al., 1974). In contrast, it was reported that the abnormal glucagon secretion of human diabetics could not be corrected by administration of large doses of exogenous insulin (Unger et al., 1972). On the basis of these results, as well as their summary of a series of studies in which somatostatin was administered to diabetic humans and animals, Unger and Orci (1975) postulated that diabetes mellitus was a bihormonal disease, characterized by primary abnormalities of both insulin and glucagon secretion. They stated that "the major consequence of absolute or relative insulin lack is glucose underutilization and that absolute or relative glucagon excess is the principal factor in the over-production of glucose in diabetes."

Although this is a very appealing theory, more recent experimental data raise serious questions about its validity. Thus, recent studies from Unger's group (Raskin et al., 1975) indicate that administration of insulin can significantly lower glucagon levels in hyperglycemic subjects with both adult- and juvenile-onset diabetes. These results are certainly consistent with the notion that the hyperglucagonemia is secondary to the insulin deficiency and not the cause of the diabetes. Furthermore, when Sherwin et al. (1976) produced hyperglucagonemia (three to six times basal levels) by glucagon infusions, they could not demonstrate a significant effect on glucose homeostasis in normal subjects, nondiabetic obese subjects, adult-onset diabetic patients, or juvenile-onset diabetics receiving insulin replacement. In contrast, a significant hyperglycemic response could be produced by administering glucagon to juvenile-onset diabetic patients in whom insulin had been withdrawn. They concluded that glucagon-induced hyperglycemia occurs only in the presence of severe insulin deficiency, and that hyperglucagonemia in diabetes is a consequence of insulin deficiency. Finally, Barnes et al. (1975) and Barnes and Bloom (1976) have indicated that hyperglycemia occurs in the absence of glucagon in totally pancreatectomized diabetics. They also found that the glucagon levels do not significantly change nor are they correlated with glucose and ketone levels, when insulin-dependent diabetics are followed for several hours after their usual morning insulin dose is omitted.

Thus, it seems to us that significant doubt has been raised concerning the thesis that there is a primary abnormality of glucagon secretion in human diabetes. It is our view that the evidence favors the notion that hyperglucagonemia is secondary to insulin deficiency and has its major effects on glucose homeostasis in patients who are absolutely insulin-deficient. Furthermore, since absolute hyperglucagonemia seems to be confined to patients with severe insulin deficiency, it seems unlikely that increased levels of glucagon play a significant role in the insulin resistance of nonketotic diabetics with either fasting hyperglycemia or chemical diabetes. Indeed, we are unaware of any evidence that suggests that any known circulating insulin antagonist is reponsible for the insulin resistance in patients with chemical diabetes.

Tissue responsiveness to insulin. Insulin exerts it biologic effects on target tissues by binding to specific receptors on the plasma membrane and initiating a complex series of metabolic events. Obviously, resistance to the action of insulin could result from an abnormality, or series of abnormalities, at any step in this overall process. It is our belief that the primary insulin resistance of patients with chemical diabetes is due to a basic defect in cellular responsiveness to insulin. Furthermore, we believe that a significant proportion of the secondary insulin resistance of insulin-deficient patients with nonketotic diabetes may be due to an acquired abnormality of tissue responsiveness to insulin. Unfortunately, relatively little information is available for evaluating either of these suggestions.

Insulin Receptors. Studies from our laboratory (Olefsky and Reaven, 1974, 1976a, 1976b) have indicated that there is a decrease in the binding of radiolabeled insulin to specific insulin receptors on circulating mononuclear leukocytes obtained from nonketotic, nonobese diabetic patients with significant fasting hyperglycemia. This decrease in the binding of insulin was found to be secondary to a decrease in the total number of insulin receptors, without any change in the affinity of insulin for its receptors. This observation has recently been confirmed by Goldstein et al. (1975). At present there are no published data concerning the binding of insulin in nonobese patients with chemical diabetes. However, unpublished observations from our laboratory indicate that there is decreased insulin binding in adults with chemical diabetes, comparable to that described in patients with significant fasting hyperglycemia (Olefsky and Reaven, 1977). We think it possible that in patients with chemical diabetes this defect in binding could account for insulin resistance. On the other hand, the role that the abnormal binding seen in patients with fasting hyperglycemia plays in the genesis of insulin resistance is unclear. Furthermore, whether this decreased binding is a primary phenomenon or is secondary to the diabetic state is not completely resolved. In this regard, we did not find a decrease in insulin binding to circulating mononuclear leukocytes obtained from patients whose diabetes was secondary to the insulin deficiency of chronic pancreatitis (Olefsky and Reaven, 1974).

On the other hand, reduction of fasting hyperglycemia with chlorpropamide was found to lead to a significant increase in the number of insulin receptors in mononuclear cells of nonobese, nonketotic diabetic patients (Olefsky and Reaven, 1976a). There are several possible interpretations of the latter finding, but one alternative is that the decrease in number of insulin receptors is secondary to the diabetic state and that any successful treatment will lead to a return toward a normal number of receptors. Obviously, considerably more information is needed concerning the efficacy of insulin binding in various kinds of diabetic subjects, as well as the correlation between insulin binding and insulin resistance, before we can define the role played by defects in insulin binding in the insulin resistance of nonketotic diabetes. (For another viewpoint on this subject, the reader is referred to Chap. 8.)

Intracellular Events. In an earlier section we reviewed the evidence demonstrating that *in vitro* insulin-mediated glucose uptake was decreased in adipose tissue obtained from nonketotic diabetic subjects. This decrease in glucose uptake could be secondary to a decrease in the binding of insulin to its receptors, an abnormality in the cell membrane components responsible for transmitting the receptors' action, an intrinsic defect in the glucose transport system, or any number of abnormalities in intracellular glucose metabolism. In the latter regard, Galton and his colleagues have published a series of papers attempting to define defects in adipose tissue metabolism that occur distal to the glucose transport system (Galton and Wilson, 1970, 1971; Galton et al., 1971; Page and Galton, 1975). These authors have studied adipose tissue from control subjects and adult-onset diabetics. The various abnormalities they have described are all consistent with the notion that phosphofructokinase may play a regulatory role in human adipose tissue and that the abnormalities of glucose uptake seen in this tissue from diabetic subjects may be secondary to an intracellular deficiency of this enzyme.

These observations remain to be confirmed, and the role that such abnormalities may play in the hyperglycemia and insulin resistance of adult patients with nonketotic diabetes remains to be clarified. For example, it appears that the decreased adipose tissue phosphofructokinase levels in diabetics can be returned to normal by treatment with insulin or hypoglycemic drugs (Galton and Wilson, 1971). Thus, the abnormality noted may be secondary to the diabetic state, and not a primary lesion. However, even in this instance it could play a role in the secondary resistance of the nonketotic diabetic patient. In any event, it seems apparent that such attempts to identify abnormalities of intracellular glucose metabolism must be carried out in an effort to define the mechanism of insulin resistance in patients with nonketotic diabetes.

GLUCOCORTICOIDS

It is well recognized that excess endogenous or exogenous glucocorticoids will lead to impairment of carbohydrate metabolism, and this is often referred to as "steroid diabetes." This phenomenon is illustrated in patients with Cushing's syndrome. In such subjects carbohydrate tolerance is often impaired and the pattern of this abnormality is usually that of simple glucose intolerance. Thus, the fasting blood sugar values in patients with Cushing's syndrome are not usually elevated and the abnormalities in carbohydrate tolerance are generally limited to those which can be elicited only through the stress of a large glucose challenge. In a minority of patients with Cushing's syndrome fasting hyperglycemia develops, and it is generally found that diabetes mellitus predated the onset of adrenocortical hyperfunction in these subjects. Analogous results are seen in patients who receive exogenous glucocorticoids. Thus, if a patient has normal carbohydrate tolerance to begin with, glucocorticoid administration will usually lead to some degree of deterioration in his ability to respond to a glucose load (Fajans and Conn, 1954). Although the development of fasting hyperglycemia or frank diabetes is unusual, patients with either chemical or overt diabetes prior to glucocorticoid therapy may develop severe posttherapy diabetes.

When glucocorticoids are administered to nondiabetic human subjects, some deterioration of glucose tolerance can be noted in most patients within 12 hr (Fajans and Conn, 1954). In only a minority of subjects will this deterioration lead to abnormal glucose tolerance by standard criteria. When corticoid administration is prolonged, the changes in glucose tolerance tend to return to pretreatment levels (Bastenie et al., 1954; Cahill, 1971), and when the effects of chronic corticoid administration on glucose tolerance are examined, only very minor changes in a small percentage of patients can be found (Conn and Fajans, 1956; McKiddie et al., 1968). In nondiabetic subjects the degree of impairment of glucose tolerance is related to the preexisting ability to dispose of the glucose challenge. As Fajans and Conn (1954) have demonstrated, this phenomenon forms the rationale for the cortisone glucose tolerance test.

Analysis of glucose tolerance tests after treatment with glucocorticoids reveals considerably increased plasma insulin values at each time point, while only mild to moderate increases in glucose concentration are observed (Berger et al., 1966; Perley and Kipnis, 1966a). This pattern of glucose intolerance—increased glucose concentrations in the face of increased insulin concentrations—is characteristic of an insulin-resistant state. Thus, glucocorticoids can cause some degree of hyperglycemia associated with hyperinsulinemia, and therefore the hyperglycemia is due to insulin resistance rather than insulin deficiency.

Mechanism of Insulin Resistance

Insulin has two major effects on *in vivo* glucose homeostasis: it promotes glucose uptake and utilization by insulin-sensitive tissues, and it inhibits the production of glucose by the liver. Therefore, the hyperglycemia observed in the glucocorticoid-induced insulin-resistant state could be due to decreased glucose utilization, increased glucose production, or both.

Increased Glucose Production

First let us consider the matter of glucose overproduction. This has been studied in several laboratories, and it has been concluded that glucocorticoids increase the ability of the liver to produce glucose (Haynes, 1962; Ninomiya et al., 1965; Eisenstein et al., 1966; Cahill, 1971; Issekutz and Allen, 1972).

For example, Issekutz and Allen (1972) used [2-^{3}H] glucose to study hepatic glucose output in prednisone-treated dogs. They found that 1–5 days of treatment resulted in a marked increase in basal hepatic glucose output and that this increased glucose production could be attributed to enhanced gluconeogenesis. This increase in hepatic glucose output could be due to an inherent increase in hepatic capacity to produce glucose or to increased availability of gluconeogenic substrates. Evidence for both mechanisms exists. Thus, as reviewed by Landau (1965), *in vivo* administration of glucocorticoids leads to induction of the gluconeogenic enzymes glucose-6-phosphatase, fructose-1,6-diphosphatase, and PEP carboxykinase. Glucocorticoids also increase the release of certain gluconeogenic amino acids (Wise et al., 1973) and lactate (Issekutz and Allen, 1972) from peripheral tissues, thereby increasing the availability of these substrates to the liver. It has been suggested that the increased concentration of hepatic gluconeogenic enzymes noted *in vivo* is a result of substrate induction (Cahill, 1971; Issekutz and Allen, 1972). However, it can be demonstrated *in vitro* that dexamethasone directly induces the synthesis of gluconeogenic enzymes (Wicks et al., 1974), and this effect obviously cannot be due to substrate induction. Thus, it seems likely that both substrate availability and increased hepatic capacity to produce glucose are involved in the glucocorticoid-induced increase in hepatic glucose production.

Glucagon is another factor that may be related to the effects of glucocorticoids in the *in vivo* setting. Marco et al. (1973) have found that in humans glucocorticoid administration leads to an increase in basal plasma glucagon levels, while Wise et al. (1973) have shown an increase in glucagon levels during alanine infusion following glucocorticoid treatment. The ability of glucagon to promote hepatic glucose output is well known and could clearly augment the increase in hepatic glucose production (Exton et al., 1972; Issekutz and Borkow, 1973). Consequently, in the intact organism, increased plasma glucagon levels are also likely to be involved in leading to glucocorticoid-induced increases in hepatic glucose production.

Decreased Glucose Utilization

Now let us consider the ability of glucocorticoids to decrease glucose utilization. Studies by Owen and Cahill (1973) in intact humans have shown that acute administration of glucocorticoids leads to an overall decrease in glucose utilization. These *in vivo* observations are supported by a large number of *in vitro* studies in which glucocorticoids lead to decreases in glucose utilization by muscle (Riddick et al., 1962; Kipnis and Stein, 1964), adipose (Fain et al., 1963; Yorke, 1967), dermal (Plager and Matsui, 1966), and lymphoid (Munck, 1971) tissue. Thus, there is much evidence that is consistent with the hypothesis that glucocorticoids decrease glucose utilization. This subject has recently been reviewed by Munck (1971). However, decreased cellular glucose utilization is a rather general observation, and further studies concerning the mechanism of this effect have been carried out. For example, it is well established that, *in vitro*, corticosteroids can decrease the ability of adipocytes (Leboeuf et al., 1962; Fain et al., 1963; Fain, 1964; Blecher, 1966; Czech and Fain, 1972) and skeletal muscle (Riddick et al., 1962; Kipnis and Stein, 1964) to oxidize glucose. Initially, it was found that corticosteroids could decrease adipocyte glucose oxidation in the absence of insulin (basal oxidation), but that this effect could be overcome by high concentrations of insulin (Leboeuf et al., 1962; Fain, 1964; Yorke, 1967). This led to the hypothesis that there were two distinct glucose transport systems: a basal system and an insulin-sensitive system, and that only the basal glucose transport system was sensitive to glucocorticoid inhibition (Leboeuf et al., 1962; Fain, 1964; Yorke, 1967). An alternate hypothesis to explain these observations was suggested by Czech and Fain (1972). These workers pointed out that glucose oxidation reflects glucose transport only at low rates of transport, while at higher rates of glucose influx intracellular oxidative pathways become rate-limiting. Thus, under basal conditions, glucose transport would be rate-determining for glucose oxidation, while in the presence of high levels of insulin, transport would be great enough to saturate the intracellular oxidative pathways. Furthermore, in studies in which dexamethasone did not inhibit insulin-stimulated glucose oxidation (Leboeuf et al., 1962; Fain, 1964; Yorke, 1967), high glucose concentrations and maximal doses of insulin were employed—conditions under which glucose transport is probably not rate-limiting for glucose oxidation. Therefore, Czech and Fain (1972) predicted that if glucocorticoids only inhibited the glucose transport system, then decreased glucose oxidation should be seen under basal conditions but not in the presence of high concentrations of insulin. These workers provided evidence for this hypothesis by showing that at low glucose levels and at submaximal insulin concentrations, dexamethasone does inhibit oxidation, and that this inhibitory effect can only be overcome at maximal doses of insulin.

More direct evidence for this idea has been provided by two more recent studies (Livingston and Lockwood, 1975; Olefsky, 1975). When glucose transport was specifically measured in adipocytes, treatment with glucocorticoids *in vitro* led to a decrease in both basal and insulin-stimulated glucose transport (Livingston and Lockwood, 1975; Olefsky, 1975). This effect was characterized by a decrease in the V_{max} of the transport system with no change in K_m in both basal and insulin-stimulated states (Olefsky, 1975). Lastly, under conditions of high rates of glucose influx, where transport is no longer rate-limiting, no effect of dexamethasone on glucose oxidation was observed (Olefsky, 1975). Even though Bernstein and Kipnis (1973) have demonstrated a decrease in hexokinase activity secondary to glucocorticoids, this effect does not appear to influence the overall rates of cellular glucose oxidation.

Insulin Receptors

Although the *in vitro* observations described above appear to explain the decrease in overall glucose utilization seen with glucocorticoid administration (Owen and Cahill, 1973), additional factors exist in the *in vivo* situation. For example, we have found that administration of dexamethasone to rats leads to a decrease in the ability of isolated hepatocytes and adipocytes to bind insulin (Olefsky et al., 1975b). Analysis of this insulin-binding defect reveals that this decrease is due to both a decrease in the number of insulin receptors per cell and a decrease in the affinity of the receptor for insulin. Comparable results have been reported by Kahn et al. (1973b) and Goldfine et al. (1973), who found decreased insulin binding to liver plasma membranes from dexamethasone-treated rats or from animals with ACTH-secreting tumors, respectively.

The mechanism of this effect, however, is not entirely clear. For example, glucocorticoid treatment results in hyperinsulinemia, and the hypothesis that hyperinsulinemia can lead to a decrease in insulin receptors has already been discussed. Therefore, it is possible that, *in vivo*, the initial effect of excess glucocorticoid is to inhibit the glucose transport system. This could then lead to insulin resistance and hyperinsulinemia. The resulting hyperinsulinemia could then cause down regulation of insulin receptors with subsequent worsening of the insulin-resistant state. On the other hand, dexamethasone treatment also causes a decrease in the affinity of the receptor for insulin (Olefsky et al., 1975b), and this effect cannot be attributed to hyperinsulinemia. Therefore, even if hyperinsulinemia causes the decrease in insulin receptors, one still must postulate an additional primary or secondary effect of glucocorticoids on the affinity of the insulin receptor to bind insulin. Regardless of the mechanism of this latter phenomenon, it seems likely that, *in vivo,* the effect of excess glucocorticoids to decrease glucose utilization is due to a combination of decreased insulin binding and decreased activity of the glucose transport system.

UREMIA

Glucose Intolerance in Renal Insufficiency

Carbohydrate intolerance was first recognized in uremic subjects in the early 1900s (Hopkins, 1915; Myers and Bailey, 1916; Hamman and Hirschman, 1917; Williams and Humphreys, 1919). Although this abnormality probably exists to some extent in most patients with renal insufficiency, its severity has been greatly overestimated by methods for measuring glucose that do not discriminate between glucose- and nonglucose-reducing substances (Hutchings et al., 1966; Cerletty and Engbring, 1967; Spitz et al., 1970; Powell and Djuh, 1971). For example, we (Reaven et al., 1974) have found a 40 mg/dl mean difference between true plasma glucose concentrations and

values of total reducing substances in patients with end-stage renal insufficiency. This figure corresponds to the 36 mg/dl difference between true
plasma glucose and total reducing substances reported by Hutchings et al.
(1966). Given this difference, it is easy to see how patients with end-stage
renal failure can be reported to have an increased incidence of diabetes
mellitus if total reducing substances are measured. For example, a true plasma
glucose concentration in excess of 145 mg/dl 2 hr after an orally administered
load is considered to be abnormal (Report of the Committee on Statistics of
the American Diabetes Association, 1969). Therefore, a patient with end-stage
renal failure would have to have a 2 hr true plasma glucose value of less than
105 mg/dl to not be classified as having chemical diabetes if glucose was
measured by a nonspecific method.

The likelihood of overestimating the incidence of glucose intolerance in
uremia is also present when one is dealing with the plasma glucose response to
an acute glucose load administered intravenously. In this instance, the
normality of the response is determined by graphing the fall in plasma glucose
concentration on semilog paper and computing the fractional disappearance
rate (k value). For example, we have shown (Reaven et al., 1974) that the
simple addition of 40 mg/dl (the difference between true glucose and total
reducing substances) to each value obtained during an intravenous glucose
tolerance test resulted in a fall in mean k in normal subjects from 1.67% to
1.21%. Approximately half of the patients now had a k value considered to be
diagnostic of mild diabetes. Thus, in this instance the use of an improper
method to measure plasma glucose concentration in patients with end-stage
renal failure could have led to the false conclusion that more than 50% of
uremic subjects have abnormal glucose tolerance.

On the other hand, studies in which specific methods for measuring
plasma glucose concentrations were used have demonstrated that uremic
subjects do have an increased incidence of abnormal responses to either an
acute iv or orally administered glucose challenge (Westervelt and Schreiner,
1962; Hutchings et al., 1966; Cerletty and Engbring, 1967; Horton et al.,
1968; Davidson et al., 1969; Orskov and Christensen, 1971). Furthermore, the
degree of abnormality of glucose response is correlated with the degree of
azotemia (Reaven et al., 1974). It therefore appears that end-stage renal
insufficiency leads to deterioration in glucose tolerance. However, it also
appears that the deterioration is relatively moderate, affecting only the plasma
glucose response to an acute iv or orally administered glucose challenge. In
addition, as noted above, determination of plasma glucose concentrations by
methods that measure total reducing substances will lead to an overestimation
of the degree of glucose intolerance in these patients.

Insulin Response in Renal Insufficiency

Most studies have indicated that both fasting and postglucose challenge
plasma immunoreactive insulin (IRI) levels in patients with chronic renal

failure, are equal to or greater than those in normal subjects (Hampers et al., 1966, 1968; Hutchings et al., 1966; Cerletty and Engbring, 1967; Briggs et al., 1967; Horton et al., 1968; Davidson et al., 1969; Lowrie et al., 1970; Spitz et al., 1970; Orskov and Christensen, 1971). The fact that insulin levels are, if anything, greater than normal in these patients demonstrates that their glucose intolerance occurs in spite of an increase in pancreatic insulin secretion. This has often been taken to mean that resistance to the action of insulin must be responsible for the hyperglycemia. However, it is not possible to assume that the plasma IRI response to glucose provides a direct estimate of the pancreatic secretion rate in patients with chronic renal failure. Indeed, given the fact that insulin removal is delayed in patients with renal insufficiency (Rubenstein and Spitz, 1968; Silvers et al., 1969; Swenson et al., 1971), elevated plasma insulin levels may represent delayed insulin catabolism secondary to the loss of renal parenchyma as well as increased pancreatic secretion.

We have attempted to separate these two possible effects by studying the insulin response to a constant infusion of glucose in dogs with both ureters diverted into the vena cava. In this manner uremia was produced without loss of renal mass, and we were able to determine the insulin response under conditions in which the renal excretory system remained intact. The results of these studies (Swenson et al., 1973) indicated that higher steady-state plasma glucose levels were attained in all dogs after the production of azotemia. These results provide further support for the notion that glucose intolerance occurs in uremia. However, there was no difference in the insulin response before and after uremia. Thus, the impairment in glucose response that occurs in acute uremia is not associated with an increase in insulin response when there has been no loss of renal parenchyma. These results suggest that elevated concentrations of plasma insulin in uremic subjects may be due to a defect in insulin removal, and they need not be indicative of an increase in insulin secretion.

Indeed, it could be argued that these results indicate that the insulin response is actually decreased in uremia. Thus, since uremia resulted in glucose intolerance, increased amounts of insulin should have been secreted to prevent this occurrence. More direct evidence in support of the view that uremia suppresses the insulin response has been offered by Hampers et al. (1966, 1968), who point out that the early insulin response to an acute iv-administered glucose load is depressed in patients with uremia. However, in a later study by the same group (Lowrie et al., 1970), no differences in the early insulin response to an iv-administered glucose challenge were seen between normal subjects and patients with renal insufficiency. Moreover, a normal early insulin response to iv-administered glucose has been reported in other studies (Hutchings et al., 1966; Horton et al., 1968).

Thus, there is little evidence indicating that the glucose intolerance of azotemia is due to a primary defect in insulin secretion, and in most instances actual increases in plasma insulin concentrations are observed. However, such rises in plasma insulin concentration need not mean that there is an associated increase in pancreatic insulin response. It appears from the above considerations that the actual insulin secretion in patients with renal insufficiency is comparable to that of normal subjects. It therefore still seems reasonable to consider the possibility that the glucose intolerance of the uremic patient is secondary to resistance to the action of endogenous insulin. Nevertheless, the fact that the pancreatic response is not increased in absolute terms, in spite of the glucose intolerance, raises the possibility that uremia inhibits the normal compensatory response of the pancreas to hyperglycemia. Obviously, this latter argument is based on the notion that the plasma insulin response is a linear function of the coexisting plasma glucose response. Although this may appear to be a reasonable assumption, there is considerable evidence suggesting the contrary (Hales and Randle, 1963; Castro et al., 1970; Peterson and Reaven, 1971; Olefsky et al., 1973b).

Evidence for Insulin Resistance in
Renal Insufficiency

The glucose intolerance observed in patients with renal insufficiency could be due either to a decrease in insulin secretion or to insulin resistance. Since there is little evidence to support the view that there is an absolute decrease in insulin secretion in patients with uremia, resistance to insulin-mediated glucose uptake would appear to be primarily responsible for the glucose intolerance in these patients. Direct evidence for this thesis can be found in a variety of studies which indicate that the ability of exogenous insulin to acutely lower plasma glucose concentration is impaired in uremic subjects (Perkoff et al., 1958; Westervelt and Schreiner, 1962; Hampers et al., 1966; Cerletty and Engbring, 1967; Horton et al., 1968; Spitz et al., 1970). We recently reevaluated the ability of insulin to promote glucose uptake in uremic subjects in a somewhat different fashion (Swenson et al., 1973). These studies were carried out in dogs, made uremic by surgical diversion of both ureters into the vena cava. Insulin resistance was estimated by our method in which glucose, insulin, epinephrine, and propranolol are constantly infused (Shen et al., 1970). By this approach, endogenous insulin secretion and hepatic glucose output are inhibited, similar circulating insulin concentrations are produced in all subjects, and the height of the ensuing steady-state plasma glucose concentration becomes a direct estimate of insulin resistance. These studies were performed before and 4 days after uremia had been produced by bilateral ureteral diversion in nine dogs. Steady-state plasma glucose concentrations were higher after uremia had developed in each dog, despite comparable steady-state plasma insulin levels. More specifically, these dogs had developed insulin resistance.

It therefore seems clear that insulin resistance exists in uremia. There is also evidence to suggest that this resistance involves the action of insulin on both peripheral tissues and liver. In this regard, Westervelt (1968, 1969, 1970) has shown that insulin-stimulated forearm glucose uptake was only 25% of normal values in uremic subjects. Phosphorus uptake was also decreased when forearms of uremic subjects were perfused with insulin. The ability of insulin to increase forearm lactate production was also attenuated in these subjects, but the amount of lactate produced per mol of glucose utilized was the same. The latter observation suggests that intracellular mechanisms for glucose catabolism are intact in uremia and that the defect lies at the transport step. These results strongly suggest that there is resistance to insulin-stimulated glucose uptake in uremia.

Evidence for an abnormality in hepatic responsiveness to the action of insulin has come primarily from the work of Cohen and collaborators (1962, 1967, 1968) who, on the basis of a variety of experimental observations, suggested that there was an abnormality of hepatic glucose uptake in uremia. They believed that a decrease in hepatic glycogen content would lead to a defect in both glycogenolysis and gluconeogenesis and play a role in both the glucose intolerance and hypoglycemic unresponsiveness of uremia. It should be pointed out that not all investigators share this view. Normal glycogen content has been reported in livers of uremic patients (Dzurik and Brixova, 1968) and rats with either acute or chronic experimental uremia (Boucot et al., 1958, 1960). Furthermore, incorporation of glucose into glycogen has been found to be normal in chronically uremic rats (Cummings and Zottu, 1960). Thus, it is clear that final conclusions concerning the site (or sites) of the insulin resistance in uremia remain to be clarified.

Mechanism of Insulin Resistance in Renal Insufficiency

Resistance to insulin-mediated glucose uptake in uremic patients could theoretically be due to the secretion of an abnormal form of insulin by these patients. However, there is no experimental support for this notion. The fact that these patients are also resistant to the action of exogenous insulin makes this an unlikely possibility. Therefore, the insulin resistance must be secondary to the presence of a circulating insulin antagonist and/or to an intrinsic defect in the cellular response to insulin associated with the uremic syndrome. Since there is essentially no information available at this time concerning the second possibility, we will devote the remainder of this section to considering the causal role that various circulating insulin antagonists might play in the insulin resistance of uremia.

Renal insufficiency is characterized by the retention of many substances, and it is possible that one or more of these is responsible for the insulin antagonism. For example, metabolic acidosis has been shown to produce glucose intolerance (Guest et al., 1952). However, we have directly measured the effect of acidosis on insulin resistance by the constant infusion method described earlier and found this effect to be a modest one (Weisinger et al., 1972). Thus, the increase in insulin resistance produced by lowering serum pH to 7.05 ± 0.04 (mean ± SEM) with ammonium chloride was only 25% of that produced following bilateral ureteral diversion. Furthermore, in the case of bilateral ureteral diversion, the pH only fell to 7.30 ± 0.02. This demonstration of the relatively minor effect of severe metabolic acidosis on insulin resistance is consistent with studies on uremic patients in which it has been difficult to show a correlation between the degree of acidemia and the degree of glucose intolerance (Hampers et al., 1966; Spitz et al., 1970; Westervelt and Schreiner, 1962).

Another circulating factor that has been implicated in the insulin resistance of uremia is growth hormone. Growth hormone is well recognized as a diabetogenic factor, and several studies have shown a significant correlation between degree of azotemia and elevation in fasting growth hormone levels (Horton et al., 1968; Wright et al., 1968; Spitz et al., 1970; Orskov and Christensen, 1971; Reaven et al., 1974). Such observations raise the possibility that elevated concentrations of growth hormone could be responsible for the glucose intolerance and insulin resistance of uremia. On the other hand, it has also been pointed out that there is no correlation between degree of glucose intolerance and growth hormone concentration (Horton et al., 1968; Wright et al., 1968; Spitz et al., 1970). Thus, the ultimate role played by excessive growth hormone in the glucose intolerance of uremia remains to be clarified.

More recently, excessive secretion of parathyroid hormone has been suggested as a possible cause of glucose intolerance and insulin resistance in patients with renal failure (Lindall et al., 1971). Since secondary hyperparathyroidism is a common finding in patients with renal insufficiency, and hyperparathyroidism seems to lead to insulin resistance and increased insulin secretion (Kim et al., 1971), the possibility that increased circulating levels of parathyroid hormone and/or hypocalcemia may play a role in the development of insulin resistance of uremia must be evaluated. In this regard, recent studies by Amend and associates (1975) of six patients with chronic renal failure, before and after parathyroidectomy for secondary hyperparathyroidism, suggest that elevated parathyroid hormone levels do not act as insulin antagonists. This conclusion is consistent with our studies, in which we could not document a significant effect of elevated parathyroid hormone levels on insulin resistance in patients with primary hyperparathyroidism (Ginsberg et al., 1975a). Furthermore, Amend et al. found that hypercalcemia, not hypocalcemia, resulted in a decrease in normal tissue sensitivity to insulin. This finding is somewhat surprising in light of the results of Lisch et al. (1973), who found that the ability of insulin to promote glucose uptake was increased when hypocalcemic patients with chronic renal failure were made eucalcemic. The reason for this apparent discrepancy concerning the role of hypocalcemia in the insulin resistance of uremia is not clear, and it is obvious that further studies must be done to fully evaluate the possible role of hyperparathyroidism and/or hypocalcemia.

The circulating factor that has received the greatest attention recently as the cause of the insulin resistance in uremia is glucagon. The possibility that excessive glucagon levels might contribute to glucose intolerance seemed to be unlikely following the initial report of normal glucagon concentration in patients with uremia (Tchobroutsky et al., 1969). However, subsequent studies have repeatedly confirmed the presence of fasting hyperglucagonemia in patients with chronic renal failure (Daubresse et al., 1976; Kuku et al., 1976; Sherwin et al., 1976). Nevertheless, the fact that there are increased levels of glucagon in patients with chronic uremia does not mean that the insulin resistance of these patients is due to hyperglucagonemia. This is particularly relevant since the results of Kuku et al. (1976) clearly indicate that the predominant form of plasma glucagon in patients with renal failure was of an intermediate size (MW ± 9,000), consistent with its being proglucagon. The role that this accumulation of proglucagon may play in the glucose intolerance of uremia obviously cannot be clarified until we have a better idea of its biological activity. Until we have such information, it is difficult to evaluate the significance of the finding that undialyzed patients with renal failure are abnormally sensitive to the hyperglycemic effects of exogenous glucagon (Sherwin et al., 1976). Although it is clear that increased glucagon levels may play a role in the insulin resistance of uremia, it is also clear that a good deal of additional work is needed to evaluate this possibility.

Finally, many other possible causes of insulin resistance in azotemia have been suggested, including urea itself, retention of other toxic metabolites, and decreased total body potassium concentration. All of these alternatives require further study before they can be evaluated as possible circulating antagonists to insulin. It is also possible that there is no one circulating factor that is uniquely responsible for the insulin resistance of uremia, and that several factors contribute. Indeed, it is also possible that none of these circulating factors play a substantial role as insulin antagonists, and that the defect causing the insulin resistance is at the cellular level. This is an alternative that we are currently investigating.

CONCLUSION

In this review we have summarized the evidence that obesity, nonketotic diabetes, glucocorticoid excess, and uremia are characterized by insulin resistance. We have also focused on the mechanisms for this insulin resistance insofar as this information is available. It should be obvious at this point that insulin resistance is a rather general term, which is loosely used to describe situations in which the effects of insulin are subnormal. Clearly, different mechanisms for "insulin resistance" occur in the different situations described, and even within a single abnormal physiological state a single cause for decreased insulin responsiveness may not exist. Thus, the mechanisms for insulin resistance are as complex as insulin action itself, and decreased insulin effectiveness can be due to single or multiple abnormalities located at any step of the pathway of insulin action.

REFERENCES

Alford, F. P., Martin, F. I. R. and Pearson, M. J. 1971. *Diabetologia* 7:173.

Amatruda, J. H., Livingston, J. N. and Lockwood, D. H. 1975. *Science* 188:264.

Amend, W. C., Jr., Steinberg, S. M., Lowrie, E. G., Lazarus, J. M., Soeldner, J. S., Hampers, C. L. and Merrill, J. P. 1975. *J. Lab. Clin. Med.* 86:435.

Aguilar-Parada, E., Eisentraut, A. M. and Unger, R. H. 1969. *Am. J. Med. Sci.* 257:415.

Archer, J. A., Gorden, P., Gavin, J. R., III, Lesniak, M. and Roth, J. 1973. *J. Clin. Endocrinol. Metab.* 36:627.

Archer, J. A., Gorden, P. and Roth, J. 1975. *J. Clin. Invest.* 55:166.

Bagdade, J. D., Bierman, E. L. and Porte, D., Jr. 1967. *J. Clin. Invest.* 46:1549.

Bar, R. S., Gorden, P., Roth, J., Kahn, C. R. and De Meyts, P. 1977. *J. Clin. Invest.*, in press.

Barnes, A. J. and Bloom, S. R. 1976. *Lancet* 1:219.

Barnes, A. J., Bloom, A., Crowley, M. F., Tuttlebee, J. W., Bloom, S. R., Alberti, K. G. M. M., Smythe, P. and Turnell, D. 1975. *Lancet* 2:734.

Bastenie, P. A., Conard, V. and Franckson, J. R. M. 1954. *Diabetes* 3:205.

Bearn, A. G., Billing, B. H. and Sherlock, S. 1951. *Lancet* 2:698.

Benson, S. and Talun, R. S. 1965. *Diabetes* 14:549.

Berger, S., Downey, J. I., Traisman, H. S. and Metz, R. 1966. *N. Engl. J. Med.* 274:1460.

Berkowitz, D. 1964. *J. Am. Med. Assoc.* 187:399.

Bernstein, R. S. and Kipnis, D. M. 1973. *Diabetes* 22:923.

Berson, S. A. and Yalow, R. S. 1962. *Ciba Found. Colloq. Endocrinol.* 14:182.

Berson, S. A. and Yalow, R. S. 1965. *Diabetes* 14:549.

Bilbrey, G. L., Faloona, G. R., White, M. G. and Knochel, J. P. 1974. *J. Clin. Invest.* 53:841.

Birnbaumer, L., Pohl, S. L. and Kaumann, A. J. 1974. *Adv. Cyclic Nucleotide Res.* 4:239.

Bjorntorp, P. 1966. *Acta Med. Scand.* 179:229.

Blecher, M. 1966. *Endocrinology* 79:541.

Bornstein, J. and Lawrence, D. D. 1951. *Br. Med. J.* 2:1541.

Bornstein, J. and Trewhella, P. 1950. *Aust. J. Exp. Biol. Med. Sci.* 28:569.

Boucot, N. G., Guild, W. R. and Merrill, J. P. 1958. *Am. J. Physiol.* 192:30.

Boucot, N. G., Nurser, E. K. and Merrill, J. P. 1960. *Am. J. Physiol.* 198:797.

Braaten, J. T., Faloona, G. R. and Unger, R. H. 1974. *J. Clin. Invest.* 53:1017.

Bray, G. A., Davidson, M. B. and Drenick, E. J. 1972. *Ann. Intern. Med.* 77:797.

Briggs, J. D., Buchanan, K. D., Luke, R. G. and McKiddie, M. T. 1967. *Lancet* 1:462.

Buchanan, K. D. and Mawhinney, W. A. A. 1973. *Diabetes* 27:797.

Buchanan, K. D. and McCarroll, A. M. 1972. *Lancet* 2:1394.

Buchanan, K. D. and McKiddie, M. T. 1967. *Diabetes* 16:466.

Cahill, G. F. 1971. *The human adrenal cortex*, p. 205. New York: Harper & Row.

Castro, A., Scott, J. P., Grettie, D. P., McFarlane, D. and Bailey, R. E. 1970. *Diabetes* 19:842.
Cerasi, E. 1967. *Acta Endocrinol.* 55:163.
Cerasi, E. and Luft, R. 1967. *Acta Endocrinol.* 55:278.
Cerletty, J. M. and Engbring, N. H. 1967. *Ann. Intern. Med.* 66:1097.
Chiles, R. and Tzagournis, M. 1970. *Diabetes* 19:458.
Cohen, B. D. 1962. *Ann. Intern. Med.* 57:204.
Cohen, B. D. and Horowitz, H. I. 1968. *Am. J. Clin. Nutr.* 21:407.
Cohen, B. D., Galloway, J., McMahon, R. E., Culp, H. W., Root, M. A. and Henniquer, K. J. 1967. *Am. J. Med. Sci.* 254:608.
Conn, J. W. and Fajans, S. S. 1956. *Metabolism* 5:114.
Cuatrecasas, P. 1974. *Annu. Rev. Biochem.* 43:169.
Cummings, N. G. and Zottu, S. M. 1960. *Am. J. Physiol.* 198:1079.
Czech, M. P. 1976. *J. Clin. Invest.* 57:1523.
Czech, M. P. and Fain, J. N. 1972. *Endocrinology* 91:518.
Czech, M. P. and Richardson, D. K. 1976. *Abstr. 58th Annu. Meet. Endocr. Soc.*, p. 93, no. 71.
Danowski, T. S., Khurana, R., Nolan, S., Stephan, T., Gegick, C., Chae, S. and Vidalan, C. 1973. *Diabetes* 22:808.
Daubresse, J. C., Lerson, G., Plamteux, G., Rorive, G., Luyckx, P. S. and LeFebvre, P. J. 1976. *Eur. J. Clin. Invest.* 6:159.
Davidson, J. and Haist, R. 1958. *Lancet* 2:656.
Davidson, M. B., Lowrie, E. G. and Hampers, C. L. 1969. *Metabolism* 18:387.
Di Girolamo, M. and Rudman, D. 1968. *Endocrinology* 82:1133.
Duckworth, W. C. and Kitabachi, A. E. 1972. *Am. J. Med.* 53:418.
Dzurik, R. and Brixova, E. 1968. *Experientia* 24:552.
Ehrlich, R. M. and Bambers, G. 1964. *Diabetes* 13:177.
Eisenstein, A. B., Spencer, S., Flatness, S. and Brodsky, A. 1966. *Endocrinology* 79:182.
Exton, J. H., Friedmann, N., Wond, E. H., Brineaux, J. P., Corbin, J. D. and Park, C. R. 1972. *J. Biol. Chem.* 247:3579.
Fain, J. N. 1964. *J. Biol. Chem.* 239:958.
Fain, J. N., Scow, R. O. and Chernick, S. S. 1963. *J. Biol. Chem.* 238:54.
Fajans, S. S. and Conn, J. W. 1954. *Diabetes* 3:296.
Farrant, P. C., Neville, R. W. J. and Stewart, G. A. 1969. *Diabetologia* 5:198.
Felig, P., Wahren, J., Hendler, R. and Brundin, T. 1974. *J. Clin. Invest.* 53:582.
Field, J. B. 1962. *Annu. Rev. Med.* 13:249.
Forgue, M. and Freychet, P. 1975. *Diabetes* 24:715.
Frankel, B. J., Gerich, J. E., Hagura, R., Fanska, R. E., Gerritsen, G. C. and Grodsky, G. M. 1974. *J. Clin. Invest.* 53:1637.
Freeman, C., Karoly, K. and Adelman, R. C. 1973. *Biochem. Biophys. Res. Commun.* 54:1573.
Freychet, P. and Forgue, M. 1975. *Diabetes* 24:715.
Freychet, P., Laudat, M. H., Laudat, P., Rosselin, G., Kahn, C. R., Gorden, P. and Roth, J. 1972. *FEBS Lett.* 25:339.
Frohman, L. A., Goldman, J. K. and Bernardis, L. L. 1972. *Metabolism* 21:1133.
Galton, D. J. and Wilson, J. P. D. 1970. *Clin. Sci.* 38:661.
Galton, D. J. and Wilson, J. P. D. 1971. *Clin. Sci.* 41:545.
Galton, D. J., Wilson, J. P. D. and Kissebah, A. H. 1971. *Eur. J. Clin. Invest.* 1:399.

Gammeltoft, S. and Gliemann, J. 1973. *Biochim. Biophys. Acta* 320:16.

Gavin, J. R., III, Gorden, P., Roth, J., Archer, J. W. and Buell, O. 1973. *J. Biol. Chem.* 248:2202.

Gavin, J. R., III, Roth, J., Neville, D. M., Jr., DeMeyts, P. and Buell, D. N. 1974. *Proc. Natl. Acad. Sci. U.S.A.* 71:84.

Ginsberg, H., Olefsky, J. M. and Reaven, G. M. 1974. *Diabetes* 23:674.

Ginsberg, H., Olefsky, J. M. and Reaven, G. M. 1975a. *Proc. Soc. Exp. Biol. Med.* 148:942.

Ginsberg, H., Kimmerling, G., Olefsky, J. M. and Reaven, G. M. 1975b. *J. Clin. Invest.* 55:454.

Gliemann, J., Gammeltoft, S. and Vinten, J. 1975. *J. Biol. Chem.* 250:3368.

Goldfine, I. D., Kahn, C. R., Neville, D. M., Jr., Roth, J., Garrison, M. M. and Bates, R. W. 1973. *Biochem. Biophys. Res. Commun.* 53:852.

Goldstein, S., Blecher, M., Binder, R., Perrino, P. V. and Recant, L. 1975. *Endocr. Res. Comm.* 2:367.

Gorden, P. and Roth, J. 1970. *J. Clin. Invest.* 48:2225.

Gorden, P., Hendricks, C. M. and Roth, J. 1974. *Diabetologia* 10:469.

Grey, W. and Kipnis, D. M. 1971. *N. Engl. J. Med.* 285:827.

Guest, G. M., Mackler, B. and Knowles, H. C., Jr. 1952. *Diabetes* 1:276.

Hales, C. N. and Randle, P. J. 1963. *Lancet* 1:790.

Hamman, L. and Hirschman, I. I. 1917. *Arch. Intern. Med.* 20:761.

Hampers, C. L., Soeldner, J. S., Doak, P. B. and Merrill, J. P. 1966. *J. Clin. Invest.* 45:1719.

Hampers, C. L., Soeldner, J. S., Gleason, R. E., Bailey, G. L., Diamond, J. A. and Merrill, J. P. 1968. *Am. J. Clin. Nutr.* 21:414.

Hansen, A. P. 1970. *J. Clin. Invest.* 49:1467.

Hansen, A. P. 1971. *J. Clin. Invest.* 50:1806.

Hansen, A. P. 1973a. *J. Clin. Endocrinol. Metab.* 36:638.

Hansen, A. P. 1973b. *Diabetes* 22:619.

Hansen, A. P. and Johansen, K. 1970. *Diabetologia* 6:27.

Harrison, L. C., Martin, F. I. R. and Melick, R. A. 1976. *J. Clin. Invest.* 58:1435.

Haynes, R. C., Jr. 1962. *Endocrinology* 71:399.

Heller, N., Kalant, N. and Hoffman, M. M. 1958. *J. Lab. Clin. Med.* 52:394.

Hewing, R., Liebermeister, H., Daweke, H., Gries, F. A. and Gruneklee, D. 1973. *Diabetologia* 9:197.

Himsworth, H. 1936. *Lancet* 1:127.

Hopkins, A. H. 1915. *Am. J. Med. Sci.* 149:254.

Horton, E. S., Johnson, C. and Lebovitz, H. E. 1968. *Ann. Intern. Med.* 68:63.

Hoshi, M. and Shreeve, W. W. 1973. *Diabetes* 22:16.

Houssay, B. A. and Anderson, E. 1949. *Endocrinology* 45:627.

Hutchings, R. H., Hegstrom, R. M. and Scribner, B. H. 1966. *Ann. Intern. Med.* 65:275.

Issekutz, B. and Allen, M. 1972. *Metabolism* 21:48.

Issekutz, B. and Borkow, I. 1973. *Metabolism* 22:39.

Johansen, K. and Hansen, A. P. 1969. *Br. Med. J.* 2:356.

Johansen, K. and Hansen, A. P. 1971. *Diabetes* 20:239.

Kahlenberg, A. and Kalant, N. 1964. *Can. J. Biochem.* 42:1623.

Kahn, C. R., Neville, D. M., Jr. and Roth, J. 1973a. *J. Biol. Chem.* 248:244.

Kahn, C. R., Goldfine, I. D., Neville, D. M., Jr., Roth, J., Bates, R. W. and Garrison, M. M. 1973b. *Endocrinology* 93:A-168 (abstract).

Kalant, H., Csorba, T. R. and Heller, N. 1963. *Metabolism* 12:1100.

Kalkhoff, R. K., Kim, H. J., Cerletty, J. and Ferrou, C. A. 1971. *Diabetes* 20:83.

Karam, J. H., Grodsky, G. M. and Forsham, P. H. 1963. *Diabetes* 12:197.

Karam, J. H., Pavlatos, F. C., Grodsky, G. M. and Forsham, P. H. 1965. *Lancet* 1:286.

Katsilambros, N. Y., Abdel Rahman, Y., Minz, M., Fussganger, K. E., Schroder, K. E., Straub, K. and Pfeiffer, E. F. 1970. *Horm. Metab. Res.* 2:286.

Katzen, H. M. and Glitzer, M. S. 1968. In *Carbohydrate metabolism and its disorders,* eds. F. Dickens, P. J. Randle, and W. J. Whelan, vol. 2, pp. 265–287. New York: Academic Press.

Kim, H., Kalkhoff, R. K., Costrini, N. V., Cerletty, J. M. and Jacobson, M. 1971. *J. Clin. Invest.* 50:2596.

Kimmerling, G., Javorski, W. C., Olefsky, J. M. and Reaven, G. M. 1976. *Diabetes* 25:673.

Kipnis, D. M. and Stein, M. G. 1964. *Ciba Found. Colloq. Endocrinol.* 15:156.

Kjeldsen, H., Hansen, A. P. and Lundbaek, K. 1975. *Diabetes* 24:977.

Knittle, J. L. and Ginsberg-Fellner, F. 1972. *Diabetes* 21:754.

Kobayashi, M. and Meek, J. C. 1976. *Abstr. 58th Annu. Meet. Endocr. Soc.,* p. 299, no. 484.

Kono, T. and Barham, F. W. 1971. *J. Biol. Chem.* 246:6210.

Kosaka, K., Harura, R., Odagiri, R., Saito, F. and Kuzuya, T. 1972. *J. Clin. Endocrinol. Metab.* 35:655.

Kosmakos, F. C. and Roth, J. 1976. *Abstr. 58th Annu. Meet. Endocr. Soc.,* p. 69, no. 26.

Kreisberg, R. A., Boshell, B. R., DiPlacido, J. and Roddam, R. F. 1967. *N. Engl. J. Med.* 276:314.

Kuku, S. F., Ziedler, A., Emmanouel, D. S., Katz, A. I. and Rubenstein, A. H. 1976. *J. Clin. Endocrinol. Metab.* 42:173.

Landau, B. R. 1965. *Vitam. Horm.* 23:1.

Laube, H., Fussganger, R., Maier, V. and Pfeiffer, E. F. 1973. *Diabetologia* 9:400.

Leboeuf, B., Renold, A. E. and Cahill, G. F., Jr. 1962. *J. Biol. Chem.* 237:988.

Lesko, L., Marinetti, G. and Campbell, R. submitted.

Lindall, A., Carmena, R., Cohen, S. and Comty, C. 1971. *J. Clin. Endocrinol. Metab.* 32:653.

Lisch, H. J., Bolzano, K., Patsoh, J., Sailer, S. and Braunsteiner, H. 1973. *Diabetologia* 9:467.

Livingston, J. N. and Lockwood, D. H. 1974. *Biochem. Biophys. Res. Commun.* 61:989.

Livingston, J. N. and Lockwood, D. H. 1975. *J. Biol. Chem.* 250:8353.

Livingston, J. N., Cuatrecasas, P. and Lockwood, D. H. 1972. *Science* 177:626.

Lowrie, E. G., Soeldner, J. S., Hampers, C. L. and Merrill, J. P. 1970. *J. Lab. Clin. Med.* 76:603;

Luke, R. G., Dinwoolie, A. J., Linton, A. L. and Kennedy, A. C. 1964. *J. Lab. Clin. Med.* 64:731.

Marinetti, G. V., Schlatz, L. and Reilly, K. 1972. *Insulin action,* vol. 1, p. 224. New York: Academic Press.

Marco, J., Calle, C., Roman, D., Diaz-Fierros, M., Villanueva, M. L. and Valverde, I. 1973. *N. Engl. J. Med.* 288:128.
McKiddie, M. T., Jasani, M. K., Buchanan, K. D., Boyle, J. A. and Buchanan, W. W. 1968. *Metabolism* 17:730.
Meir, J. M., McGarry, J. D., Faloona, G. R., Unger, R. H. and Foster, D. W. 1972. *J. Lipid Res.* 13:228.
Melani, F., Rubenstein, A. and Steiner, D. 1970. *J. Clin. Invest.* 49:497.
Molnar, G. D., Taylor, W. F., Langworthy, A. and Fatourechi, V. 1972. *J. Clin. Endocrinol.* 34:837.
Muller, W. A., Faloona, G. R., Aguilar-Parada, E. and Unger, R. H. 1970. *N. Engl. J. Med.* 283:109.
Munck, A. 1971. *Perspect. Biol. Med.* 14:265.
Myers, V. C. and Bailey, C. V. 1916. *J. Biol. Chem.* 24:147.
Ninomiya, R., Forbath, N. F. and Hetenyi, G. 1965. *Diabetes* 14:729.
Olefsky, J. M. 1975. *J. Clin. Invest.* 56:1499.
Olefsky, J. M. 1976a. *J. Clin. Invest.* 57:842.
Olefsky, J. M. 1976b. *J. Clin. Invest.* 57:1165.
Olefsky, J. M. 1976c. *J. Clin. Invest.* 58:1450.
Olefsky, J. M. 1977. *Endocrinology* 100:1169.
Olefsky, J. M. and Reaven, G. M. 1974. *J. Clin. Invest.* 54:1323.
Olefsky, J. M. and Reaven, G. M. 1975. *Endocrinology* 96:1486.
Olefsky, J. M. and Reaven, G. M. 1976a. *Am. J. Med.* 60:98.
Olefsky, J. M. and Reaven, G. M. 1976b. *J. Clin. Endocrinol. Metab.* 43:232.
Olefsky, J. M. and Reaven, G. M. 1977. *Diabetes,* in press.
Olefsky, J. M., Farquhar, J. W. and Reaven, G. M. 1973a. *Diabetes* 22:507.
Olefsky, J. M., Batchelder, T., Farquhar, J. W. and Reaven, G. M. 1973b. *Metabolism* 22:1277.
Olefsky, J. M., Reaven, G. M. and Farquhar, J. W. 1974. *J. Clin. Invest.* 53:64.
Olefsky, J., Crapo, P. A., Ginsberg, H. and Reaven, G. M. 1975a. *Metabolism* 24:495.
Olefsky, J. M., Johnson, J., Liu, F., Jen, P. and Reaven, G. M. 1975b. *Metabolism* 24:517.
Olefsky, J., Bacon, V. C. and Baur, S. 1976. *Metabolism* 24:179.
Orskov, H. and Christensen, N. J. 1971. *Scand. J. Clin. Lab. Invest.* 27:51.
Owen, O. E. and Cahill, G. F. 1973. *J. Clin. Invest.* 52:2596.
Page, M. A. and Galton, D. J. 1975. *Clin. Sci. Mol. Med.* 49:27.
Perkoff, G. T., Thomas, C. L., Newton, J. D., Sellman, J. C. and Tyler, F. H. 1958. *Diabetes* 7:375.
Perley, M. and Kipnis, D. M. 1966a. *N. Engl. J. Med.* 274:1237.
Perley, M. and Kipnis, D. M. 1966b. *Diabetes* 15:867.
Perley, M. and Kipnis, D. M. 1967. *J. Clin. Invest.* 46:1954.
Peterson, D. T. and Reaven, G. M. 1971. *Diabetes* 20:729.
Plager, J. E. and Matsui, N. 1966. *Endocrinology* 78:1154.
Powell, J. B. and Djuh, Y-Y. 1971. *Am. J. Clin. Pathol.* 56:8.
Pupo, A. A., Ursich, M. J. M., Iamaguchi, E. and Vasconcellos, F. G. 1976. *Diabetes* 25:161.
Rabinowitz, D. 1970. *Annu. Rev. Med.* 21:241.
Rabinowitz, D. and Zierler, K. L. 1962. *J. Clin. Invest.* 41:2173.
Raskin, P., Fujita, Y. and Unger, R. H. 1975. *J. Clin. Invest.* 56:1132.
Reaven, G. M. and Miller, R. 1968. *Diabetes* 17:560.
Reaven, G. M. and Olefsky, J. M. 1974. *J. Clin. Endocrinol. Metab.* 38:151.

Reaven, G. M., Shen, S. W., Silvers, A. and Farquhar, J. W. 1971. *Diabetes* 20:416.

Reaven, G. M., Weisinger, J. R. and Swenson, R. S. 1974. *Kidney Int.* 6:S63.

Report of the Committee on Statistics of the American Diabetes Association. 1969. Standardization of the oral glucose tolerance test. *Diabetes* 18:299.

Riddick, F. A., Reisler, D. M. and Kipnis, D. M. 1962. *Diabetes* 11:171.

Robinson, C. A., Jr., Boshell, B. R. and Reddy, W. J. 1972. *Biochim. Biophys. Acta* 290:84.

Roth, J. 1973. *Metabolism* 22:1059.

Roth, J., Glick, S. M., Yalow, R. S. and Berson, S. A. 1963. *Metabolism* 12:577.

Roth, J., Gorden, P. and Pastan, I. 1968. *Proc. Natl. Acad. Sci. U.S.A.* 61:138.

Rubenstein, A. H. and Spitz, E. 1968. *Diabetes* 17:161.

Rubenstein, A., Cho, S. and Steiner, D. 1968. *Lancet* 1:1353.

Salans, L. B. and Dougherty, J. W. 1971. *J. Clin. Invest.* 50:1399.

Samaan, N. and Fraser, R. 1963. *Lancet* 2:311.

Samols, E., Tyler, J. M. and Kajinuma, H. 1971. *Excerpta Med. Int. Congr. Ser.* no. 231, p. 636.

Savage, P. J., Dippe, S. E., Bennett, P. H., Gorden, P., Roth, J., Rushforth, N. B. and Miller, M. 1975. *Diabetes* 24:362.

Schteingart, D. E., Gregerman, R. I. and Conn, J. W. 1963. *Metabolism* 12:484.

Seltzer, H. S., Allen, E. W., Herron, A. L., Jr. and Brennan, M. T. 1967. *J. Clin. Invest.* 46:323.

Shaw, W. N. and Chance, R. E. 1968. *Diabetes* 17:737.

Shen, S. W., Reaven, G. M. and Farquhar, J. W. 1970. *J. Clin. Invest* 49:2151.

Sherwin, R. S., Bastl, C., Finkelstein, F. O., Fisher, M., Black, H., Hendler, R. and Felig, P. 1971. *J. Clin. Invest.* 57:722.

Sherwin, R. S., Fisher, M., Hendler, R. and Felig, P. 1976. *N. Engl. J. Med.* 294:455.

Silvers, A., Swenson, R. S., Farquhar, J. W. and Reaven, G. M. 1969. *J. Clin. Invest.* 48:1461.

Sims, E. A. H., Goldman, R. F., Gluck, C. M., Horton, E. S., Kelleher, P. C. and Rowe, D. W. 1968. *Trans. Assoc. Am. Physicians* 81:153.

Smith, M. and Levine, R. 1964. *Med. Clin. North Am.* 48:1387.

Soll, A. H., Kahn, C. R., Neville, D. M., Jr. and Roth, J. 1974. *J. Biol. Chem.* 249:4127.

Soll, A. H., Kahn, C. R., Neville, D. M., Jr. and Roth, J. 1975a. *J. Clin. Invest.* 56:769.

Soll, A. H., Kahn, C. R. and Neville, D. M., Jr. 1975b. *J. Biol. Chem.* 250:4702.

Spitz, I. M., Rubenstein, A. H., Bersohn, I., Abrahams, C. and Lowy, C. 1970. *Q. J. Med.* 154:201.

Steiner, D. F., Hallund, O., Rubenstein, A., Cho, S. and Bayliss, C. 1968. *Diabetes* 17:725.

Steinke, J., Camerini, P., Marble, A. and Renold, A. 1961. *Metabolism* 10:707.

Stocks, A. E. and Martin, F. I. R. 1969. *Br. Med. J.* 4:397.

Swenson, R. S., Silvers, A., Peterson, D. T., Kohatsu, S. and Reaven, G. M. 1971. *J. Lab. Clin. Med.* 77:829.

Swenson, R. S., Peterson, D. T., Eshleman, M. and Reaven, G. M. 1973. *Kidney Int.* 4:267.

Tchobroutsky, G., Rosselin, G., Assan, R. and Derot, M. 1969. *Diabetologia* 5:25.

Tchobroutsky, G., Kopf, A., Eschwege, E. and Assan, R. 1973. *Diabetes* 22:825.

Unger, R. H. and Orci, L. 1975. *Lancet* 1:14.

Unger, R. H., Aguilar-Parada, E., Muller, W. A. and Eisentraut, A. M. 1970. *J. Clin. Invest.* 49:837.

Unger, R. H., Madison, L. L. and Muller, W. A. 1972. *Diabetes* 21:301.

University Group Diabetes Program. 1970. *Diabetes* 19:747.

Vallence-Owen, J., Hurlock, B. and Pease, N. W. 1955. *Lancet* 2:583.

Vigneri, R., Squatrito, S., Pezzino, V., Filletti, S., Branca, S. and Polosa, P. 1976. *Diabetes* 25:167.

Weir, G. C., Knowlton, S. D., Atkins, R. F., McKennan, K. X. and Martin, D. B. 1976. *Diabetes* 25:275.

Weisinger, J., Swenson, R. S., Greene, W. G., Taylor, J. B. and Reaven, G. M. 1972. *Diabetes* 21:1109.

Westervelt, F. B. 1968. *Am. J. Clin. Nutr.* 21:423.

Westervelt, F. B. 1969. *J. Lab. Clin. Med.* 74:79.

Westervelt, F. B. 1970. *Arch. Intern. Med.* 126:856.

Westervelt, F. B., Jr. and Schreiner, G. E. 1962. *Am. Intern. Med.* 57:266.

Wicks, W. D., Barnett, C. A. and McKibbin, J. B. 1974. *Fed. Proc.* 33:1105.

Williams, J. R. and Humphreys, E. M. 1919. *Arch. Intern. Med.* 23:537.

Wise, J. K., Hendler, R. and Felig, P. 1973. *J. Clin. Invest.* 52:2774.

Wright, A. D., Lowy, C., Fraser, T. R., Spitz, I. M., Rubenstein, A. H. and Bersohn, I. 1968. *Lancet* 2:798.

Yalow, R. S. and Berson, S. A. 1960. *J. Clin. Invest* 39:1157.

Yalow, R. S., Glick, S. M., Roth, J. and Berson, S. A. 1965. *Ann. N.Y. Acad. Sci.* 131:357.

Yalow, R. S., Goldsmith, S. J. and Berson, S. A. 1969. *Diabetes* 18:402.

Yde, H. 1969. *Acta Med. Scand.* 186:499.

Yde, H. 1970. *Acta Endocrinol.* 64:339.

York, D. A., Steinke, J. and Bray, G. A. 1972. *Metabolism* 21:277.

Yorke, R. E. 1967. *J. Endocrinol.* 39:329.

Zierler, K. and Rabinowitz, D. 1963. *Medicine* 42:385.

Chapter 8

RELATIONSHIP OF ADIPOSITY AND DIET TO THE ABNORMALITIES OF CARBOHYDRATE METABOLISM IN OBESITY

Lester B. Salans and Samuel W. Cushman

Department of Medicine
Dartmouth Medical School
Hanover, New Hampshire

INTRODUCTION

Obesity is a disorder in which the ingestion of calories in excess of those being utilized by the organism results in an excessive expansion of the adipose tissue mass. This disorder is often accompanied by abnormalities in systemic carbohydrate and lipid metabolism and in the secretion and action of insulin, alterations thought to reflect the "diabetogenic" effects of obesity (Paullin and Sauls, 1922; Ogilvie, 1935; Salans et al., 1970). For example, glucose intolerance is common in obese individuals even in the absence of clinically manifest diabetes mellitus. Moreover, in patients and animals with established diabetes, hyperglycemia worsens with increasing adiposity. Abnormalities of lipid metabolism, as reflected by hypertriglyceridemia, hypercholesterolemia, and increased plasma levels of nonesterified fatty acids, may also accompany obesity (Farquhar et al., 1975; Angel, 1975), but these relationships are less well established than those for obesity and carbohydrate metabolism. These alterations in systemic carbohydrate and lipid metabolism occur in spite of an increased rate of secretion of insulin from the islets of Langerhans and elevated plasma levels of this hormone; inappropriately elevated concentrations of plasma insulin relative to glucose, both in the fasting state and following oral or intravenous glucose challenge, are well documented in obese patients with or without glucose intolerance.

The studies summarized in this chapter that were undertaken in this laboratory were performed with the excellent technical assistance of Ms. Mary Jane Zarnowski and Mrs. Ruth Segal. Special thanks is given to Mrs. Tara Mitchell for her help in preparing this manuscript. These studies were conducted with support from U.S. Public Health Service research grants AM13321 and 5 R01 AM 10254, and grants from the Hitchcock Foundation, Weight Watchers, and the American Diabetes Association.

These observations and the additional demonstration of a diminished hypoglycemic response of the obese individual to exogenously administered insulin (Franckson et al., 1966) have led to the concept that the tissues of the obese are relatively "resistant" to the action of insulin. The diminished response to insulin at the tissue level is postulated to result in a compensatory increase in the rate of insulin secretion from the pancreas, and hyperinsulinemia; the feedback mechanism operating between insulin-resistant tissues and the B-cell remains to be defined. The degree of tissue resistance to insulin and the extent of pancreatic compensation determine whether glucose homeostasis is maintained or glucose intolerance and hyperglycemia develop.

Since the expanded adipose tissue mass is the most characteristic abnormality of obesity, this tissue has received major investigative attention as the primary site of the postulated insulin resistance, and the tissue responsible for the systemic derangements of carbohydrate metabolism associated with this disorder. The observation that glucose tolerance and plasma insulin levels are frequently restored to normal with weight loss and reduction in the size of adipose tissue mass in spontaneously obese subjects (Newburgh, 1942; Salans et al., 1968) would appear to support this hypothesis; in addition, these abnormalities in systemic metabolism can be induced in nonobese, nondiabetic individuals through experimental weight gain and increased adiposity (Sims et al., 1968). Nevertheless, tissues other than adipose tissue are equally, or more, intimately involved in the regulation of glucose homeostasis, and any explanation for the insulin-resistant state and the altered carbohydrate metabolism of obesity must take into account the metabolic state of skeletal muscle and the liver. Moreover, factors other than tissue resistance to insulin may contribute to the development and perpetuation of the abnormalities of glucose metabolism, insulin secretion, and insulin action in obesity; most prominent among these is the nutritional state of the organism. Both dietary composition and total caloric intake, for example, profoundly influence systemic glucose metabolism and insulin secretion (Cahill et al., 1966; Grey et al., 1970; Brunzell et al., 1971; Grey and Kipnis, 1971; Salans and Cushman, 1973). Increased ingestion of calories and turnover of metabolic fuels are themselves associated with increased requirements for insulin and changes in the general metabolic state of an organism. The obese individual not only ingests excessive total calories, but also tends to consume diets containing excessive quantities of carbohydrate; increased caloric and/or carbohydrate intake could contribute directly and significantly to the glucose intolerance and hyperinsulinemia of obesity. The metabolic abnormalities accompanying obesity may therefore reflect not only an increased adipose tissue mass and the alteration of metabolic function in this and other tissues, but dietary factors as well. A potential role for altered physical activity in these metabolic abnormalities of obesity remains to be investigated in depth (Bjorntorp, 1975).

During the past several years, this laboratory has conducted a detailed series of investigations into the nature of the metabolic abnormalities of obesity at both the cellular and systemic levels. *In vitro* studies of tissue function have focused primarily on adipose tissue and cells as a model for elucidating the biochemical nature of these abnormalities at the cellular level. Investigations of systemic metabolism have centered on the plasma concentrations of glucose and insulin, and on glucose tolerance. The possible role of an expanded adipose tissue mass and of the diet in the development and perpetuation of these metabolic abnormalities has been examined. The discussion to follow will review the most pertinent of these studies, concentrating on the diabetogenic effects of obesity, and particularly on glucose intolerance and hyperinsulinemia. Initially, the characteristics of *in vitro* glucose metabolism in adipose tissue obtained from obese and nonobese humans and experimental animals will be reviewed; these characteristics will be related to glucose metabolism in the intact organism, as reflected in plasma parameters of systemic function. Attention will then turn to the influence of diet on the metabolic character of this tissue, and of the organism as a whole. Finally, preliminary studies of glucose metabolism in the skeletal muscle and liver of obese subjects will be summarized. This chapter will attempt to review in detail neither the important studies of other investigators that have contributed to our understanding of the relationship between obesity and carbohydrate metabolism, nor the studies dealing with the association of obesity and abnormal lipid metabolism.

ADIPOSE TISSUE

General Characteristics of Adipose Tissue Metabolism

For many years, adipose tissue was considered an inert reserve of fat, functioning only in thermal insulation and bodily protection. The pioneering studies of Wertheimer and Shapiro (1948), however, clearly demonstrated the high levels of metabolic activity in this tissue and established the central role played by adipose tissue in the regulation of carbohydrate and lipid metabolism in the mammalian organism; the adipose cells comprising this tissue contain a full complement of enzymes and subcellular organelles and respond to a wide variety of humoral, hormonal, neural, and nutritional factors (Renold and Cahill, 1965).

The primary function of adipose tissue is the storage of metabolic fuel as triglyceride; in humans, adipose tissue represents the major caloric reservoir of the body. Storage and mobilization of triglyceride by the specialized adipose cells of this tissue are active metabolic processes involving lipogenic and lipolytic functions. The lipogenic function consists of *de novo* long-chain fatty acid synthesis from glucose and esterification of these fatty acids, as well as those of exogenous origin derived from lipoprotein, with α-glycerophosphate to form triglyceride (Fig. 1). These activities are stimulated by increased

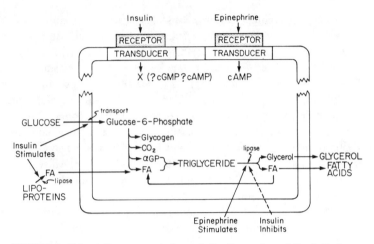

FIGURE 1 Schematic representation of the lipogenic and lipolytic functions of the adipose cell and their regulation by insulin and epinephrine.

substrate availability, but more specifically by insulin; indeed, insulin is essential for the normal conversion of carbohydrate to fat in the adipose cell. Lipolytic function, on the other hand, comprises the breakdown of stored triglyceride by a specific "hormone-sensitive" lipase, and subsequent release from the cell of glycerol and fatty acids. Hormone-stimulated lipolysis is inhibited by insulin and the prostaglandins, and stimulated by a variety of hormones including epinephrine, norepinephrine, ACTH, glucagon, and growth hormone.

Integration of these lipogenic and lipolytic functions occurs at several levels. At the plasma membrane, each hormone binds to its specific receptor (recognition), triggering a sequence of events (activation) that culminates in the modulation of specific metabolic activities of the cell (translation). Epinephrine, for example, enhances lipolysis through interaction with its receptor, stimulation of membrane-bound adenyl cyclase activity, transient elevation of the cyclic AMP levels, deinhibition of a protein kinase, and conversion of the hormone-sensitive lipase from an inactive to an active form through phosphorylation. Insulin, on the other hand, enhances lipogenesis, at least in part, by stimulating glucose transport; the mechanism of action of insulin, however, is unknown. Insulin may antagonize the effects of the lipolytic hormones by inhibiting adenyl cyclase activity, by stimulating the activity of a specific cyclic AMP phosphodiesterase, or by some as yet unidentified mechanism. The potential roles of guanyl cyclase and cyclic GMP in the regulation of adipose cell function remain to be established. Calcium appears to play a role in the mechanism of insulin action. It is postulated that insulin interacts with its membrane receptor, resulting in the activation of a membrane enzyme system, which catalyzes the production of a second messenger. This factor alters the subcellular distribution of calcium, which in turn influences the various intracellular kinases and phosphatases that control the enzymes of the metabolic pathways regulating lipogenesis and lipolysis (McDonald et al., 1976). Intracellularly, the availability of α-glycerophosphate for esterification relative to the rate of triglyceride breakdown by way of lipolysis appears to determine whether fatty acids are released from or remain stored within the cell.

The balance between the triglyceride storage and mobilization functions of the adipose cell, and therefore the size of the adipose tissue mass, depends on the overall supply of calories to the organism relative to the organism's metabolic requirements for energy. In obesity, caloric intake exceeds caloric expenditure; triglyceride storage in adipose tissue, therefore, exceeds its mobilization and the adipose depot is enlarged. As noted above, and reviewed in detail elsewhere in this volume, expansion of the adipose tissue mass occurs through increasing adipose cell size and/or number; all forms of obesity are characterized, however, by a certain degree of adipose cellular enlargement (Hirsch and Knittle, 1970; Salans et al., 1973).

Investigations of the possible relationship between the expanded adipose tissue mass and the altered state of systemic carbohydrate metabolism and insulin secretion in obesity have largely focused on studies of the influence of adipose cell size on the metabolic function of the adipose tissue. This approach has been based on the following considerations: (1) adipose cellular enlargement is common to all types of obesity (Hirsch and Knittle, 1970; Salans et al., 1973); (2) weight loss and gain, at least in adult life, are achieved solely by changes in adipose cell size (Salans et al., 1971); (3) weight loss and reduction in adipose cell size in spontaneously obese subjects are associated with a restoration to normal of the abnormalities of carbohydrate metabolism and insulin secretion (Salans et al., 1968); (4) experimental weight gain and loss in lean individuals, accompanied by increasing and decreasing adipose cell size, respectively, are associated with a reversible induction of these systemic abnormalities (Salans et al., 1974); and (5) the severity of these systemic abnormalities in obesity appears to correlate more closely with adipose cell size than total cell number (Bjorntorp et al., 1970). The metabolic activity of the adipose tissue of a large number of nonobese and obese animals and humans has been studied *in vitro* as a function of adipose cell size, and the relationship between this activity and measurements of plasma glucose and insulin concentration in the same experimental subjects examined. The results obtained in this laboratory indicate that the *in vitro* metabolic character of adipose tissue is indeed influenced by its cellular character, and that alterations in the metabolic function of this tissue occur in both obese animals and humans.

Glucose Metabolism

In general, the metabolism of glucose in adipose tissue fragments obtained from laboratory animals and humans can be directly related to the number of adipose cells in those fragments. Indeed, adipose cells isolated from adipose tissue almost entirely retain the quantitative and qualitative metabolic character of the intact tissue itself (Rodbell, 1964). At the same time, however, several parameters of glucose metabolism in this tissue are influenced by the size of its constituent cells; cell size–related alterations in metabolic function can be observed in both intact adipose tissue and isolated adipose cells.

When adipose tissue is obtained from rats ingesting diets of similar carbohydrate, fat, and protein composition, and during similar growth states, increasing adipose cell size in the absence of insulin is associated with unchanging rates of glucose oxidation, increasing rates of glucose carbon incorporation into triglyceride glycerol, and decreasing rates of *de novo* fatty acid synthesis from glucose (Fig. 2). On the other hand, the stimulation of each of these metabolic parameters by insulin decreases with adipose cellular enlargement when studied under these same conditions (Fig. 2). Virtually identical relationships between cell size and glucose metabolism are observed when cells of different size are obtained from rats of different body weight and age, or from different fat depots within the same rats (Salans and Dougherty, 1971). In addition, comparable metabolic patterns in lean, young and older, obese rats have been reported from several other laboratories (Zinder et al., 1967; DiGirolomo et al., 1974; Olefsky, 1976a; Czech, 1976a).

A similar phenomenon is observed in human adipose cells of different size obtained from patients under comparable nutritional conditions. Thus, when tissue is obtained from subjects during periods of weight maintenance and ingestion of diets of similar composition, increasing adipose cell size is associated with unchanging basal rates of glucose oxidation, and slightly increasing basal rates of glucose carbon incorporation into triglyceride glycerol (Fig. 3). On the other hand, the stimulation of glucose oxidation by insulin decreases while that of triglyceride glycerol production from glucose remains low and unchanged with cellular enlargement (Fig. 3). Significant rates of *de novo* fatty acid synthesis from glucose have not been demonstrated, however, in human adipose cells of any size, even in the presence of insulin, when

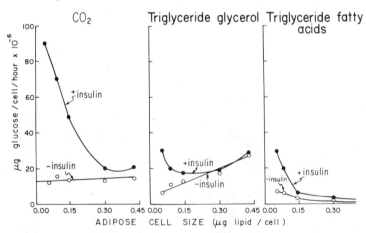

FIGURE 2 Relationship between adipose cell size and glucose metabolism in rat epididymal adipose cells. Basal and insulin (100 μU/ml) stimulated [1-^{14}C] glucose incorporation into CO_2, triglyceride glycerol, and triglyceride fatty acids by adipose cells isolated from the epididymal fat of rats ranging widely in age and body weight.

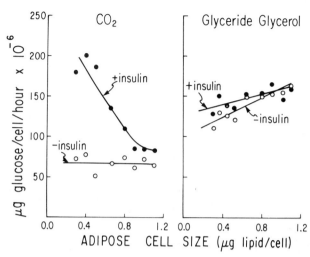

FIGURE 3 Relationship between adipose cell size and basal and insulin-stimulated glucose metabolism in human adipose tissue. Values represent the means of triplicate determinations of individual patients.

tissue is obtained from adult subjects during periods of weight maintenance (Hirsch and Goldrick, 1964; Salans et al., 1974).

Figure 4 illustrates that the relationships just described between glucose metabolism in human adipose tissue and the size of its constituent fat cells are a direct reflection of the degree of obesity of the subjects from whom tissue is obtained. When adipose tissue is removed from patients on weight maintenance diets of similar caloric composition, that of obese individuals oxidizes glucose in the absence of insulin at rates that are similar to those observed in the tissue of nonobese controls, in spite of the large difference in mean adipose cell size between the two groups (Fig. 4a). The capacity of a maximally stimulating concentration of insulin to enhance this metabolic function, however, is diminished in the tissue of the obese subjects. Figure 4b indicates that although the basal rate of glucose carbon incorporation into triglyceride glycerol is slightly increased in adipose tissue from obese, compared to nonobese, individuals, no difference in the capacity of insulin to stimulate this parameter of glucose metabolism is observed.

Similar studies of the metabolism of human adipose tissue from nonobese and obese subjects have been reported from other laboratories; the results of these various studies, however, are often more discordant than similar. Thus, the stimulation of glucose metabolism by insulin in human adipose tissue from obese, relative to nonobese, individuals may be decreased (Smith, 1971), increased (Bjorntorp, 1966), or unchanged (Davidson, 1975). The reported effects of obesity on basal glucose metabolism in human adipose tissue are similarly variable; basal glucose oxidation and incorporation of

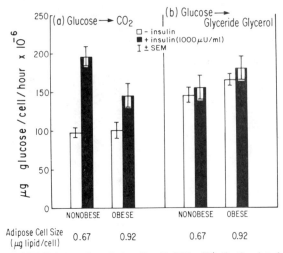

FIGURE 4 Basal and insulin (1,000 μU/ml)-stimulated [1-^{14}C] glucose incorporation into (a) CO_2 and (b) glyceride glycerol by fragments of human adipose tissue from nonobese and obese patients during periods of ingestion of weight maintenance diets of identical composition. Each value is the mean ± SEM of several individuals.

glucose carbons into triglyceride glycerol and fatty acids in the enlarged adipose cells from obese subjects may be greater than or equal to that in the smaller cells from nonobese subjects. While an explanation for these discrepancies remains to be found, recent studies in experimental animals and humans, discussed in detail in subsequent paragraphs of this chapter, indicate that the *in vitro* metabolic function of adipose tissue is influenced not only by its cellular character, but also by the nutritional and growth state (weight gain, weight loss) and the physical activity of the organism at the time the tissue is obtained for examination (Salans and Dougherty, 1971; Salans and Cushman, 1975; Bray, 1969, 1972). Such factors may have directly contributed to the discrepancies just described. In view of the potential role of factors other than adipose cell size, comparative studies of adipose tissue metabolism in both humans and experimental animals must be carried out under conditions of carefully controlled dietary intake and growth.

The studies in this laboratory described above were so conducted, and they demonstrate that obesity and adipose cellular enlargement in rat and human are accompanied by specific alterations in basal and insulin-stimulated glucose metabolism in the adipose tissue. It is of interest to observe, in addition, that these cell size–associated metabolic alterations in the adipose tissue can be reversed through weight loss and reduction of adipose cell size, and induced through weight gain and adipose cellular enlargement. Figure 5a illustrates, for example, that the metabolic alterations in adipose cells from spontaneously obese subjects are reversible through weight loss, and reduction in the adipose tissue mass and size of the tissue's constituent adipose cells; experimental subjects must be consuming weight maintenance diets, however, at the time of study at each body weight (Salans and Cushman, 1975). Figure 5b further illustrates that similar alterations in glucose metabolism can be induced in the adipose tissue of nonobese individuals through experimental weight gain and increased adipose cell size. The reversible induction of these changes in metabolic function with weight gain and loss, and increasing and decreasing adipose cell size, are likewise observed in the laboratory rat (Salans and Cushman, 1975). These observations suggest that the altered *in vitro*

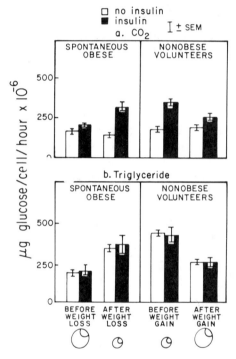

FIGURE 5 Effect of weight loss and gain on glucose metabolism of human adipose tissue *in vitro*. Basal and insulin (1,000 μU/ml)-stimulated [1-^{14}C] glucose incorporation into (a) CO_2 and (b) triglyceride by fragments of human adipose tissue from obese patients before and after weight loss and nonobese volunteers before and after weight gain. All studies were done during periods of weight maintenance. Each value is the mean ± SEM of several individuals (Salans and Cushman, 1975).

glucose metabolism of adipose tissue may represent adaptive, rather than primary, changes in adipose cell function.

Increasing adipose cell size with its accumulating intracellular triglyceride store is accompanied by an expansion of the adipose cell's surface area and, presumably, plasma membrane. The cytoplasmic mass of the cell, relegated to the peripheral portion of its volume surrounding the large, central lipid droplet, also increases with cellular enlargement, as reflected in an increasing intracellular water space (Foley et al., 1976a; DiGirolomo and Owens, 1974); it does not increase, however, as rapidly as the cell's surface area. When the metabolism of adipose cells of increasing size is examined as a function of changing cellular geometry, most of the metabolic alterations occurring with cellular enlargement described in the preceding discussion can be related to one or another structural parameter and therefore appear to reflect the normal consequence of the process by which adipose cells grow (Cushman and Salans, 1973b). Such observations provide further support for the concept that the altered *in vitro* glucose metabolism of adipose tissue in obesity represents adaptive, rather than primary, changes in adipose cell function.

Lipolysis

The lipolytic character of adipose tissue also appears to be influenced by the size of its constituent adipose cells (Cushman and Salans, 1973a; Salans and Cushman, 1975). The basal rate of lipolysis in isolated rat adipose cells, as reflected in glycerol release, increases with increasing cell size, and is paralleled by increasing fatty acid release in the absence, but not in the presence, of glucose (Fig. 6). Increasing adipose cell size is also associated with a

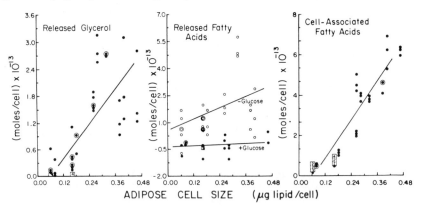

FIGURE 6 Relationship between adipose cell size and basal lipolysis in rat epididymal adipose cells. Adipose cells of various sizes were isolated from the distal portions of the epididymal fat pads of rats ranging widely in age and body weight, and incubated for 60 min at 37°C in KRB buffer containing 3.0 g bovine albumin per 100 ml, 0.0 or 1.0 mg/ml glucose, but no hormones. Each point represents the mean of triplicate determinations of individual experiments (Salans and Cushman, 1975).

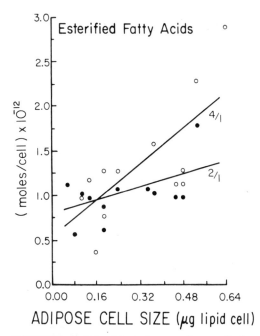

FIGURE 7 Relationship between adipose cell size and esterification of exogenous fatty acids in rat epididymal adipose cells. Cells were isolated as described in Fig. 6 and incubated for 30 min in KRB buffer containing 0.5 mg/ml glucose, and fatty acids at a molar ratio to albumin of 2/1 (●) or 4/1 (○). Each point represents the mean of triplicate values of individual experiments (Salans and Cushman, 1975).

progressive elevation of cell-associated, presumably intracellular, nonesterified fatty acids (CAFA). The enhanced basal rate of lipolysis associated with adipose cellular enlargement is accompanied, as illustrated in Fig. 2, by a marked decrease in the rate of *de novo* fatty acid synthesis from glucose; the capacity for reesterifying preformed fatty acids, however, as measured by the incorporation of glucose carbons into triglyceride glycerol (Fig. 2) or calculated from the ratio of total fatty acids produced (sum of released fatty acids and CAFA) to released glycerol, increases with increasing cell size. Moreover, the capacity for esterifying exogenous fatty acids also increases with cellular enlargement, particularly when cells are exposed to high extracellular concentrations of fatty acid (Fig. 7). These observations suggest, then, that increasing adipose cell size is associated with increasing basal lipolytic activity and a shift away from glucose lipogenesis to increased esterification of preformed fatty acids; the net effect, in the absence of a lipolytic stimulus, is an increased turnover of triglyceride within the enlarged adipose cell. The relationship between altered basal lipolytic activity and altered cellular geometry further suggests that changes in lipolysis also reflect the natural consequences of adipose cell growth (Cushman and Salans, 1973b).

Maximally epinephrine-stimulated lipolysis, or glycerol release, in the presence of glucose increases only modestly with increasing adipose cell size, but is accompanied by markedly increasing fatty acid release with epinephrine-elevated CAFA levels (Fig. 8). Reesterification in the large adipose cells appears to account for a considerably smaller proportion of the theoretical quantity of fatty acids produced by lipolysis than in the smaller cells, as reflected by an increasing ratio of total fatty acids measured to released glycerol (Fig. 7). The net metabolic effect of increasing cell size is an increase in the efficiency of lipolysis and a relative decrease in reesterification. Enlargement of the adipose cell, under conditions of similar nutritional intake

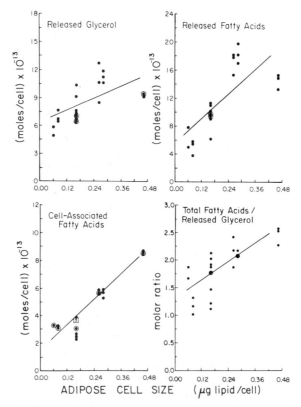

FIGURE 8 Relationship between adipose cell size and epinephrine-stimulated lipolysis and total fatty acid/glycerol ratio in rat epididymal adipose cells. Adipose cells of different sizes were isolated and incubated in the presence of glucose for 20 min as described in Fig. 6 (Salans and Cushman, 1975).

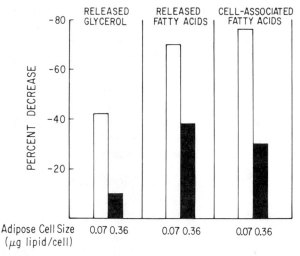

FIGURE 9 Relationship between adipose cell size and the antilipolytic effect of insulin on rat epididymal adipose cells. "Percent decrease" refers to the effect (antilipolytic) of insulin in decreasing epinephrine-stimulated glycerol release. Small and large cells were isolated from the epididymal fat pads of rats of varying age and body weight, and incubated as described in Fig. 6 in the presence of 1.0 mg/ml glucose, 0.25 µg/ml epinephrine, and (□) 0 or (■) 100 µU/ml insulin (Salans and Cushman, 1975).

and growth, is, therefore, accompanied by increasing epinephrine-stimulated lipolytic activity, increasing net triglyceride mobilization, and increasing intracellular fatty acid levels, alterations which again can be related to altered cellular geometry (Cushman and Salans, 1973b). It should, however, be noted that while the maximal capacity for lipolysis increases with increasing adipose cell size, as just described, the enlarged adipose cell is less sensitive to the effect of epinephrine than the small cell, as reflected in the greater concentration of hormone required to produce a half-maximal response (S. W. Cushman and L. B. Salans, in preparation).

Increasing adipose cell size in the rat is also accompanied by a decreasing antilipolytic effect of insulin (Fig. 9). The inhibition of epinephrine-stimulated glycerol and fatty acid release and the reduction of epinephrine-elevated CAFA levels by insulin are diminished in large, compared to small, cells. The association between adipose cellular enlargement and increasing basal and epinephrine-stimulated triglyceride turnover is, therefore, paralleled by a decreasing response to, and antilipolytic effect of, insulin. Increasing CAFA levels accompany all these cell size-related metabolic alterations.

Study of the relationship between adipose cell size and the lipolytic function of this cell in rats have also been carried out in other laboratories.

Several reports describe increasing basal and epinephrine-stimulated glycerol and fatty acid release with increasing adipose cell size (Zinder and Shapiro, 1971), while others describe rates of epinephrine- and norepinephrine-stimulated glycerol release in large cells that are equal to, or less than, those observed in small cells (Hartman et al., 1971). A similar lack of agreement is present in studies comparing the lipolytic character of the adipose tissue of obese and nonobese humans (Goldrick and McLoughlin, 1970; Bray, 1975). The factors responsible for these discrepancies remain to be defined but may, once again, reside in differences in the nutritional, growth, and physical activity states of the animals and patients studied.

Mechanism of Altered Insulin Action
in Enlarged Adipocytes

Many, if not all, of the alterations in basal metabolic function, both glucose metabolism and lipolysis, of the adipose cell with enlargement can be related to altered cellular structure and/or geometry and, therefore, appear to reflect the natural consequences of the process by which the adipose cell grows with accumulating intracellular triglyceride. Alterations in the maximal capacity for a lipolytic response to epinephrine with increasing adipose cell size appear to be likewise explicable. The decreasing sensitivity to lipolytic hormones, on the other hand, has been related, by other investigators, either to increasing cyclic AMP phosphodiesterase activity in the absence of altered hormone binding, as in the case of epinephrine, or to a combination of increasing phosphodiesterase activity and decreasing hormone binding, as in the case of glucagon (Livingston et al., 1974; DeSantis et al., 1974); these observations remain, however, to be confirmed.

The decreasing lipogenic and antilipolytic responses to insulin with adipose cellular enlargement are presently the subject of intensive investigation in this laboratory and elsewhere; to date, attention has been primarily focused on the altered capacity of insulin to stimulate glucose metabolism in the enlarged adipose cell. Each of the as yet hypothetical steps in the mechanism of action of insulin—binding to receptor, stimulation of glucose transport, and enhancement of glucose metabolism—has been examined in isolated rat adipose cells as a function of increasing adipose cell size. Similar, but preliminary, studies have been carried out with human adipose tissue fragments or isolated adipose cells.

Specific equilibrium insulin binding to the enlarged adipose cells of genetically obese mice is reportedly decreased relative to binding to the smaller cells of lean controls (Freychet et al., 1972); insulin binding to the enlarged adipose cells of obese humans and old, obese male rats may, however, either be decreased (Olefsky, 1976a, 1976b) or remain unchanged (Livingston et al., 1972) relative to binding to the smaller cells of respective controls. Studies in this laboratory fail to demonstrate any reduction in equilibrium insulin binding to isolated rat and human adipose cells with adipose cellular enlargement; to the contrary, increasing cell size appears to be associated with increasing insulin binding to rat adipose cells (Cushman and Salans, 1975b) and a tendency, although not statistically significant, toward increasing binding to human adipose cells (J. Horton et al., in preparation). The increase in equilibrium insulin binding, especially at hormone concentrations in the physiological range, may be related to the adipose cell's expanding surface area and plasma membrane with increasing cell size; indeed, studies in this laboratory indicate that insulin binding per unit cell surface area is similar among adipose cells of widely different size, suggesting once again an alteration that may be related to normal cell growth. However, in view of the complicated nature of the insulin binding process, including negative site-site interactions and/or multiple independent binding sites, alterations in the affinity and/or number of insulin binding sites remain to be distinguished. Nevertheless, studies in this laboratory demonstrate under all circumstances increasing insulin binding per cell and unchanged insulin binding per unit surface area, alterations that do not parallel and cannot explain the decreasing metabolic response to insulin with adipose cell enlargement.

Studies of glucose transport activity in adipose cells through the use of nonmetabolizable glucose analogs have been hampered by the extremely small cytoplasmic mass (roughly 3-5%) of this cell type, even in the largest cells examined (Crofford and Renold, 1965; Gliemann et al., 1972). A new method has, therefore, been recently developed in this laboratory, employing L-arabinose, a nonmetabolizable pentose that traverses the plasma membrane of the adipose cell by way of the glucose transport system, but does so at a relatively low rate because of its low affinity for the carrier (Foley et al., 1976a). Preliminary observations obtained with this new method indicate that increasing rat adipose cell size is associated with increasing basal and submaximally insulin-stimulated glucose transport activity proportional to the cell's expanding surface area (Foley et al., 1976b); maximally insulin-stimulated transport activity, on the other hand, remains roughly constant on a per cell basis. Under all circumstances, the enlarged adipose cell's capacity for glucose transport far exceeds the quantities of glucose actually taken up and metabolized, suggesting that (1) alterations in glucose metabolism beyond transport must be responsible for the decreasing rates of insulin-stimulated glucose utilization with increasing adipose cell size, and (2) glucose transport activity, the well-established rate-limiting site of insulin action in small rat adipose cells (Crofford and Renold, 1965), may no longer represent the rate-limiting step in glucose utilization in the enlarged adipose cell of older animals. Moreover, these studies fail to demonstrate alterations in the sensitivity of the glucose transport to insulin, the concentration of insulin required to produce a half-maximal response, with adipose cellular enlargement; this observation closely parallels that demonstrating no decrease in insulin binding to the enlarged cell.

Studies of the concentration-dependent stimulation of several parameters of glucose metabolism by insulin provide further evidence for metabolic alterations beyond the glucose transport step in adipose cells of increasing size. Figure 10 demonstrates the lack of effect of cell size on the sensitivity of human adipose cells to the stimulation by insulin of glucose oxidation; virtually identical results have been obtained with rat adipose cells (L. B. Salans and S. W. Cushman, in preparation). Since CO_2 production represents a roughly constant proportion of the total glucose metabolized, a decreasing maximal response to insulin in the absence of altered sensitivity to hormone concentration reflects an effect of adipose cellular enlargement on the cell's capacity for glucose metabolism and not on the mechanism of insulin action. Similar relationships are observed between adipose cell size and the concentration-dependent stimulation by insulin of *de novo* fatty acid synthesis from glucose and the incorporation of glucose carbons into triglyceride glycerol (L. B. Salans and S. W. Cushman, in preparation).

A Model of the Effects of Cell Size
on Adipose Cell Function

While the lipogenic and lipolytic functions of the adipose cell may be conveniently considered for investigative purposes as separate activities, each controlled by its respective hormonal stimuli, overall net adipose cell function reflects the balance between these two antagonistic activities (Jeanrenaud, 1968; Vaughan, 1961; Renold and Cahill, 1965; Whipple, 1965). *In vitro*

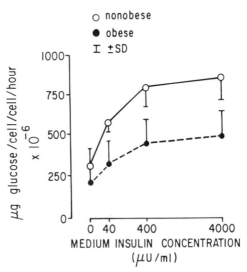

FIGURE 10 Influence of spontaneous obesity on the insulin dose-glucose oxidation response of human adipose tissue. Values represent the mean ± SD of several nonobese and obese subjects (Salans et al., 1974).

studies in the presence of controlled hormonal and substrate environments offer considerable insight into the mechanisms regulating adipose cell function; nevertheless, the adipose cell *in vivo* is continuously exposed to an environment simultaneously containing a variety of hormones and substrates, varying only in the relative concentrations of each. The physiologically important lipolytic hormones appear to influence adipose cell function through stimulation of the membrane-bound adenyl cyclase system and, ultimately, the "hormone-sensitive lipase." Insulin, on the other hand, is thought to stimulate lipogenesis from glucose primarily through its enhancement of glucose transport activity; the step(s) inhibited by insulin in the activation of lipolysis by lipolytic agents and the reported effects of insulin on specific intracellular lipogenic pathways remain to be established.

Evidence from a variety of sources suggests that a key determinant of net adipose cell function under any given set of hormonal and substrate conditions lies in the relative rates of nonesterified fatty acid production through lipolysis, and fatty acid reesterification through combination with α-glycerophosphate (Vaughan, 1961; Renold and Cahill, 1965; Whipple, 1965; Jeanrenaud, 1968). Cell-associated, probably intracellular, nonesterified fatty acids appear, in turn, to represent the balance among lipolytic activity, reesterification, and fatty acid release (Angel et al., 1971a; Cushman et al., 1973); alterations in CAFA levels accompany alterations in many of the metabolic activities of the adipose cell, including glucose metabolism, lipolysis, ATP production and utilization, and α-aminoisobutyric acid and potassium uptake (Angel et al., 1971b; Cushman et al., 1973; Heindel et al., 1974). The capacity of the adipose cell for α-glycerophosphate synthesis and CAFA levels may, therefore, be crucial to the mechanism integrating lipolysis and lipogenesis; alterations in these two potential regulatory factors may, in turn, contribute significantly to the changing net metabolic function of the adipose cell with increasing cell size.

Alterations in both the lipogenic and lipolytic activities of the adipose cell occur during the normal growth of the mammalian organism and in obesity. Adipose cellular enlargement is accompanied, in the absence of glucose, by increasing basal lipolytic activity, fatty acid release, and CAFA levels, and in the presence of glucose, by increasing basal lipolytic activity, triglyceride glycerol production, fatty acid reesterification, and CAFA levels and decreasing *de novo* fatty acid synthesis (Salans and Dougherty, 1971; DiGirolomo et al., 1974; Salans and Cushman, 1975; Czech, 1976a; S. W. Cushman and L. B. Salans, in preparation). These basal metabolic activities of the enlarged adipose cell parallel, in many respects, those observed in small cells during the normal lipolytic response to a maximally stimulating concentration of epinephrine, when lipolytic rates and CAFA levels are high. At the same time, basal glucose transport activity in the adipose cell increases with increasing cell size (Livingston et al., 1974; Foley et al., 1976b); thus, basal lipolytic activity and triglyceride glycerol production from glucose increase together and do so in the presence of increasing glucose transport activity.

Total basal glucose uptake and metabolism, on the other hand, do not increase with adipose cellular enlargement, due primarily to the fact that the rate of *de novo* fatty acid synthesis markedly decreases (Salans and Dougherty, 1971; Cushman and Salans, 1973a, 1973b; DiGirolomo et al., 1974; L. B. Salans and S. W. Cushman, in preparation). This pattern is remarkably similar to that observed when small adipose cells actively synthesizing fatty acids under conditions of rapid glucose uptake are exposed to a lipolytic stimulus; total glucose uptake and metabolism may be reduced, or remain unchanged, while triglyceride glycerol production is enhanced and fatty acid synthesis is inhibited (S. W. Cushman and L. B. Salans, in preparation). Furthermore, when small adipose cells are exposed to increasing glucose concentrations in the absence of hormones, *de novo* fatty acid synthesis increases rapidly and total glucose uptake and metabolism continue to increase as the concentration associated with near maximal rates of triglyceride glycerol production is surpassed; in large adipose cells, no such increase in fatty acid synthesis is observed and total glucose utilization rises only as long as the rate of triglyceride glycerol production does (DiGirolomo et al., 1974; Czech, 1976a; L. B. Salans and S. W. Cushman, in preparation). Finally, the results of preliminary glucose countertransport experiments in this laboratory appear to indicate, albeit indirectly, that free glucose does indeed accumulate in the intracellular space of enlarged, but not small, adipose cells under basal conditions in the presence of high extracellular glucose concentrations (Foley et al., 1976b). These observations suggest that (1) the enlarged adipose cell's maximal capacity for α-glycerophosphate synthesis, even in the presence of high extracellular glucose concentrations, is not sufficient to reesterify all the fatty acids produced by the relatively high basal rate of lipolysis, (2) CAFA levels are, therefore, elevated and fatty acid synthesis is inhibited, and (3) the glycolytic pathway for glucose metabolism becomes saturated and glucose transport activity no longer represents the rate-limiting step in net glucose uptake.

Additional evidence supporting the hypothesis that the enlarged adipose cell's capacity for α-glycerophosphate synthesis is limited is provided by studies of glucose metabolism and lipolysis in the presence of maximally stimulating concentrations of insulin and epinephrine. In small adipose cells at low glucose concentrations, insulin stimulates both triglyceride glycerol and fatty acid production from glucose, as well as glucose oxidation; in large cells at the same low glucose concentrations, insulin continues to stimulate triglyceride glycerol production, but its effect on fatty acid synthesis and CO_2 production is blunted (L. B. Salans and S. W. Cushman, in preparation). At higher glucose concentrations, the stimulation of glucose metabolism by insulin in enlarged adipose cells disappears completely, while stimulation of fatty acid synthesis and glucose oxidation becomes the predominant effect of insulin in small cells (DiGirolomo et al., 1974; Czech, 1976b; L. B. Salans and

S. W. Cushman, in preparation). Inhibitory effects of insulin on basal lipolysis are not demonstrable in either the absence or the presence of glucose (Salans and Cushman, 1975; S. W. Cushman and L. B. Salans, in preparation); lipolytic activity and CAFA levels, then, accompany increasing adipose cell size even in the presence of insulin. In large adipose cells, where the capacity for α-glycerophosphate synthesis is low relative to the high basal rate of lipolysis, saturation of this pathway occurs at relatively low rates of glucose uptake whether insulin is present or not; in turn, even maximal rates of α-glycerophosphate synthesis are not sufficient to fulfill the enlarged cell's reesterification requirements, CAFA accumulate, and fatty acid synthesis, glucose uptake, and oxidation are inhibited. Indeed, Czech (1976b) has recently reported the results of metabolic crossover studies in the presence of insulin suggesting a decrease in the activities of α-glycerophosphate dehydrogenase (α-GPD) and phosphofructokinase in large, compared to small, adipose cells; Bray (1975) has demonstrated similarly reduced α-GPD activities in homogenates of human adipose tissue removed from obese, compared to lean, subjects.

While insulin stimulates glucose metabolism primarily through a direct effect on carbohydrate transport and therefore availability, epinephrine appears to stimulate glucose metabolism indirectly through its effect on lipolytic activity. Maximally stimulating concentrations of epinephrine enhance triglyceride glycerol production, fatty acid reesterification, and lipolysis in both small and large adipose cells at both low and high glucose concentrations. While epinephrine-stimulated lipolysis increases with increasing adipose cell size, epinephrine-stimulated triglyceride glycerol production and fatty acid reesterification decrease, particularly in the presence of a high glucose concentration (Cushman and Salans, 1973a, in preparation). Moreover, glucose markedly enhances the maximal rate of epinephrine-stimulated lipolysis and fatty acid reesterification in small, but not in large, adipose cells (S. W. Cushman and L. B. Salans, in preparation). While CAFA levels in the presence of epinephrine are higher in large than in small cells, glucose reduces epinephrine-elevated CAFA only in the smaller cells (S. W. Cushman and L. B. Salans, in preparation). Thus, the rate of α-glycerophosphate synthesis is determined by the rate of lipolysis in the presence, as well as the absence, of epinephrine, and epinephrine-stimulated lipolytic activity is, in turn, modulated by the CAFA levels achieved. In small adipose cells, where the capacity for triglyceride glycerol production is high relative to the capacity for lipolytic activity, glucose availability in the presence of epinephrine permit rapid rates of fatty acid reesterification, reduced CAFA levels, and enhanced lipolytic activity. In large adipose cells, where the capacity for α-glycerophosphate synthesis is low relative even to the basal rate of lipolysis, glucose availability has little effect on epinephrine-stimulated metabolic activity. A low maximal capacity for α-glycerophosphate production from glucose relative to the rate of lipolysis, leading to elevated CAFA levels, may then very well explain the observed alterations in the net function of the enlarged adipose cell in the presence, as well as the absence, of hormones.

Most of the alterations in the function of the adipose cell with enlargement appear, therefore, to reflect the altered relationships among individual metabolic pathways within the cell; these relationships represent the major determinant of net metabolic function under any given set of environmental conditions. Nevertheless, several apparent alterations in the mechanism of hormone action are also observed in the enlarged adipose cell. For example, while the decreasing stimulation of glucose metabolism by insulin with increasing adipose cell size is probably due to the altered metabolic relationships described above and not to a reduction in the cell's capacity for glucose transport, the magnitude of the stimulation of glucose transport activity relative to the basal rate at each concentration of insulin does decrease with adipose cellular enlargement (Livingston et al., 1974; Czech, 1976a; Foley et al., 1976b; Olefsky, 1976a). The inhibition of epinephrine-stimulated lipolytic activity at a maximally stimulating concentration of insulin also decreases (Salans and Cushman, 1975). Increasing equilibrium insulin binding and unchanging sensitivities to insulin in either multiple parameters of glucose metabolism or glucose transport activity suggest that the interaction of insulin with the enlarged cell's expanded plasma membrane and the generation of the corresponding translational signal(s) are unperturbed by increasing adipose cell size (Cushman and Salans, 1975b; Foley et al., 1976b; L. B. Salans and S. W. Cushman, in preparation). Inhibition of insulin-mediated glucose transport activity itself, on the other hand, would be reflected in just such an effect of cell size on the capacity, but not sensitivity, of the adipose cell to respond to insulin. While the factor responsible for such inhibition remains to be established, elevated CAFA levels parallel the inhibited stimulation of glucose transport activity by insulin and therefore represent a potential mediator of this effect of adipose cell size. The decreasing capacity of insulin to inhibit epinephrine-stimulated lipolysis with adipose cellular enlargement might be explained in a similar fashion.

In contrast to the alterations in the response to insulin, the maximal lipolytic response to epinephrine increases with increasing adipose cell size, especially in the absence of glucose, while the enlarged cell's sensitivity to epinephrine is decreased. Both the maximal response and sensitivity to glucagon, on the other hand, are reportedly decreased (Manganiello and Vaughan, 1972; Livingston et al., 1974; S. W. Cushman and L. B. Salans, in preparation). The effects of adipose cell size on the response to glucagon and epinephrine have been attributed, at least partially, to increasing cyclic AMP phosphodiesterase activity (DeSantis et al., 1974); a decrease in glucagon binding to the enlarged cell's plasma membrane may account, in addition, for part of the defect in glucagon response (Livingston et al., 1974). The observation that nonesterified fatty acids inhibit adenyl cyclase activity (Fain and Shepard, 1975) suggests that the elevated CAFA levels in the enlarged adipose cell may play a direct role in this cell's altered sensitivity to lipolytic hormones. The well-known capacity of the adenyl cyclase system for generating cyclic AMP far in excess of that required for maximal lipolytic activity suggests that even the inhibited cyclase could potentially mediate a maximal response in the presence of sufficiently high concentrations of epinephrine.

The altered metabolic function of the adipose cell with increasing size and accumulating triglyceride stores may very well, therefore, reflect the natural consequence of the process by which this cell grows during the normal development of an organism or in obesity. As will be discussed in detail below, however, other factors such as dietary composition and total caloric intake are also capable of influencing net adipose cell function. Adipose cell structure-function relationships probably define a basic physiological framework within which this cell adapts to a variety of externally controlled environmental factors.

Relationship between Adipose Tissue and Cell Function *in Vitro* and Systemic Metabolism

The alterations in adipose cell function observed *in vitro* with increasing cell size and obesity are paralleled by similar alterations in the systemic metabolism of carbohydrate and lipid in the organism as a whole. Thus, at a time when an impairment in the ability of insulin to influence glucose metabolism in the enlarged adipose cells of spontaneously obese subjects is observed *in vitro,* the ability of insulin to influence glucose metabolism in the whole organism is also impaired, as reflected in glucose intolerance and hyperinsulinemia (Fig. 11) and a decreased hypoglycemic response to insulin (Salans et al., 1968). Furthermore, the increasing *in vitro* rates of lipolysis and triglyceride turnover and the shift from glucose lipogenesis to preformed fatty acid uptake and esterification with adipose cellular enlargement appear to parallel the reported increase in systemic fatty acid flux (Flatt, 1972) and hypertriglyceridemia (Farquhar et al., 1975), in obese subjects.

The same systemic manifestations of disordered glucose metabolism and insulin secretion and action are observed in experimental human obesity (Fig. 12) (Sims et al., 1968), and at the same time the capacity of insulin to influence the *in vitro* glucose metabolism of their enlarged adipose cells is impaired (Salans et al., 1974). In addition, weight loss in both spontaneous and experimental obesity is associated with an improvement in glucose tolerance and a fall in plasma insulin concentrations, concomitant with a restoration to normal of the *in vitro* metabolic character of the adipose tissue and a reduction in adipose cell size (Salans et al., 1968). These observations, then, lend support to, but do not prove, the concept that the altered metabolic state of the obese individual may reflect changes in the metabolic state of the expanded adipose tissue mass and its constituent, enlarged adipose cells. Since the alterations in systemic metabolism are not only reversible in obese subjects with weight loss, but also inducible in nonobese subjects

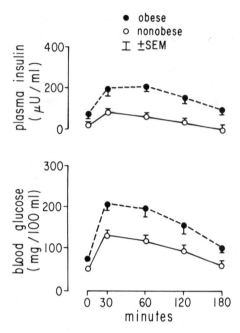

FIGURE 11 Influence of spontaneous obesity on the blood glucose and plasma insulin response to an acute oral glucose challenge. The values represent the mean blood glucose and plasma insulin concentrations of ten nonobese (o) and ten obese (•) patients during oral glucose tolerance tests.

through weight gain, they too, like the altered *in vitro* metabolism of adipose tissue, may represent adaptive rather than primary changes in metabolic function.

The experimental results presented above and their discussion clearly demonstrate the rationale for functionally relating the systemic metabolic disorders, expanded adipose tissue mass, and adipose cellular enlargement characteristic of the obese state. Recent awareness of the complex inter-dependence among a variety of tissues in regulating the flow of metabolic fuels and of the variety of factors regulating cellular function has, however, raised significant doubts relative to the simplicity of this view. The potentially major roles of muscle and liver in the abnormalities of systemic metabolism and of diet in the alterations of adipose tissue function and systemic metabolism in obesity must, therefore, be considered.

SKELETAL MUSCLE AND LIVER

Estimates of the distribution of an oral glucose load to various tissues of fasting humans indicate that roughly 85% is taken up by the liver and only a very small proportion delivered to the peripheral tissues, including the adipose tissue (Rabinowitz, 1970). Thus, quantitatively, the impaired glucose metabolism of adipose tissue in obesity may be relatively unimportant in the metabolic derangement of the organism as a whole. Nevertheless, these studies of tissue glucose utilization were undertaken in subjects in the fasting state and in response to relatively small and acute oral glucose challenges. Whether significantly more glucose escapes the liver and becomes available to the adipose tissue of obese subjects ingesting their usual diets containing excessive amounts of calories and carbohydrates remains to be determined; under such circumstances, alterations in glucose metabolism in the expanded adipose tissue mass may very well contribute significantly to the altered systemic metabolic state.

The bulk of the evidence to date, however, supports the concept that the altered metabolic function of the enlarged adipose tissue mass, and specifically the impaired capacity of insulin to influence glucose metabolism in the enlarged adipose cell, cannot directly account for the glucose intolerance, hyperinsulinemia, and insulin resistance of the obese individual. Indeed, caloric

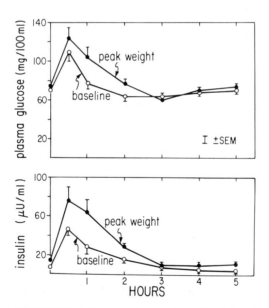

FIGURE 12 Influence of experimentally induced obesity on the plasma glucose and insulin responses to an acute oral glucose challenge. The values represent the mean ± SEM plasma glucose and insulin concentrations during oral glucose tolerance tests in 11 normal subjects before (o) and after (●) weight gain by increasing all elements of the diet (Horton et al., 1975).

restriction in the obese individual is associated with a rather prompt and significant reduction in plasma glucose and insulin concentrations, long before a substantial change in body weight and adiposity is observed. The alterations in systemic glucose metabolism and insulin secretion appear more likely to reflect metabolic alterations in tissues that are quantitatively more directly involved in glucose homeostasis, such as skeletal muscle and, in particular, liver.

In spontaneous obesity in humans, an impairment in the capacity of insulin to stimulate glucose metabolism in forearm muscle tissue of obese individuals has been observed (Fig. 13). In addition, the inhibition of branched-chain amino acid release from skeletal muscle by insulin is also impaired in obese, compared to nonobese, subjects (Felig et al., 1969, 1971). These alterations, like those observed in adipose tissue, are reversible through weight loss (Horton et al., 1974). Moreover, as demonstrated in Fig. 14, a similar impairment in insulin's capacity to stimulate glucose uptake in the forearm muscle of nonobese subjects can be induced through weight gain. Thus, the skeletal muscle of obese individuals appears to share with adipose tissue a reversible and inducible reduction in the capacity of insulin to influence glucose metabolism; this tissue may, therefore, contribute at least as directly as the adipose tissue to the deranged metabolic state of the obese individual.

Recent studies in lean and obese humans have also demonstrated that the normal inhibition of splanchnic glucose output by insulin is reduced in

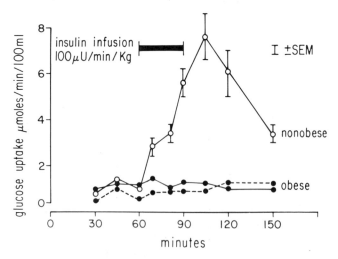

FIGURE 13 Comparison of basal and insulin-stimulated arterial-deep venous glucose concentration differences across forearm muscle in two obese and five nonobese individuals studied during periods of weight maintenance (Horton et al., 1974).

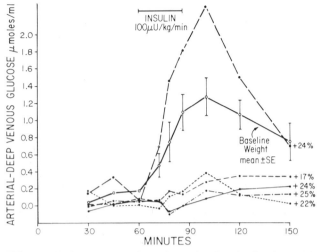

FIGURE 14 Comparison of basal and insulin-stimulated arterial-deep venous glucose concentration differences across forearm muscle in five normal subjects before and after weight gain by increasing all elements of the diet. All individuals were studied during periods of weight maintenance. The lighter lines represent the individual responses after gains of 17–25% above the initial weight (Horton et al., 1975).

obesity (Felig et al., 1974); these observations establish the liver as an additional site of impaired insulin action. In view of the predominant quantitative contribution of the liver to glucose homeostasis, the glucose intolerance observed in obesity is most likely the direct consequence of such an impairment of insulin action in the liver. While studies are not available on the effects of weight loss or gain on hepatic glucose output, the reversibility and inducibility of alterations in insulin's action on liver function might be predicted.

A direct quantitative role for the expanded adipose tissue mass and its altered metabolic state in the development and perpetuation of abnormal systemic carbohydrate and lipid metabolism in obesity seems, therefore, unlikely; an indirect role has not, however, been ruled out. Indeed, the relative stability of an organism's ultimate body weight, once achieved, suggests the presence of some as yet unidentified signal(s) indicating the size and functional state of the adipose tissue mass (Stern and Hirsch, 1972). The alterations in adipose tissue and cell metabolic activity in obesity may therefore be reflected in corresponding alterations in this signaling mechanism, and thereby influence indirectly the metabolic function of other tissues such as muscle, the liver, and the pancreatic B-cell. The existence of such a mechanism and the nature of its signal(s) remain to be established. Since the alterations in glucose metabolism in skeletal muscle and the liver are, or are very likely to be, both reversible in obese individuals through weight loss and inducible in nonobese subjects through weight gain, they too, like the altered *in vitro* metabolism of adipose tissue, may represent adaptive, rather than primary, changes in metabolic function.

DIETARY INFLUENCES

In addition to an expanded adipose tissue mass and enlarged adipose cells, obesity is characterized by the intake of large numbers of calories. The diet of the obese individual is excessive, however, not only in total calories, but also in carbohydrate; the profound influence of both the quantity and quality of calories being ingested on systemic glucose metabolism and insulin secretion is well established (Cahill et al., 1966; Kipnis, 1972; Salans and Cushman, 1973). The altered glucose metabolism and hyperinsulinemia of obesity are, therefore, possibly a consequence of these dietary factors rather than, or in addition to, "insulin antagonism" at the tissue level. With excessive caloric intake, the rates of fat and protein synthesis and of carbohydrate disposition are greatly enhanced; an increase in the rate of insulin secretion is required for these purposes. Indeed, in experimental animals, excessive ingestion either of total calories or of carbohydrate is associated with hyperplasia of the islets of Langerhans and an increase in circulating insulin levels (Renold et al., 1975). A potential role for such dietary factors in the altered metabolic state of the obese individual must, therefore, at least be considered. Indeed, some investigators have postulated that the insulin resistance of obesity may represent an adaptive mechanism protecting the obese individual from a hypoglycemic reaction consequent to excessive caloric and/or carbohydrate intake (Grey and Kipnis, 1971).

Detailed investigations of the effects of varying total caloric intake and dietary composition on the metabolic character of the adipose tissue, skeletal muscle, and systemic carbohydrate metabolism of nonobese and obese experimental animals and humans have, therefore, been undertaken. The evidence for a relationship between the size of the adipose depot and its constituent fat cells, and the *in vitro* metabolism of these cells and of the organism as a whole, described in the preceding paragraphs, was derived from studies in laboratory animals and experimental patients possessing widely different adipose tissue masses and adipose cell sizes, but in whom the state of nutrition was similar. As described below, however, these relationships are considerably influenced by alterations in the nutritional state of the organism.

Influence of Total Caloric Intake on Adipose Tissue and Systemic Glucose Metabolism

Variations in total caloric intake profoundly affect the metabolic character of the adipose tissue of both experimental animals and humans (Salans and Cushman, 1975) Adipose cells prepared from rats fed diets sufficiently restricted in calories to induce weight loss oxidize glucose at basal rates that are markedly reduced compared to those observed in cells from normally fed control animals of the same age (Fig. 15 A and B). Moreover, insulin completely fails to stimulate glucose oxidation in the adipose cells from the calorically restricted animals in spite of their markedly reduced cell size compared to controls. Refeeding such calorically restricted animals for 1 wk, on the other hand, raises the basal rate of glucose metabolism in their adipose cells to levels significantly greater than those observed in larger cells obtained from continuously *ad libitum*-fed controls (Fig. 15, A and C). At the same time, the stimulation of glucose metabolism by insulin in the adipose cells from the refed animals is not only greater than that in the much smaller cells from the starved animals (Fig. 15, B and C), but also equal to or greater than that observed in the somewhat smaller cells from younger *ad libitum*-fed animals (not illustrated). The adipose cells from rats fed diets that are calorically restricted, but contain sufficient calories to maintain constant body weight, also demonstrate reduced basal and insulin-stimulated rates of glucose metabolism when compared to the larger cells from normally fed control animals of the same age (Fig. 15, A and D).

These effects of varying total caloric intake on the metabolic character of rat adipose tissue have also been observed in humans. Thus, when adipose tissue is obtained from nonobese adult subjects ingesting excessive calories as a balanced diet in amounts sufficient to produce weight gain, the rates of glucose oxidation in both the absence and the presence of insulin are significantly greater than those observed in tissue containing cells of slightly smaller size, obtained from these same subjects ingesting weight maintenance diets (Fig. 16, a and b). Similarly, when adipose tissue is obtained from obese individuals during active weight gain induced by the ingestion of excessive calories as a balanced diet, the basal rate of glucose metabolism and response

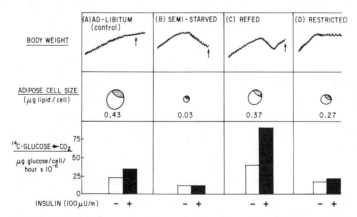

FIGURE 15 Influence of total caloric intake on basal and insulin (100 μU/ml)-stimulated glucose oxidation by rat adipose cells of various sizes isolated from the epididymal fat pads of animals ingesting varying amounts of calories (Salans and Cushman, 1975).

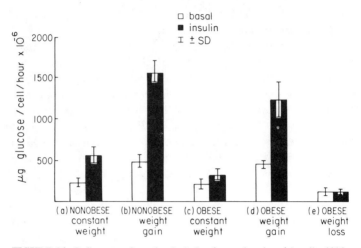

FIGURE 16 Influence of total caloric intake on basal and insulin (400 μu/ml)-stimulated glucose oxidation by fragments of human adipose tissue isolated from nonobese and obese individuals ingesting varying amounts of calories. Values represent the mean ± SD of several individuals (Salans et al., 1974).

to insulin in these large adipose cells are greater than those observed in the smaller cells from nonobese and obese subjects at constant body weight (Fig. 16, a, c, and d). The basal rate of glucose metabolism in adipose tissue from obese subjects during caloric restriction is very low, and no response to insulin is observed even though these cells are smaller than those obtained during ingestion of excess or weight maintenance numbers of calories (Fig. 16, c–e).

These effects of variations in total caloric intake on the metabolic character of adipose tissue *in vitro* appear to be paralleled, at least in part, by similar changes in the systemic metabolism of glucose in the organism as a whole; only a limited number of studies of systemic metabolic function are available, however, during the process of active weight gain or loss (Cahill et al., 1966). For example, periods of starvation and active weight loss are associated, in both obese and nonobese subjects, with a diminished glucose tolerance. Ingestion of a weight maintenance regimen following attainment of a reduced body weight in previously obese subjects, on the other hand, is associated with an improved response to oral glucose relative to that observed during weight maintenance at the initial elevated body weight. It should be recalled once again, however, that caloric restriction alone in obese patients is accompanied by improved glucose tolerance and reduced plasma insulin concentrations during periods of subsequent weight maintenance, even before significant weight and adipose tissue are lost. Similar information regarding glucose tolerance during periods of active weight gain are not readily available. Enhanced glucose tolerance might be expected, however, to accompany weight gain during increased caloric intake in spite of the decreased tolerance to glucose once stable experimental obesity has been achieved.

Influence of Dietary Composition on Adipose Tissue and Systemic Glucose Metabolism

The metabolic character of the adipose tissue of humans and experimental animals is also influenced by the quality or the composition of dietary calories being ingested. Changing from a weight maintenance, low-carbohydrate diet to an isocaloric diet containing a high ratio of carbohydrate to fat, at a time when the size of the adipose tissue mass and its constituent adipose cells remains constant, is associated in both obese and nonobese subjects with an increase in the basal rate of glucose carbon incorporation into CO_2 and glyceride glycerol, as well as an enhanced stimulation of these two metabolic parameters by insulin (Fig. 17). In fact, the response to insulin in

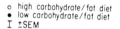

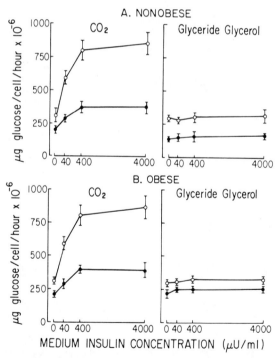

FIGURE 17 Comparison of glucose oxidation by human adipose tissue isolated from obese and nonobese individuals ingesting isocaloric diets of different composition. Studies were done during periods of weight maintenance (Salans et al., 1974).

the large adipose cells obtained from obese individuals ingesting a high-carbohydrate diet may be equal to, or even greater than, that of the smaller cells obtained from nonobese individuals ingesting isocaloric, low-carbohydrate diets (Fig. 18). Among adipose tissue samples obtained from subjects consuming a diet of given composition, however, adipose cell size continues to be inversely correlated with the capacity of insulin to stimulate glucose metabolism (Salans et al., 1974). Dietary composition, therefore, profoundly influences the metabolic character of human adipose tissue, and its control becomes critical in comparisons of the metabolic character of adipose cells from nonobese and obese individuals. These observations may explain, at least in part, some of the disparity among results of studies of basal and insulin-stimulated glucose metabolism in human adipose tissue, obtained in different laboratories.

A similar effect of dietary composition on the metabolic character of rat adipose tissue has been demonstrated. The adipose tissue of rats fed isocaloric diets of differing caloric composition varies markedly in basal glucose metabolism and the response to insulin, according to the carbohydrate and/or fat content of the antecedent diet (Cushman and Salans, 1975a). For example, ingestion of a diet containing, by calories, 20% protein, 70% carbohydrate, and 10% fat increases the basal and insulin-stimulated rates of glucose oxidation compared to those observed in adipose cells of the same size obtained from animals ingesting isocaloric diets containing 20% protein, 30%

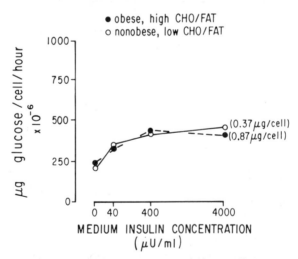

FIGURE 18   Effect of insulin on the rate of $[1\text{-}^{14}C]$ glucose incorporation into CO_2 by adipose tissue from nonobese volunteers (o) ingesting a diet containing a low ratio of carbohydrate to fat and by adipose tissue from obese patients (•) ingesting a high carbohydrate, low fat diet. Both diets provided sufficient calories to maintain constant body weight. Each point represents the mean ± SEM of several individuals (Salans et al., 1974).

carbohydrate, and 50% fat. Similar effects of a high-carbohydrate diet on the production of total triglyceride and triglyceride glycerol and fatty acids from glucose have also been observed in rat adipose cells. These. alterations in insulin-stimulated glucose metabolism induced in rat adipose cells by manipulating the composition of the diet appear to occur, however, in the absence of any change in the specific equilibrium binding of insulin to these cells (Cushman and Salans, 1975a). Indeed, the lack of effect of dietary composition on insulin binding is paralleled by the maintenance of the normal sensitivity of the adipose cell to insulin; the effect of dietary carbohydrate is, instead, on the adipose cell's capacity to metabolize glucose in the presence of insulin.

The composition of the diet also influences the systemic metabolism of the intact organism, as reflected in the concentrations of glucose and insulin in the plasma and the character of the glucose tolerance. The nature of these effects, however, has been the source of controversy. An increase in the ratio of carbohydrate to fat in the diet of nonobese and obese subjects ingesting isocaloric, weight maintenance diets has been reported to improve (Brunzell et al., 1971) or to impair (Grey and Kipnis, 1971) glucose tolerance, and the plasma insulin concentrations observed during the response to an acute oral glucose challenge in these subjects have been reported to be decreased, unchanged, or increased with increasing dietary carbohydrate intake. The factors responsible for these differences remain to be identified, but may reside in the quantity of glucose administered as a test load, the nature of the antecedent diet, and whether the individual is studied during a period of weight maintenance or slight weight gain or loss. If, on the other hand, plasma glucose and insulin concentrations are measured hourly over a 24 hr period of normal meal consumption, ingestion of diets containing a high ratio of carbohydrate to fat is associated with higher plasma concentrations of both glucose and insulin throughout all but the early morning hours, compared to those observed during ingestion of isocaloric low-carbohydrate, high-fat diets (Salans and Cushman, 1973); 24 hr measurements in response to a normal pattern of feeding behavior may, therefore, be a better indicator of the influence of dietary composition on plasma glucose and insulin levels than is the oral glucose tolerance test. The enhancement of basal glucose metabolism and the response to insulin in adipose tissue obtained during ingestion of high-carbohydrate meals, in spite of the elevated plasma glucose and insulin concentrations accompanying such a dietary regimen, also suggest that the systemic abnormalities of glucose metabolism in obesity may be as much (if not more) a reflection of dietary factors as of an increased and metabolically altered adipose tissue mass.

Influence of Diet on Skeletal Muscle and the Liver

Recent studies indicate that variations in dietary composition may influence insulin's capacity to stimulate glucose uptake in human forearm muscle in a manner similar to that observed in adipose tissue *in vitro* (Horton et al., 1974), further indicating an important role for dietary factors in the regulation of tissue function in general. Studies of the influence of diet on hepatic glucose output and its regulation by insulin in humans have not been undertaken. Effects of the quantity and quality of ingested calories on these functions of the liver, however, seem likely. Indeed, the metabolic alterations in skeletal muscle and the liver, like those in adipose tissue, may very well represent adaptive responses to dietary factors, rather than abnormalities associated with obesity *per se*. This hypothesis remains to be tested.

SUMMARY

Evidence presented in the preceding paragraphs indicates that both the degree of adiposity and the quantity of total caloric and carbohydrate intake influence glucose metabolism in the organism as a whole and in its tissues, and that both dietary factors and alterations in the function of the adipose tissue, as well as other tissues of the body, contribute to the diabetogenic metabolic derangements in obesity.

An impairment in the capacity of insulin to influence certain characteristics of the glucose metabolism in the adipose tissue, skeletal muscle, and liver of obese humans and experimental animals can be demonstrated. Whether these alterations at the tissue level are primary reflections of obesity *per se* and can be modified by variations in dietary intake and physical activity or represent the development of tissue insulin resistance as an adaptive response to a primary abnormality in feeding behavior remains to be determined. The available evidence, however, appears to support the hypothesis that the alterations in adipose tissue and skeletal muscle function in obesity are not primary defects, but rather reflections of tissue adaptation to its nutrient environment.

Adipose tissue has been used as a model in examining the nature of these adaptive changes in tissue metabolism in more detail. Studies of this tissue indicate that during the stage of developing obesity—that is, during intake of calories in excess of those being utilized—the lipogenic function of the adipose cell is increased; at the same time, the lipolytic function of the cell is diminished. The imbalance in activity appears to be the consequence of increased substrate delivery to the cell under these conditions. During this phase of active weight gain, the adipose cell readily responds to insulin. These metabolic changes in the adipose tissue in response to excess caloric intake are exaggerated further when the calories are composed primarily of carbohydrate. As the adipose cell enlarges with accumulating triglyceride, and especially following the attainment of a steady state of obesity, certain adaptive changes occur. The lipolytic activity of the enlarged adipose cell is enhanced, although greater concentrations of epinephrine are required to produce a maximal response, and the capacity of insulin to influence glucose metabolism and lipolysis is diminished—adaptations that might be expected to prevent further storage of metabolic fuel as triglyceride and to enhance net mobilization of calories from, and contraction of, the adipose tissue mass. These adaptations, however, are overcome by the obese individual's continued ingestion of large quantities of food and the delivery of excess lipogenic substrate in the form of glucose and lipoproteins to the adipose cell. In contrast, however, to what is observed during the phase of developing obesity, where glucose represents a good lipogenic substrate for the adipose cell, the enlarged adipose cell appears to have only a limited capacity for glucose lipogenesis in the individual who has achieved a steady state of obesity. This is consistent with the observation that in humans at constant body weight, the adipose tissue mass accounts for only a very small fraction of the total glucose utilized by the body in the fasting state. Under these circumstances, the major lipogenic substrate becomes fatty acids of lipoprotein origin, present in excess in the overeating obese subject. However, as demonstrated above, during the ingestion of a diet containing large quantities of carbohydrate, and with the consequent delivery of excess glucose to the cell, the altered metabolism of glucose in the enlarged adipose cell can be overcome. The regulation of adipose tissue function in obesity appears, therefore, to depend more on the adipose cell's nutrient than its hormonal environment; similar adaptive mechanisms are likely to be operative in skeletal muscle and the liver as well.

REFERENCES

Angel, A. 1975. In *Obesity in perspective,* ed. G. Bray. DHEW Publ. No. (NIH) 75-708, p. 265.

Angel, A., Desai, K. S. and Halperin, M. L. 1971a. *J. Lipid Res.* 12:104–111.

Angel, A., Desai, K. S. and Halperin, M. L. 1971b. *J. Lipid Res.* 12:203–213.

Bjorntorp, P. 1966. *Acta Med. Scand.* 179:229.

Bjorntorp, P. 1975. In *Obesity in perspective,* ed. G. Bray. DHEW Publ. No. (NIH) 75-708, p. 397.

Bjorntorp, P., Gustafson, A. and Tibbin, G. 1970. In *Atherosclerosis, Proceedings of the Second International Symposium,* ed. R. J. Jones, p. 374. Berlin: Springer-Verlag.

Bray, G. A. 1969. *J. Clin. Invest.* 48:1413.

Bray, G. A. 1972. *J. Clin. Invest.* 51:537.

Bray, G. A. 1975. In *Obesity in perspective,* ed. G. Bray. DHEW Publ. No. (NIH) 75-708, p. 253.

Brunzell, J. D., Lerner, R. L., Hazzard, W. R., Porte, D., Jr. and Bierman, E. L. 1971. *N. Engl. J. Med.* 284:521.

Cahill, G. F., Jr., Herrera, M. G., Morgan, A. P. and Kipnis, D. W. 1966. *J. Clin. Invest.* 45:1751.

Crofford, O. B. and Renold, A. E. 1965. *J. Biol. Chem.* 240:14.

Cushman, S. W. and Salans, L. B. 1973a. *Fed. Proc.* 32:940a.

Cushman, S. W. and Salans, L. B. 1973b. *Clin. Res.* 21:620A.

Cushman, S. W. and Salans, L. B. 1975a. *Clin. Res.* 23:317a.

Cushman, S. W. and Salans, L. B. 1975b. *Endocrinology* 85:92.

Cushman, S. W., Heindel, J. J. and Jeanrenaud, B. 1973. *J. Lipid Res.* 14:632.

Czech, M. P. 1976a. *J. Clin. Invest.* 57:1523.
Czech, M. P. 1976b. *Abstr. 58th. Annu. Meet. Endocr. Soc.,* p. 92.
Davidson, M. B. 1975. *Diabetes* 24:1086.
DeSantis, R. A., Gorenstein, T., Livingston, J. N. and Lockwood, D. H. 1974. *J. Lipid Res.* 15:33.
DiGirolomo, M. and Owens, J. 1974. *Diabetes* 23 (Suppl. 1):370.
DiGirolomo, M., Howe, M. D., Esposito, J., Thurman, L. and Owens, J. L. 1974. *J. Lipid Res.* 15:332.
Fain, J. N. and Shepard, R. E. 1975. *J. Biol. Chem.* 250:6586.
Farquhar, J. W., Olefsky, J., Stern, M. and Reaven, G. M. 1975. In *Obesity in perspective,* ed. G. Bray. DHEW Publ. No. (NIH) 75-708, p. 313.
Felig, P., Marliss, E. and Cahill, G. F., Jr. 1969. *N. Engl. J. Med.* 281:811.
Felig, P., Horton, E. S., Runge, C. F. and Sims, E. A. H. 1971. Paper presented at the annual meeting of the Endocrine Society.
Felig, P., Wahren, J., Hendler, R. and Brundin, T. 1974. *J. Clin. Invest.* 53:582.
Flatt, J. P. 1972. *Am. J. Clin. Nutr.* 25:1189.
Foley, J. E., Cushman, S. W. and Salans, L. B. 1976a. *Fed. Proc.* 35:419.
Foley, J. E., Cushman, S. W. and Salans, L. B. 1976b. *Clin. Res.* 24:360A.
Franckson, J. R. M., Malaise, W., Arnould, Y., Rasio, E., Ooms, H. A., Balasse, E., Conrad, V. and Bastenie, P. A. 1966. *Diabetologia* 2:96.
Freychet, P., Laudat, M. G., Laudat, P., Rosselin, G., Kahn, C. R., Gorden, P. and Roth, J. 1972. *FEBS Lett.* 25:339.
Gliemann, J., Osterlind, K., Vinten, J. and Gammeltoft, S. 1972. *Biochim. Biophys. Acta* 286:1.
Goldrick, R. B. and McLoughlin, G. M. 1970. *J. Clin. Invest.* 49:1213.
Grey, N. and Kipnis, D. M. 1971. *N. Engl. J. Med.* 285:827.
Grey, N. J., Goldring, S. and Kipnis, D. M. 1970. *J. Clin. Invest.* 49:881.
Hartman, A. D., Cohen, A. I., Richane, C. J. and Hsu, T. 1971. *J. Lipid Res.* 12:498.
Heindel, J. J., Cushman, S. W. and Jeanrenaud, B. 1974. *Am. J. Physiol.* 226:16.
Hirsch, J. and Goldrick, R. B. 1964. *J. Clin. Invest.* 43:1776.
Hirsch, J. and Knittle, J. L. 1970. *Fed. Proc.* 29:1516.
Horton, E. S., Danforth, E., Jr., Sims, E. A. H. and Salans, L. B. 1974. In *Obesity,* eds. W. L. Burland, P. D. Samuel and J. Yudkin, p. 217. London: Churchill Livingstone.
Horton, E. S., Danforth, E., Jr., Sims, E. A. H. and Salans, L. B. 1975. In *Obesity in perspective,* ed. G. Bray. DHEW Publ. No. (NIH) 75-708, p. 331.
Jeanrenaud, B. 1968. *Rev. Physiol. Biochem. Exp. Pharmacol.* 60:57.
Kipnis, D. M. 1972. *Diabetes* 21:606.
Livingston, J. N., Cuatrecasas, P. and Lockwood, D. H. 1972. *Science* 177:626.
Livingston, J. N., Cuatrecasas, P. and Lockwood, D. H. 1974. *J. Lipid Res.* 15:26.
Manganiello, V. and Vaughan, M. 1972. *J. Lipid Res.* 13:12.
McDonald, J. M., Burns, D. E. and Jarett, L. 1976. *Biochem. Biophys. Res. Commun.* 71:114.
Newburgh, L. H. 1942. *Ann. Intern. Med.* 17:935.
Ogilvie, R. F. 1935. *Q. J. Med.* 4:345.
Olefsky, J. M. 1976a. *J. Clin. Invest.* 57:842.
Olefsky, J. M. 1976b. *J. Clin. Invest.* 57:1165.
Paullin, J. E. and Sauls, H. C. 1972. *South. Med. J.* 15:249.

Rabinowitz, D. 1970. *Annu. Rev. Med.* 21:241.

Renold, A. E. and Cahill, G. F., Jr. 1965. In *Handbook of physiology*, Sect. 5: *Adipose tissue.* Washington, D.C.: American Physiological Society.

Renold, A. E., Rabinovitch, A., Kikuchi, M., Gutzeit, A. H., Amherdt, M. and Orci, L. 1975. In *Obesity in perspective*, ed. G. Bray. DHEW Publ. No. (NIH) 75-708, p. 289.

Rodbell, M. 1964. *J. Biol. Chem.* 239:375.

Salans, L. B. and Cushman, S. W. 1973. *Clin. Res.* 21:636.

Salans, L. B. and Cushman, S. W. 1975. In *Obesity in perspective*, ed. G. Bray. DHEW Publ. No. (NIH) 75-708, p. 245.

Salans, L. B. and Dougherty, J. W. 1971. *J. Clin. Invest.* 50:1399.

Salans, L. B., Knittle, J. L. and Hirsch, J. 1968. *J. Clin. Invest.* 47:153.

Salans, L. B., Knittle, J. L. and Hirsch, J. 1970. In *Diabetes mellitus: Theory and practice,* eds. M. Ellenberg and H. Rifkin, p. 424. New York: McGraw-Hill.

Salans, L. B., Horton, E. S. and Sims, E. A. H. 1971. *J. Clin. Invest.* 50:1005.

Salans, L. B., Cushman, S. W. and Weismann, R. E. 1973. *J. Clin. Invest.* 52:929.

Salans, L. B., Bray, G. A., Cushman, S. W., Danforth, E., Jr., Glennon, J. A., Horton, E. S. and Sims, E. A. H. 1974. *J. Clin. Invest.* 53:848.

Sims, E. A. H., Goldman, R. F., Gluck, C. M., Horton, E. S., Kelleher, P. C. and Rowe, D. W. 1968. *Trans. Assoc. Am. Physicians* 81:153.

Smith, U. 1971. *J. Lipid Res.* 12:65.

Stern, J. S. and Hirsch, J. 1972. In *Handbook of physiology*, Sect. 7: *Endocrinology,* Vol. 1: *Endocrine pancreas*, p. 641. Washington, D.C.: American Physiological Society.

Vaughan, M. 1961. *J. Lipid Res.* 2:293.

Wertheimer, E. and Shapiro, B. 1948. *Physiol. Rev.* 28:451.

Whipple, H. E. 1965. *Ann. N.Y. Acad. Sci.* 131:1.

Zinder, O. and Shapiro, B. 1971. *J. Lipid Res.* 12:91.

Zinder, O., Arad, R. and Shapiro, B. 1967. *Isr. J. Med. Sci.* 3:787.

Chapter 9

SIZE AND NUMBER OF ADIPOCYTES AND THEIR IMPLICATIONS

Judith S. Stern
Department of Nutrition
University of California
Davis, California

Patricia R. Johnson
Rockefeller University, New York, New York
and Department of Biology, Vassar College
Poughkeepsie, New York

INTRODUCTION

Until the 1950s, adipose tissue was the neglected tissue of the mammalian system. It was considered to be only the passive recipient of calories consumed in excess of immediate metabolic needs. When adipose mass expands excessively the result is an obese animal or person. The cause was attributed to the individual's inability to control the amount of calories consumed. Several advances occurred thereafter which altered radically the conceptualization of the role of adipose tissue in normal mammalian metabolism and in the major pathology associated with this tissue—obesity.

A burst of *in vitro* studies of the tissue's metabolic activity established that adipose tissue was highly sensitive to many hormonal signals and that its two major functions, lipid deposition and lipid mobilization, were "fine tuned" by numerous hormonal signals (Wertheimer and Shafrir, 1960; Winegrad, 1962). It soon became clear that insulin played a major part in determining the rate at which lipid deposition occurred (Winegrad and Renold, 1958), while the catecholamines were the primary hormonal stimulus to lipid mobilization (Rizack, 1961). Growth hormone (Fain and Scow, 1965), thyroxin (Challoner, 1969), ACTH (White and Engel, 1958), cortical steroids (Fain et al., 1965), TSH (Vaughan, 1960), and also glucagon (Vaughan, 1960) were found to influence the net rate of lipid mobilization from adipose tissue.

This work was supported by National Institutes of Health grant AM 18899.

Thus, adipose tissue came to be viewed as a highly active, carefully regulated metabolic mass, rather than as a passive storage depot.

In 1964, Rodbell published a method for isolating the lipid-laden white adipose cell from its connective tissue matrix, using the enzyme collagenase. Cells isolated in this manner retain the ability to take up substrate from the incubation medium, to release free fatty acids and glycerol, and to respond to hormonal signals in a manner similar to the tissue response. Thus, it became possible to relate adipose tissue activity to the activity of the adipocyte within the tissue.

In 1968, Hirsch and Gallian presented a new method for the determination of size and number of adipocytes in a given adipose depot of humans and other animals. Prior to the introduction of this rapid counting technique, studies of the morphology of adipose tissue were based on histological techniques. With histological techniques, individual fat cells are sized and counted directly from serial sections using a calibrated eyepiece. The main advantage of these techniques is that adipocytes may be observed directly embedded in their tissue matrix. The methods are quite tedious, however, and relatively few cells are used for actual sizing and counting.

Measurements of total DNA in isolated adipocytes have also been used as an index of adipose cell number, since the DNA content of adipocytes is relatively constant; that is, approximately 6.7 pg/cell (Hollenberg and Vost, 1968). A major shortcoming of this method is that 70–80% of adipose tissue DNA is not derived from fat cells, but from blood vessels, fibrous tissue, and mast cells, the precise percentage depending on the age of the animal (Hollenberg and Vost, 1968). Thus a small amount of contamination by nonadipocyte DNA can lead to large errors in determinations of adipocyte numbers.

The protein content of isolated fat cells has also been used as a measure of fat cell number. Protein content of rat fat cells is also relatively constant over a wide range of fat cell sizes (0.589–0.599 pg/cell) except in very small cells of young rats (0.540 pg/cell) (Hill et al., 1972). No estimation of the distribution of cell sizes is possible when using this method. In addition, protein content per cell must be corrected for adherent collagenase and albumin used in the isolation procedures. For both DNA and protein determinations, adipocytes must first be isolated, since DNA and protein determinations on whole adipose tissue do not necessarily reflect the number of adipocytes in the tissue.

In the Hirsch and Gallian (1968) method a number of the disadvantages of the above techniques were overcome. Adipose tissue is fixed with osmium tetroxide, which combines with lipid in the adipocyte. Fat cells are separated from nonadipocytes by serial filtration through nylon mesh and counted electronically in a particle counter. This procedure allows for the rapid determination of fat cell number and size distribution by counting thousands of cells. Cell size is calculated as the average lipid content per cell. Total fat cell number in humans is determined indirectly. Total body fat is calculated from indirect measures such as total body water or body density. Total cell number is calculated by dividing total body fat by average fat cell size. In other animals, the various adipose depots are carefully dissected and total fat and fat cell size are determined directly. Total fat cell number is the sum of the cell numbers determined for the individual depots. The major disadvantage of the osmium fixation method is that very small fat cells containing less than 0.01 μg triglyceride are not counted; therefore, underestimation of cell number occurs in tissue from very young animals or from animals that have undergone severe starvation. Furthermore, no information is obtained about the *in situ* distribution of cell sizes.

Utilization of the Hirsch and Gallian method quickly established that the size of any given adipose tissue mass in humans or other animals was the product of the mean size of the adipocytes and the number of adipocytes present in the tissue. For example, Hirsch and Knittle (1970) reported that nonobese individuals have an average cell size of 0.6 μg of triglyceride per cell and an average cell number of 25 billion. It could be shown that adipocyte size varies over a wide range and is responsive to numerous manipulations in the adult animal, while adipocyte number is essentially determined early in development and remains quite resistant to attempts to change it in the adult (Hirsch and Han, 1969; Salans et al., 1971; Stern and Greenwood, 1974). It became possible to assess obesity and other diseases, such as diabetes, that are often associated with altered adipose tissue stores, in terms of alterations in both the size and the number of adipocytes. The metabolic activity and hormonal responsiveness of the tissue could be expressed on a per unit cell basis, and the factors that influenced adipocyte size could be dissected from those that influenced adipocyte replication. At this time, it is clear that before we can thoroughly understand obesity and diabetes, or their interrelationship, we must understand the implications of adipocyte size and number, and how these are regulated in the normal animal.

DEVELOPMENT OF ADIPOSE TISSUE CELLULARITY IN HUMANS AND OTHER ANIMALS

Mammalian tissues and organs normally grow in a predictable manner, so that at the time of maturity the mass of each person is stable and represents an unchanging portion of the total body mass. The mature size of the organ is achieved through the processes of cellular replication and cellular enlargement, which in turn are regulated by humoral factors during critical periods of development. In some tissues or organs, new cells are produced at approximately the same rate at which old cells are lost throughout the life span, the result being that the number of cells in the organ or tissue remains relatively constant (e.g., blood and liver). In other tissues, cellular replication is halted at some critical point in development and the tissue is no longer capable of cellular replacement thereafter (e.g., neurons of the central nervous system).

The status of adipose tissue in respect to its mode of growth and development has been widely debated. Studies by Hirsch, Salans, and others have presented evidence that adipose tissue cell number is fixed in the adult animal (Hirsch and Han, 1969; Bray, 1970; Salans et al., 1971, 1973; Stern et al., 1972a; Hirsch and Batchelor, 1976). As established by counting osmium-fixed fat cells from the normal rat, the epididymal fat pad appears to grow by an increase in adipocyte number and size until maturity, 12–14 wk of age (Fig. 1) (Greenwood and Hirsch, 1974). From 14 wk onward, further increases in pad size are the result of cell enlargement only. Data derived by the use of such counting techniques, however, do not distinguish between cell proliferation and cell filling. Differentiation between cell proliferation and cell filling was accomplished by measuring the incorporation of tritiated thymidine into adipocyte DNA following a pulse injection. Using this method, Greenwood and Hirsch (1974) established that the epididymal fat pad of the normal rat grows largely by an increase in adipocyte number until the third postnatal week (Fig. 2). From the third week (weaning) until about the seventh week (puberty) the pad grows by small increments in cell number and cell enlargement. From maturity onward, further increases in pad size are the result of cell enlargement only. The apparent increase in cell number from 7 to 14 wk of age is due primarily to lipid filling of preexisting cells.

These studies of Greenwood and Hirsch (1974), utilizing the appearance of labeled precursor into fat cell DNA, confirmed and extended the earlier hypothesis of Enesco and LeBlond (1962) concerning the general pattern of cellular development of adipose as well as other tissues. These critical incorporation studies, which differentiate between cell proliferation and lipid filling, have only been reported for the epididymal fat pad. Recognizing that the pattern of cell size and number change during growth, as determined by osmium fixation and Coulter counting, is similar for other adipose depots of the rat, such as the retroperitoneal and subcutaneous depots, it seems reasonable to conclude that all adipose depots grow in a similar fashion in the rat. There may, of course, be species differences. DiGirolamo and Mendlinger (1971) found that between 6 wk and 1 yr of age, the expansion of the epididymal fat pad in the guinea pig was attributable mainly to an increase in the number of fat cells. Studies by Hellman et al. (1962) and by Johnson and Hirsch (1972) suggest that the critical period for fixation of adult adipocyte numbers in the mouse may be slightly later (40–60 days) than in the rat.

Other investigators have questioned the interpretation of a critical period after which adipocyte replication ceases, and have proposed that new fat cells may appear in the adult animals (Widdowson and Shaw, 1973; Ashwell and Garrow, 1973). Ashwell et al. (1975) have presented evidence of small pockets of adipose cells in sections of tissue from adult mice; Kirtland et al. (1975) present similar evidence in adipose tissue obtained from guinea pigs, and Stiles et al. (1976) have shown very small fat cells (8 μm in diameter) in collagenase

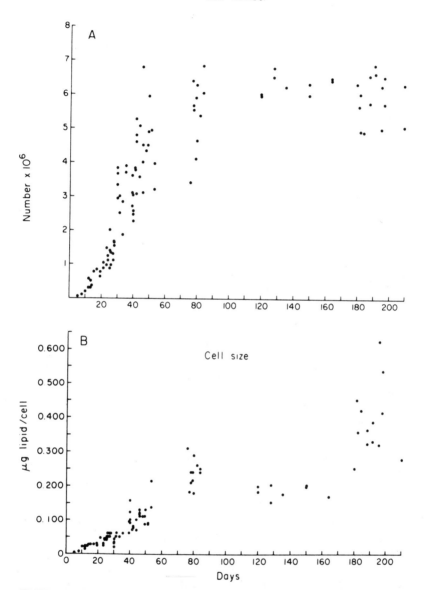

FIGURE 1 Cellularity of rat epididymal pad determined by the osmium fixation technique of Hirsch and Gallian (1968). For both cell number and cell size, each data point represents the mean pooled value for 4-12 rats (from Greenwood and Hirsch, 1974).

PROLIFERATION   PROLIFERATION

ENLARGEMENT   ENLARGEMENT   ENLARGEMENT

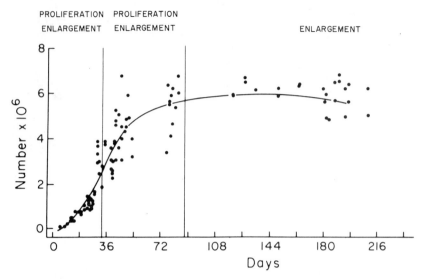

FIGURE 2 Development of adipose cell number in rat epididymal fat pad. Proliferation of adipocytes was monitored by determining specific activity changes of DNA in isolated stromal-vascular and adipocyte fractions of adipose tissue after a pulse injection of tritiated thymidine (data of Greenwood, from Winick, (1974).

digests of adipose tissue from Sprague-Dawley rats over 1 yr of age. Whether these findings represent evidence of significant cellular addition in the adult animal awaits confirmation by other investigators using techniques that measure actual DNA synthesis. It seems unlikely that major cell replication or cell loss contributes substantially to change in adipose mass in the adult, since most experimental interventions designed to alter adult adipose mass result only in cell size change.

While the critical period for adipocyte proliferation appears to be prior to weaning in the normal rat and mouse, the pattern in humans is different. Cellularity data on human infants and children are sparse. The data of Brook (1972) suggest that the early period of proliferation may be over by 1 yr of age. The body fat organ appears in the human fetus at about week 30 of gestation. It undergoes rapid proliferative growth, which continues for the first 9–12 months of extrauterine life. Brook theorizes that increases in cell number after 1 yr may represent lipid filling of preformed adipocytes. This interpretation by Brook is based on calculations of total fat from skinfold thickness data obtained from 64 healthy children undergoing elective surgery.

Knittle (1976) studied adipose tissue cellularity in nonobese children ranging in age from 2 to 16 yr. These children were between 80 and 120% of ideal body weight. Adipose tissue cellularity was determined on samples of subcutaneous fat obtained by needle biopsy by the method of Hirsch and Gallian (1968). Total body lipid was determined either by total body ^{40}K

counting or by height-weight formulas. Total body fat remained stable between 2 and 10 yr of age and increased between 10 and 16 yr of age (Fig. 3). Cell size increased in these subjects from age 10 to age 16. Cell number increased between ages 10 and 14, when the adult number of cells was achieved (see Fig. 3). These data indicate that there are two proliferative periods in normal weight individuals; the first occurs prior to the age of 2, the second is associated with puberty. Brook (1972), in contrast to Knittle (1976), interprets the data to mean that the cell number increase after 1 yr of age is simply due to lipid filling. Since these studies have relied on electronic counting of osmium-fixed cells for determination of cell number, the crucial question of whether an increase in cell number represents actual proliferation, rather than lipid filling of cells produced at an earlier time and remaining inactive with respect to lipid accumulation, is still unanswered.

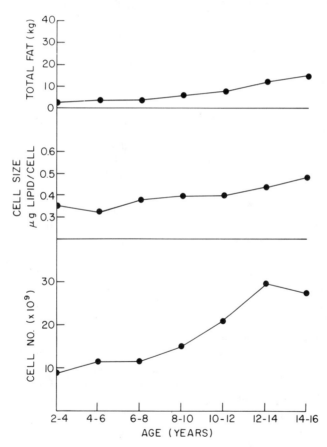

FIGURE 3 Total fat, adipose cell size, adipose and cell number in normal-weight children as a function of age (data of Knittle, 1976).

The major problem hindering a thorough understanding of the cellular growth and development of adipose tissue is the lack of a functional marker for the precursor cell to the adipocyte. The criteria currently in use for identification of the adipocyte depend on the cell containing some minimum amount of accumulated lipid. By the time the cell has filled with lipid to a detectable extent, it must be considered as "mature" in the sense that its DNA content is diploid and no further mitotic activity occurs. Mohr and Beneke (1969) demonstrated by a histochemical method an α-naphthyl esterase in a fibrocytic cell type in adipose tissue sections. Since other cells in the section that appeared morphologically similar showed a positive glycogen reaction believed to precede lipid deposition, they proposed that these cells would later become osmophilic by lipid accretion and that therefore these cells could be considered preadipocytes. Wertheimer and Shafrir (1960) had previously shown that glycogen deposition preceded fat accumulation in starved-refed rats, and had suggested that such a process occurred during the normal course of fat cell development. This study is perhaps the only one suggesting a histochemical demonstration of the preadipocyte, and it is still not possible to separate a clearly characterized preadipocyte fraction from presumptive adipose tissue.

GENERAL INFLUENCES

Among the reported and characterized mutant strains of laboratory rats and mice are a number of cases in which the phenotype includes an increased mass of adipose tissue, that is, obesity (Bray and York, 1971). In most of these cases the obese condition follows the inheritance pattern of a single Mendelian recessive gene. We have determined the adipocyte cellularity profile of a number of these mutant strains and have found that the morphology of the enlarged adipose depots falls into one of two categories: *hypertrophic* obesity, or *hypertrophic-hyperplastic* obesity (Johnson and Hirsch, 1972; Johnson et al., 1971; Robertson et al., 1974). The most common is hypertrophic obesity, in which the increased adipose mass is due only to enlargement of adipocytes (Table 1). It is seen in the yellow mouse strains (aA^y, aA^{vy}, aA^{iy}), the *dbdb* mouse, and the sand rat (*Psammomys obesus*). Hypertrophic-hyperplastic obesity, in which both cell size and cell number are increased, occurs in the obese-hyperglycemic (*obob*) mouse, the New Zealand obese (NZO) mouse, and the Zucker obese (*fafa*) rat.

Studies of the development of adiposity in the Zucker obese rat have suggested that this model continues to increase the number of adipocytes present in adipose tissue for a year, well beyond the time (3 wk) when cell number normally becomes stable in lean animals (Johnson et al., 1977). These data derived from electronic counting of osmium-fixed cells are supported by the additional finding that tritiated thymidine incorporation into adipocyte DNA occurs in 14-wk-old Zucker obese rats (Greenwood et al.,

TABLE 1 Size and Number of Adipocytes from Dorsal
Subcutaneous Fat Pad of 26-Wk-Old Male Animals[a]

Species	Type of animal	Body weight (g)	Fat cell size (μg TG/cell)	Fat cell number ($\times 10^6$)
Rat	Lean	432 ± 22	0.1621 ± 0.0141	16.380 ± 1.750
	Obese (*fafa*)	705 ± 11[b]	1.2633 ± 0.0959[b]	41.042 ± 9.000[b]
	Hypothalamic lesion (VMH)	593 ± 19[b]	1.0300 ± 0.1360[b]	18.220 ± 1.820
	Lean sand rat[c]	164 ± 24	0.3157 ± 0.1599	4.382 ± 1.522
	Obese sand rat[c]	235 ± 12[b]	0.8007 ± 0.1598[b]	6.268 ± 0.999
Mouse	Lean	29.6 ± 1.4	0.0671 ± 0.0195	2.051 ± 0.244
	Yellow-obese (*A*[y]*a*)	42.5 ± 0.7[b]	0.2809 ± 0.0314[b]	3.109 ± 0.503
	Gold thioglucose	40.7 ± 1.4[b]	0.3467 ± 0.0336[b]	2.852 ± 0.293
	Obese (*obob*)	53.6 ± 1.0[b]	0.7024 ± 0.0496[b]	2.801 ± 0.350[b]
	Obese (*dbdb*)	50.3 ± 1.7[b]	0.9256 ± 0.0624[b]	1.934 ± 0.192
	Obese (NZO)	51.2 ± 0.6[b]	0.1617 ± 0.0141[b]	8.521 ± 0.374[b]

[a]Data of Johnson and Hirsch, 1972; Johnson et al., 1971; Robertson et al., 1974.
[b]Significantly different from lean control, $p < 0.05$.
[c]Total subcutaneous depot.

1976). Thymidine kinase follows the same pattern during development as does thymidine incorporation into DNA and may be considered as an indicator of the proliferative phase of adipocyte development. In the nonobese rat, Cleary et al. (1976) have demonstrated that thymidine kinase activity in adipose tissue is elevated up to 28 days of age and drops off thereafter. In contrast, thymidine kinase activity in epididymal fat pad cells is elevated in preparations made from 14-wk-old Zucker obese animals, both male and female (Cleary et al., 1975).

We have suggested on the basis of these studies that the genetic lesion in the Zucker obese rat may involve a failure of the regulatory controls of adipocyte proliferation at a critical period in development (Johnson et al., 1977). The hypothesis that the obese Zucker rat can continue to form new adipocytes well into adulthood is further strengthened by studies in which a number of environmental stimuli have been used to manipulate cell number during various stages of this animal's life span. These studies will be discussed in the next section. Similar developmental data, unfortunately, do not exist for the other hyperplastic-hypertrophic strain, the *obob* mouse. The fact that other obese strains, such as the yellow mouse, do not show hyperplasia suggests that the underlying mechanism of adipose depot enlargement is fundamentally different, and perhaps involves regulation of net lipid accretion by acipocytes rather than proliferation of new cells.

Studies of adipose tissue cellularity in obese humans do not provide a clear morphological classification of obesity. Hirsch and Batchelor (1976) have reported data from 106 obese and 25 nonobese adults. Adipose cell size was averaged from sizes determined at three different subcutaneous sites. Adipose cell number was calculated by dividing total fat by average cell size. Cell size increased as percentage of ideal body weight increased up to 170% above normal. Beyond 170% there was little increase in cell size, which reached a maximum at about 1.0 μg triglyceride per cell. In contrast to cell size, cell number continued to increase as the severity of obesity increased ($r = + 0.74$). In general, the individuals with the largest cell numbers became obese at the earliest ages ($r = - 0.17$). The degree of obesity was greatest in the individuals who became obese earliest. In a study by Salans et al. (1973) a clearer relationship between adipose cell number and age of onset was established. They also found a correlation ($r = - 0.80$) between age of onset and adipose cell number. Individuals who became obese in childhood had higher cell numbers than those who became obese as adults. Salans et al. (1973) based their estimations of adipose cell size on six different cell size determinations in each patient, including three subcutaneous sites and three deep fat depots. Considerable variation was found between the six sites. They concluded that total adipose cell number of an individual was at best an estimation and that when number determination was based on cell size, it could vary by as much as 85%. Sjostrom and Bjorntorp (1974) also found that individuals who became obese as adults had fewer and larger fat cells. In summary, these studies lead to no absolutely clear classification of human obesity based on age of onset and hypercellularity. This may be in part because it is often difficult to assign an age of onset for adult obese humans *ex post facto,* since one must often rely on self-reports and photographs. Obviously, age of onset, hypercellularity, and severity of obesity are all interrelated. While it appears that individuals who become obese as children have more fat cells than those who become obese as adults, there are individuals of adult onset who are clearly hypercellular.

There is some evidence from the work of Knittle (1976) that development of obesity in childhood may reflect a problem in control of adipocyte proliferation. Knittle measured adipose cell size and number in obese and nonobese children at 2 yr intervals. Obese children had, on the average, larger fat cells than nonobese children, although there was some overlap. As previously discussed, fat cell number is stable in nonobese children from 2 through 11 yr of age (Fig. 3). During this same period, adipose cell number is increasing in obese children, with some obese children achieving an adult cell number as early as 4 yr of age (Fig. 4). Whether this reflects actual proliferation of adipocytes or merely lipid filling of preadipocytes awaits measurements such as determination of thymidine kinase activity.

Using cell number as a criterion, Knittle (1973) has identified at least two subgroups, by age 6, within the obese population: individuals with marked hyperplasia, often exceeding normal adult values, and individuals with a slight degree of hyperplasia. Within both groups, individuals have been identified who have either an increased or a normal cell size. Knittle goes on

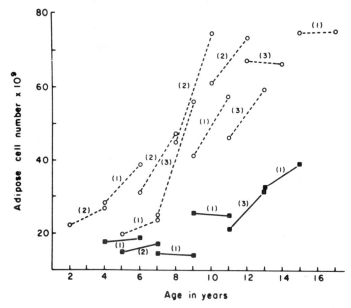

FIGURE 4 Adipose cell number in (o) obese and (■) non-obese children 2–17 yr of age. Reprinted from Knittle (1976) by permission of the M.I.T. Press, Cambridge, Massachusetts.

to speculate that children whose hypercellularity exceeds normal adult values are more likely to retain their obesity, while those with near-normal cellularity may outgrow their "baby fat."

Evidence that a genetic component contributes to obesity in the human is primarily limited to demographic data, such as those of Angel (1949) and Gurney (1936). Angel has reported that approximately half the children with one obese parent were obese, and two-thirds of the children with two obese parents were obese. Accordingly, Gurney's data show that only 9% of the children of average-weight parents were obese. Data such as these do not preclude the possibility that environmental factors are also involved in the higher incidence of obesity observed in the progeny of obese parents. For example, fatness is also correlated in husbands and wives who are genetically unrelated, yet share a similar environment (Garn et al., 1975). Family feeding patterns, particularly early in the child's life, could be a major contributing factor to the development of increased numbers of fat cells and thus to childhood obesity.

ENVIRONMENTAL INFLUENCES

A number of external environmental stimuli are known to modify the ultimate number of adipocytes found in the adult animal. The degree to which such modification occurs is highly dependent on the time in development that the stimulus acts, and to a lesser extent on the particular adipose tissue site. Environmental factors may influence adipocyte size as well. In fact, such influences on adipocyte size are the much more common phenomenon in the adult animal.

Overfeeding and Underfeeding of Young Animals

Knittle and Hirsch (1968) and Johnson et al. (1973) have shown that both preweaning over- and underfeeding do affect the ultimate number of adipose cells found in the adult rat. In the experiment of Knittle and Hirsch, Sprague-Dawley rat pups were raised in large litters (14–22 pups per dam) to limit food availability and in small litters (4 pups per dam) to maximize food availability. The normal litter size for the Sprague-Dawley rat is 8–10 pups, so we may consider that the pups raised in the large litters were underfed, while those raised in the small litters were overfed. At 3 wk of age, the rats were weaned and allowed Purina lab chow *ad libitum.* They were killed at 5, 10, 15, and 20 wk of age. At all ages studied, body weight, total body fat, epididymal adipocyte size, and epididymal adipocyte number were significantly decreased in the underfed compared to the overfed rats. Since the tritiated thymidine incorporation studies of Greenwood and Hirsch (1974) have established that the major period for adipocyte replication in the epididymal pad occurs prior to 24 days of age, these results are hardly surprising. Limited substrate availability during the period when rapid adipocyte proliferation is expected to occur must provide a signal that limits the production of adipocytes. The mechanism whereby such a signal functions is yet to be determined. Also, it is less easy to provide an explanation for the fact that the underfed rats continued to have smaller fat cells even though they were returned to *ad libitum* feeding after weaning.

In similar studies by Johnson et al. (1973), genetically obese Zucker rats and their lean littermates were used to determine whether the course of obesity could be altered by manipulating food availability during the preweaning period. Obese and nonobese rat pups were raised in large ($n = 12$-19), standard ($n = 8$), and small ($n = 3$-4) litters. At weaning (day 25) both the underfed obese and lean pups weighed less than their standard-fed controls, while the overfed pups weighed more. When the nonobese rats were killed at 26 wk of age and their adipose tissue cellularity determined, the results both confirmed and extended the earlier study of Knittle and Hirsch (Fig. 5). The underfed lean rats had 26% fewer cells than standard-fed controls, while the overfed lean rats had both 17% more cells and larger cells than standard-fed controls. These data established that the preweaning nutritional stimulus could influence the ultimate adult adipose tissue cellularity in either direction. Data were presented not only for the epididymal fat pad, but also for the retroperitoneal and subcutaneous depots. It was also possible to calculate a

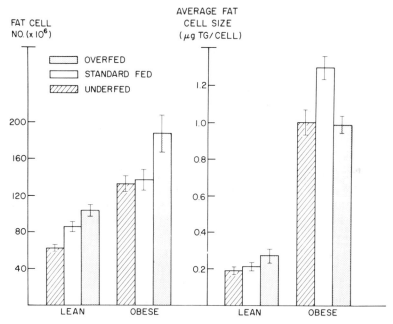

FIGURE 5 Effect of preweaning under- and overnutrition on adipose cell size and adipose cell number of 26-wk-old obese and lean Zucker rats. Rats were raised from birth until weaning (day 25) in small ($n = 3$–4), standard ($n = 8$), and large ($n = 12$–14) litters. From weaning until 26 wk of age, rats were fed *ad libitum*. Fat cell number is the sum of cell numbers in the epididymal, retroperitoneal, and subcutaneous depots. Cell size is the average cell size of the three depots. Values are means ± SEM (data of Johnson et al., 1973).

value for total adipocyte number and thus to show that the preweaning nutritional effect was not limited to the epididymal site.

When the cellularity of the obese rats was determined, however, a different picture emerged. Like their lean littermates, overfed obese rats had more adipocytes (27%) than their standard-fed controls, while underfed obese rats had no reduction in cell number when compared to standard fed controls (Fig. 5). Cell sizes were similar in the under- and overfed groups. These data strongly support the hypothesis that the Zucker obese rat is able to continue to produce adipocytes beyond the critical period of regulated proliferation seen in the normal lean animal. Once returned to *ad libitum* feeding, the underfed obese rat "caught up" with its fat cell production.

The fact that adipocyte size did not increase in the overfed obese rat is one piece of evidence that argues for the existence of a maximum adipocyte size. The very large cells of the Zucker obese rat may represent the result of maximum net lipid accumulation. When further stimulation to lipid filling occurs, the response may shift from lipid filling to cell proliferation. Such a response would result in the appearance of new and smaller fat cells in the depot population, and a lower mean cell size value would be obtained on sizing and counting. Thus, the presence of maximally filled cells may stimulate additional cell proliferation in the overfed obese Zucker rat.

Overfeeding and Underfeeding of Adults

The classic study of Sims and his colleagues clearly demonstrated that when adult men gain weight by purposefully overeating and decreasing activity, only fat cell size increases (Sims et al., 1968; Salans et al., 1971). There is no change in fat cell number. When adult rats overeat and become obese as a result of electrolytic lesions in the ventromedial area of the hypothalamus (VMH), weight gain also occurs solely by an increase in fat cell size, with no change in fat cell number (Hirsch and Han, 1969; Johnson et al., 1971). When sand rats become obese as adults only cell size increases; cell number is unchanged (Robertson et al., 1974). Similar changes have been reported for adult mice that were made obese by chemical lesioning of the VMH with gold thioglucose (GTG) (Johnson and Hirsch, 1972). While there is no change in fat cell number in GTG obese mice, there is evidence of connective tissue and blood vessel cellular proliferation in adipose tissue (Johnson and Hirsch, 1972; Rakow et al., 1971a). Most of these studies were relatively short-term. In the study of Sims et al. (1968), for example, patients were force-fed for only a few months. It is possible that adipose cell number in the adult is slow to respond to such environmental changes. Garrow (1974) has suggested that if these individuals maintained the obesity for a number of years, adipose cell number could increase; however, no studies are available to lend support to this hypothesis.

Studies in humans demonstrate that weight reduction is accomplished by decreases in fat cell size while fat cell number remains essentially unchanged (Hirsch and Knittle, 1970; Stern et al., 1972a; Salans et al., 1971; Bjorntorp and Sjostrom, 1971; Knittle and Ginsberg-Fellner, 1972). For example, Salans and colleagues (1971) demonstrated that weight reduction by adult men made obese experimentally is accomplished solely by decreases in cell size. Similarly, with food restriction in rats, depletion of the fat depot occurs by decreases in the cellular lipid content (Hirsch and Han, 1969). Hirsch and Han noted a temporary decrease in epididymal fat cell number in chronically starved rats that returned to prestarvation levels with refeeding. These authors used the osmium-fixation technique for measurements of adipose cellularity. This temporary decrease in fat cell number was probably an artifact because cells less than 25 μm in diameter are not counted by this technique. Krotkiewski and Bjorntorp (1975), using a microscopic technique developed by Sjostrom et al. (1971), measured adipose cellularity of the rat in several adipose depots after 3 and 5 days of starvation. Three days of starvation produced decreases in lipid content and cell size in three of five depots studied (Fig. 6). There were no changes in fat cell number. With more severe starvation (5 days) all depots were recruited for fat mobilization, with cell size decreased in all

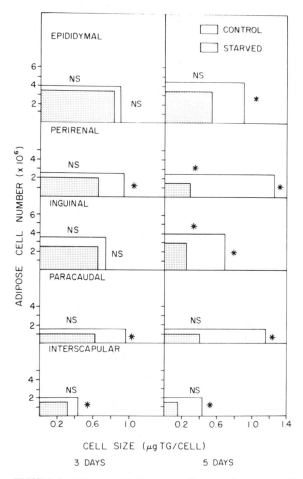

FIGURE 6 Adipose cell size and adipose cell number of different adipose tissue regions in adult rats starved for 3 or 5 days; (*) $p < 0.05$; (NS) not significant (data of Krotkiewski and Bjorntorp, 1976).

depots. In the perirenal, inguinal, paracaudal, and interscapular depots, 5 days of starvation caused a decrease in depot fat and fat cell size proportional to the characteristic cell size of that region ($r = +0.90, p < 0.05$). In epididymal fat cells, however, the cell size decrease was less than expected. Fat cell number decreased in the perirenal and inguinal depots. Although the method used by Krotkiewski and Bjorntorp (1975) does permit the measurement of smaller fat cells than the osmium-fixation method, it does not measure unfilled fat cells. It is likely that after 5 days of starvation the decrease in cell number that they report may reflect the presence of empty cells.

Total DNA content of epididymal fat pads is decreased in chronically starved mice (Rakow et al., 1971b). These data have been interpreted by some to mean that starvation does decrease adipose cell number. In this case also, limitations of the methodology have clouded the issue. Recently Rakow et al. (1971b) have shown that these decreases in total DNA (approximately 33%) were not due to a change in fat cell DNA (i.e., adipocyte number), but rather a decrease in the number of connective tissue and blood vessel cells. Similarly, the increased total DNA on refeeding is due to increased cell renewal only in connective tissue and blood vessels.

Diet Composition and Periodicity of Eating

Diet composition, as well as the amount of food available, has been shown to affect the cellularity of adipose tissue. Lau et al. (1976) fed a 7% protein diet to weanling rats for a 2 wk period and reported that adipocyte number remained below control values even when the protein-restricted rats were refed with a high-protein diet for 26 days. Knittle (1972) reported the effects of maternal caloric and protein-caloric restriction on epididymal adipose tissue cellularity in 8- and 12-wk-old rats. Maternal caloric deprivation alone produced some degree of stunting that was measurable in the offspring at 8 wk of age and was reflected by decreased adipocyte size but no difference in adipocyte number. No measure of milk production was reported, and it is likely that the differences were due to differences in the amount of milk produced and the subsequent caloric intake. The offspring of these mothers exhibited "catch-up" growth and the decrement in fat cell size had disappeared by 12 wk of age. On the other hand, the offspring of mothers that had experienced both protein (3%) and caloric restriction were more seriously stunted, in that they did not exhibit catch-up growth by 12 wk of age and had a permanently reduced number of fat cells compared to controls, as well as smaller fat cells. Again, the question of why the adipocytes remained smaller than normal in these permanently stunted animals remains unanswered, although we might speculate that dietary substrate may play a role in the determination of adipocyte membrane characteristics during critical periods of development. This question provides a rich field for future investigations.

In addition to protein, the other major dietary component known to influence adipose tissue cellularity is fat. Consumption of equicaloric diets high in fat (i.e., in excess of 10%) by laboratory rats and mice of a variety of strains results in an increased deposition of body fat (Mickelsen et al., 1955; Schemmel, 1969). It is clear in all studies reported that high-fat feeding results in an increase in mean adipocyte size for a given adipose depot. In addition, several investigators have presented evidence that adipocyte cell number also changes with high-fat feeding. Lemonnier (1972) fed male and female lean Swiss mice a high-fat (72% of calories) diet for 10 wk from the time of weaning; their dams had previously been fed the same diet from the time of mating. The mice raised from birth on the high-fat diet showed increases in cell numbers in the parametrial and retroperitoneal but not the subcutaneous and epididymal fat depots. Cell size was increased in all sizes with the exception of the retroperitoneal depot in female mice. In the same study, Lemonnier also reported that feeding the high-fat diet to lean Zucker rats from 5 months to 1 yr of age resulted in an increase in adipocyte number, but only in the retroperitoneal adipose depot. We have confirmed Lemonnier's finding in lean Zucker rats fed precisely the same high-fat diet, and noted in addition that cell number increased in the gonadal depot while cell number in the subcutaneous depot did not change (Faust et al., 1977c). There was no increase in cell number in any of the three depots in the obese rats. Furthermore, in Osborne-Mendel rats placed on a high-fat diet (70% of calories), the adipocyte number of the retroperitoneal depot increased from 14 million to 23.5 million cells after 9 wk (Faust et al., 1977c; Johnson et al., 1976). Over the same time span, the number of cells in the inguinal depot remained constant. In the Sprague-Dawley rat, the retroperitoneal pad responded to high-fat feeding by an increase in cell number (10.4 million to 19.1 million cells), but the process required a much longer period of time (5 months) (Faust et al., 1977c; Johnson et al., 1976). As in the Osborne-Mendel rat, the inguinal depot showed an increase only in cell size over the same period.

Herberg et al. (1974) reported that normally lean albino mice (NMRI strain) fed a high-fat diet (63% of calories) from weaning at 4 wk of age until 25 wk of age had an increased number of cells in both the epididymal and subcutaneous adipose depots; data for the retroperitoneal site were not reported.

In summary, these studies suggest that adipose tissue cell number may be more plastic than previously thought, although the data may be variously interpreted. In the Lemonnier mouse study, it is probable that feeding of the high-fat diet commenced prior to weaning, since the dam had access to the high-fat diet during the suckling period. Thus, pups probably consumed the diet during the period when rapid cell proliferation occurs in adipose tissue. Under this pre- and early weaning nutritional stimulus, many precursor fat cells could have been produced which continued to fill with lipid and to enter the countable pool of adipocytes at later periods during the life span. In the mouse study of Herberg et al., high-fat feeding was begun at 4 wk of age; the data of Johnson and Hirsch (1972) suggest that the period when cell number stabilizes in the normal mouse is 40–60 days. Thus, it is possible here also that high-fat feeding occurred before the end of the critical period for adipocyte proliferation. The rat data of Lemonnier (1972), Faust et al. (1977c), and Johnson et al. (1976) are more directly pertinent to the question of whether cell number can respond to manipulation in the adult, since in all of these studies the rats were clearly adult and well past the critical proliferative period. The hyperplastic response in these studies was limited to the retroperitoneal and gonadal depots, leaving open the possibility that these sites contain a reserve of preadipocytes that may fill with lipid and appear as mature adipocytes only when caloric consumption exceeds normal. It appears that adipose tissue is not a single uniform entity, but responds to challenges such as high-fat feeding in site-specific ways.

In addition to food availability and diet composition, the periodicity of eating may also effect changes in the size and number of fat cells. In the rat, meal feeding (i.e., limiting food intake to several hours per day) enhances lipogenesis and fat accumulation (Tepperman et al., 1943; Leveille, 1970). Braun et al. (1968) have reported that adult Wistar rats, limited to a feeding period of 2 hr/day, increased the number of fat cells in epididymal and parametrial adipose tissue. Their conclusion was based on an absolute increase in DNA content and an increase in $[2\text{-}^{14}C]$ thymidine incorporation into DNA of the adipose depot. In their study $[^{14}C]$ thymidine was injected intraperitoneally 1 hr before the rats were killed. Lipid-laden adipocytes were isolated and the specific activity of DNA was determined. It is unlikely that during this 1 hr period preadipocytes could proliferate and accumulate sufficient lipid to be readily harvested and identifiable as adipocytes. Previous studies by Greenwood and Hirsch (1974) indicate that this process may take up to 3 wk. Therefore it is more likely, as seen with starvation and refeeding, that this increased DNA synthesis reflects increased cellular proliferation in the stromal vascular portion of the adipose depot.

Surgical Intervention

Conventional modes of therapy for producing sustained weight loss in massively obese individuals have had a consistently poor success rate over the long term. In most cases of massive obesity hyperplasia is found in adipose depots, and the failure to sustain weight loss, once achieved, has been attributed to the fact that fat cell numbers remain elevated after weight reduction while mean fat cell size is decreased, often below normal. It has occurred to some clinical investigators that if fat cell number is an important regulated feature of the adipose depot mass, as the lipostatic theory of Kennedy (1950) would suggest, and if fat cell number is relatively constant in the adult, then the removal of adipose cells by surgical means might result in the maintenance of weight loss in the reduced obese patient. In addition, it has occurred to several investigators that the use of lipectomy as an investigative tool in animal model studies might provide a means of teasing apart the respective roles of adipocyte size, adipocyte number, and total lipid mass in the regulation of body weight. Thus the surgical removal of fat has been accomplished in humans and other animals, and the effects on adipose tissue cellularity have been reported.

Although a number of investigators have reported on adipectomy in the human (Masson, 1962; Pitanguy, 1967; Kamper et al., 1972), the rationale for these studies was essentially cosmetic and no body composition or cellularity data were reported. In one study reported by Kral (1975), however, cellularity data are presented on three female patients who underwent surgical removal of adipose tissue from three areas: the abdominal, lumbar, and femoral depots. Prior to surgery, the three patients had sustained a mean weight loss of 42.3 kg, resulting from a conventional weight loss regimen of diet and exercise. Also, they were hyperplastic, having a mean cell number of 75×10^9 cells. At surgery, 8, 15, and 12×10^9 fat cells were removed from the three patients, representing approximately 16% of their total adipose cell number. Loss of these fat cells did not prevent regain of the lost weight after the surgery, but there was apparently no recurrence of obesity at the scar sites.

These limited findings imply that cell number is not as crucial for the regulation of energy balance as cell size or total adipose mass may be. This interpretation is greatly strengthened by recent data reported by Faust et al. (1976) and by Kral (1976) on the results of lipectomy in normal rats and mice. Kral lipectomized normal adult (15-wk-old) Sprague-Dawley rats, removing approximately 24% of their total body fat from the inguinal and epididymal adipose depots. After 12 wk there was no evidence of compensatory regrowth at the site of removal, nor of compensatory hypertrophy in the remaining adipose depots. Neither was there any measurable alteration in body weight or food intake over the 12 wk period. Serum FFA, glycerol, triglyceride, cholesterol, and insulin levels were identical to the values for sham-operated controls. Faust et al. (1976) performed similar lipectomies on 16-day-old lean (Fa-) Zucker rats and normal lean adult NCS mice. After 30 and 80 days they found no evidence of local restoration of fat at the site of surgical removal in the rat or the mouse. Although there was an excess accumulation of lipid in remaining depots of the lipectomized mice 30 days after surgery, the excess was no longer apparent at 80 days. The temporary lipid accumulation correlated with some testicular disruption, which was observed at 30 days but was no longer present at 80 days. These authors, like Kral, concluded that surgical removal of fat does not lead to compensatory regrowth, at least over the short term, and that autoregulation of adipose tissue mass, if it occurs, must be related to adipocyte size rather than adipocyte number or total adipose tissue mass.

In another study, Faust et al. (1977b) observed that if Sprague-Dawley rats are lipectomized at weaning and followed for up to 7 months, total regenerative regrowth of the inguinal fat depot is found to occur. Both cell size and cell number of the dissectable subcutaneous fatty sheath are found to be equivalent in lipectomized animals and their sham-operated controls. The difference between these results and those of Kral (1976) may be explained on the basis of the different timing of the lipectomy. Kral's animals were lipectomized at 15 wk of age, which is well beyond the critical period for adipocyte proliferation, while the animals of Faust et al. (1977b) were lipectomized at 3 wk of age, which is still within the critical period for proliferative activity. It may thus be concluded that the surgical removal of fat cells during the critical period provides a sufficient stimulus for the production of precursor cells, which are capable of proliferating in numbers sufficient to restore normal cell numbers in the inguinal site. A similar regenerative response occurs neither in the epididymal pads of rats, nor in the epididymal or inguinal depots of mice. It is obvious that the factors that regulate adipose tissue growth are complex; they are at least age-, site-, and species-specific.

A kind of surgical intervention very different from lipectomy is the jejunoileal shunt now being practiced by a number of clinicians (Brill et al., 1972; Rehfield et al., 1970; Bickman, 1975) for the treatment of morbid obesity. In 15 severely obese and hyperplastic patients, Kral et al. (1976) reported that only fat cell number, in contrast to all other variables of body composition studied, remained unchanged 3 months postoperatively when a stable body weight had been achieved. The loss of body fat in these patients was related to decrements in fat cell size. Thus, the loss of weight following jejunoileal shunting, like that following reduction by more conventional means, produces no change in the number of adipocytes, but only reduction in their size through loss of lipid.

Environmental Temperature

Changes in environmental temperature have been associated with changes in food intake, activity levels, and fat deposition. As previously stated, growth of the epididymal fat pad of the postweanling rat raised at normal ambient temperature (25°C) occurs primarily by fat cell hypertrophy. In rats exposed to cold (5°C), Therriault and Mellin (1971) have reported an increase in fat cell proliferation that is dependent on the age at which cold exposure is initiated. For example, when weanling rats (50-75 g) are maintained in a cold environment (5°C) until they are 475 g in weight, the epididymal fat pads contain more than twice the number of adipocytes, which are much smaller in size (Fig. 7). Similarly, when adult rats (300 g) are placed in a cold environment until they reach 475 g, their epididymal fat pads accumulate lipid at a rate equivalent to that of rats kept in the cold from a very early age. However, growth in this case is solely due to hypertrophy rather than hyperplasia. Growth of depots other than the epididymal were not studied. Once again, this study supports the hypothesis that there are critical periods early in the life span of an animal, when environmental variables may result in changes in the proliferation of fat cells. These same variables, when applied to adult animals, may also cause changes in adipose depot size, which are expressed, however, primarily by changes in fat cell size.

Exercise

The amount of exercise engaged in by an animal or human is of major importance in regulating the fat content of the body. There have been numerous studies documenting the fact that exercise results in decreased total body fat, while forced inactivity promotes fattening (Oscai, 1973; Oscai and Holloszy, 1969; Mayer et al. 1954; Babirek et al., 1974). For example, Crews

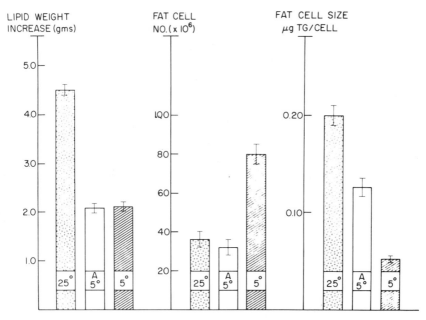

FIGURE 7 Effect of cold exposure on epididymal lipid content, fat cell number, and fat cell size in the rat. (25°) Rats were kept at 25°C throughout the experiment. (A 5°) Rats were kept at 25°C until they reached a weight of 300 g; they were then placed at 5°C (5°) Rats weighing 100 g were placed at 5°C and remained there throughout the experiment (from Therriault and Mellin, 1971).

et al. (1969) have shown that adult Sprague-Dawley rats forced to exercise are leaner and have smaller epididymal fat cells than nonexercised controls. If exercise is begun before weaning (8 days), and thus before the establishment of adult cell number in the rat, there is also a decrease in epididymal fat cell number (Oscai et al., 1972).

As in the Sprague-Dawley rat, 6-wk-old lean Zucker rats that are forced to exercise for 9 wk decrease adipose depot size by a decrease in fat cell size only (Table 2) (Stern et al., 1976). When Zucker obese rats are similarly exercised, there is a greater decrease in total lipid content of the epididymal, retroperitoneal, and subcutaneous depots. However, this decrease in lipid occurs only by a decrease in fat cell number. It is possible that in the obese rat the effect of exercising is to slow down the rate of fat cell proliferation.

We have also studied the long-term effect of early exercise on the development of adiposity in obese and lean Zucker rats (Stern and Johnson, 1977). Rats were given access to activity wheels at 16 days of age and allowed to exercise until 8 wk of age. Lean rats were more active than obese rats, running a total of 57.6×10^3 revolutions compared to 28.1×10^3 revolutions. At 8 wk of age, exercised lean and obese rats had less total fat and fewer adipocytes than their appropriate controls. Adipose cell size was decreased

TABLE 2 Effects of Forced Exercise on Adiposity in 15-Wk-Old
Genetically Obese and Lean Zucker Rats[a,b]

Group	Body weight (g)	Total fat[c] (g)	Average fat cell size[c] (μg TG/cell)	Total fat cell number[c] ($\times 10^6$)
Lean rats (Fa/-)				
Control ($n = 11$)	380.0 ± 15.9	16.14 ± 1.90	0.2882 ± 0.0348	59.459 ± 4.528
Exercised ($n = 12$)	347.9 ± 13.7	8.76 ± 0.88[d]	0.1854 ± 0.0154[e]	49.242 ± 4.187
Obese rats (*fafa*)				
Control ($n = 10$)	555.2 ± 21.7	120.21 ± 7.23	1.5680 ± 0.0860	78.372 ± 4.809
Exercised ($n = 12$)	497.9 ± 24.2[e]	86.15 ± 4.90[d]	1.3590 ± 0.0900	65.749 ± 4.108[e]

[a]Stern et al., 1976.

[b]Obese and lean 6-wk-old male Zucker rats were forced to exercise on treadmills 1,200 m/day, 6 days/wk for 9 wk.

[c]Represents the combined values from the epididymal, retroperitoneal, and total subcutaneous sites.

[d]Significantly different from control at $p < 0.01$.

[e]Significantly different from control at $p < 0.05$.

only in exercised lean rats. To assess the permanent effect of early exercise on adiposity, rats exercised until 8 wk of age were confined until 6 months of age. At autopsy, body weight and total fat were significantly elevated in formerly exercised rats compared to control rats (see Table 3). The mechanism for accelerated fat deposition in the inactive period is currently under investigation. However, it may be a phenomenon similar to the weight gain

TABLE 3 Effect of Wheel Running from 16 Days to 8 Wk of Age on
Body Weight and Adiposity in 6-Month-Old Zucker Obese and Lean Rats[a,b]

Group	Body weight (g)	Total fat[c] (g)	Average fat cell size[c] (μg TG/cell)	Total cell number[c] ($\times 10^6$)
Lean				
Control ($n = 11$)	432.0 ± 22.0	17.970 ± 1.98	0.2164 ± 0.02094	84.415 ± 5.000
Exercised ($n = 5$)	446.0 ± 10.5	30.086 ± 1.050[d]	0.4483 ± 0.0403[d]	60.910 ± 4.090[d]
Obese				
Control ($n = 12$)	705.0 ± 11.3	165.165 ± 8.097	1.2933 ± 0.0642	131.987 ± 11.240
Exercised ($n = 2$)	728.5 ± 12.2	204.969 ± 7.273[d]	1.3040 ± 0.0202	161.660 ± 3.559[e]

[a]Stern and Johnson, 1977.

[b]Values represent mean ± SEM.

[c]Represents the combined values from the epididymal, retroperitoneal, and total subcutaneous sites.

[d]Significantly different from control, $p < 0.01$.

[e]Significantly different from control, $p < 0.05$.

often observed in the aging retired athlete. Fat cell size was increased in the formerly active lean rat. Adipose cell number was permanently decreased only in formerly active lean rats. In fact, there was a significant increase of fat cell number in the formerly active obese rat, once again demonstrating the plasticity of adipose cell number in this genetically obese rodent.

HORMONAL INFLUENCES

Insulin

Although numerous hormones are intimately involved with lipid deposition and mobilization and thus with the maintenance of adipocyte size, most studies directly concerned with hormonal influences on adiposity involve insulin. There is an extensive literature linking an elevated insulin level with obesity in humans and other animals (Stern and Hirsch, 1971). Proposals by several investigators that hyperinsulinemia may be primary in the etiology of obesity are based on four types of evidence. First, nondiabetic obese humans and other animals almost uniformly have elevated fasting insulin levels (Stern and Hirsch, 1971). With weight reduction, these levels decrease to normal. Second, genetically obese rodents have been shown to have consistently elevated insulin levels, which become elevated early in life when obesity first becomes evident (Bray and York, 1971; Sneyd, 1964; Herberg et al., 1970; Coleman and Hummel, 1967; Zucker and Antoniades, 1972). Third, administration of insulin to rats has been shown by Steffens (1969), Panksepp et al. (1975), and May and Beaton (1968) to promote both hyperphagia and increased deposition in fat. Furthermore, the amount of weight gain is dose-related. Finally, when rats are lesioned in the ventromedial area of the hypothalamus (a procedure that ordinarily results in hyperphagia and obesity) and simultaneously made diabetic, they continue to be hyperphagic, but fail to become obese (Young and Liu, 1965). These observations have encouraged investigators to speculate that hyperinsulinemia per se is responsible for the disburbances in body weight seen in obesity and the establishment and maintenance of an elevated amount of adipose tissue.

The role of insulin in the establishment of adipose cell number is still being debated. Salans et al. (1972) administered insulin to young Charles River rats, ranging in age from birth to 3 wk, and to adult rats (10 wk of age) and killed the rats at different times during growth. Insulin-treated rats were fatter and had larger fat cells in the epididymal, retroperitoneal, and subcutaneous depots, but in no case was there an increase in the number of fat cells. Krotkiewski and Bjorntorp (1976) administered insulin (25 μU/kg) daily for 4 wk to adult female Sprague-Dawley rats. Adipose cell size was increased in the perirenal and subcutaneous depots, but not in the parametrial depot. There was no change in cell number due to insulin administration in any depot studied.

In contrast, Kazdova et al. (1974) administered insulin in small doses to Wistar rats for 1-6 days and found increased *in vitro* [2-^{14}C]thymidine incorporation into adipose tissue. After fractionation of the tissue with collagenase, enhanced DNA synthesis was found in both the adipocyte and stromalvascular fractions. It is possible that what Kazdova et al. were measuring in the adipocyte fraction reflected contamination by the stromal-vascular fraction. According to Greenwood and Hirsch (1974), isolated adipocytes prepared by the collagenase digestion method must be washed several times to avoid possible contamination by the stromalvascular fraction. Another possible but unlikely explanation for the discrepancy between the findings of Salans and Kazdova are strain differences, or the fact that different amounts of insulin were administered.

It is not clear whether hyperinsulinemia plays a role in the development of fat cell hyperplasia in obese animals. Hyperinsulinemia is consistently found in nondiabetic obese rodents, but hyperplasia is not uniformly present. In a previous study we reported that normalization of insulin by streptozotocin in *obob* mice did not alter the development of obesity or the fat cell hyperplasia (Batchelor et al., 1975). It is more likely that insulin levels and the establishment and/or maintenance of adipose cell size are more closely related.

There are a number of reports of significant positive correlations between adipose cell size and plasma insulin levels in humans and other animals (Stern et al., 1972a; Johnson et al., 1977; Bjorntorp and Sjostrom, 1971). Weight reduction results not only in decreases in adipose cell size, but also in decreases in plasma insulin values (Stern et al., 1972a). It is possible, as pointed out by Krotkiewski and Bjorntorp (1976), that the effects of insulin on fat cell size may be dependent on fat cell size per se. Smaller fat cells are reported to be more sensitive to insulin than larger fat cells (Zinder et al., 1967; Smith, 1971; Salans et al., 1968). Insulin injections result in similar increases in cell size in the retroperitoneal (70–90%) and epididymal (80–88%) depots, but relatively larger increases in cell size in the subcutaneous depot (100–120%), which also seems to contain smaller fat cells (Salans et al., 1972).

In a more recent developmental study with obese female Zucker rats, both fat cell size and plasma insulin reach a maximum at 14 wk of age and then decrease (Fig. 8) (Johnson et al., 1977). This sequence of events suggests that peak insulin and peak fat cell size may provide a stimulus for increased hyperplasia in the obese rat. This interpretation is further supported by measurements of thymidine kinase in adipose tissue. Thymidine kinase activity in adipose tissue in the obese rats compared to the lean controls was elevated at 14 wk of age but was not different at 26 wk of age. In addition, the cell diameter distribution data indicate the presence of a measurable population of small fat cells in subcutaneous and retroperitoneal adipose tissue at 15½ wk of age in obese rats, which is shortly after the time at which a peak mean cell size occurs in these depots. It is tempting to postulate that

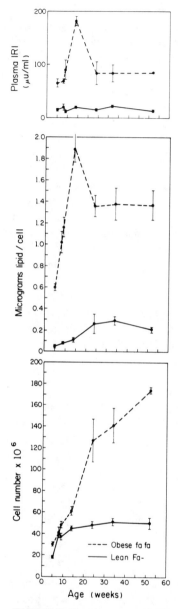

FIGURE 8 Development of plasma insulin values, adipose cell size, and adipose cell number in female obese and lean Zucker rats. (Values are means ± SEM (data of Johnson et al., 1977b).

when one population of fat cells achieves a maximum fat cell size, under the stimulus of continued high levels of substrate availability, new cells begin to appear in the depot and to accumulate lipid. The peak plasma insulin at 14 wk of age might then provide a "trigger" for further fat cell hyperplasia, but this hypothesis will require further study.

Growth Hormone

Studies of the effects of growth hormone on organs other than adipose tissue demonstrate that this hormone stimulates cellular proliferation. However, there is a paucity of literature on the effects of this hormone on adipose cellularity. Knittle et al. (1972) treated six ateliotic dwarfs with growth hormone for a period of 8 months. All patients increased in height, weight, lean body mass, and total fat. For five of the subjects, increases in total fat were a result of increases in adipose cell number. It is possible that growth hormone is involved in adipose cellular proliferation, but these data are not definitive. In contrast, in the intact animal, growth hormone administration depletes lipid stores. Batchelor and Stern (1973), for example, reported that daily administration of growth hormone to weanling male rats for 15 days leads to a depletion of epididymal fat stores. The decrease was a result of decreased epididymal cell size; fat cell number was unchanged. The effects of growth hormone on depots other than the epididymal were not studied.

Adrenal Steroids

Adrenal steroid hormones also exert powerful effects on lipid metabolism, producing changes in body weight and composition. To examine regional effects of corticosteroids on depot fat distribution, Krotkiewski and Bjorntorp (1975) administered to 6-month-old male rats for 4 wk a dose of dexamethasone (40 μg/kg-day) that produced changes in adipose tissue mass. Control rats were pair-fed to eliminate the effect of dexamethasone on decreasing food intake. Dexamethasone treatment had no effect on adipose cell number in any depot studied. Cell size was significantly decreased only in the interscapular depot and tended to be lower in the perirenal, inguinal, and paracaudal depots.

Sex Hormones

Humans and other animals vary in the amount and distribution of body fat according to sex. For example, percentage body fat is higher in women than men (Ljunggren, 1965). Nonobese men and women also show differences in adipose tissue cellularity in different subcutaneous regions. Women have more fat cells than men, while fat cell size does not significantly differ between the sexes (Sjostrom et al., 1972). A specific role of sex hormones in the development of adipose cell size and number in humans remains to be elucidated. Some data exist for other animals. Kral and Tisell (1976) have reported that castration of 16-wk-old male Sprague-Dawley rats results in significant decreases in fat cell size in the epididymal depot and a trend toward decreases in cell size in the perirenal and subcutaneous depots. Cell number was unchanged in all three depots. However, Lemonnier and Alexiu (1974) report that castration of 6-wk-old mice resulted in a twofold increase in weight and adipose cell size of the epididymal and retroperitoneal pads. Cell number was unchanged.

Administration of progesterone to female rats causes elevations in body weight that are explainable by an increase in adipose tissue weight (Krotkiewski and Bjorntorp, 1976). This increase occurs solely by increases in cell size in the three depots studied (parametrial, perirenal, and subcutaneous). Administration of progesterone also resulted in a sevenfold increase in plasma insulin levels. However, the enlargement of fat cells after progesterone treatment was probably not solely due to elevations of plasma insulin, since in insulin-treated rats fat cell enlargement occurs primarily in the subcutaneous depot (Salans et al., 1972; Krotkiewski and Bjorntorp, 1976), while in progesterone-treated rats it occurs primarily in the parametrial depot.

High doses of estrogen (120 µg/kg-month) for 10 wk decreased body weight and adipose tissue weight in female rats (Krotkiewski, 1976). Fat cell number was unchanged. The greatest fat cell size decrease occurred in the subcutaneous depot, which had the smallest cells. The least cell size decrease occurred in the parametrial depot, which had the largest cells. This is in contrast to what occurs in starvation, where the largest cells show the greatest decrease in cell size. With low doses of estrogen (60 µg/kg-month), 4 wk of treatment results in an increase in adipose tissue weight and no change in fat cell number (Krotkiewski, 1976). Fat cell size increase was greatest in the parametrial depot and may reflect a regional specificity of estrogen for adipocytes of the parametrial depot. In contrast to the effect observed with insulin administration, the largest increases in cell size occur in the depot with the smallest fat cells (Salans et al., 1972; Krotkiewski and Bjorntorp, 1976).

Adipose tissue is not uniform in its response to different hormonal stimuli. Gain or loss of body fat varies among the different antaomical regions and is dependent on the specific hormone. It is likely that some of the many hormones that affect adipose tissue development have "target sites." There is abounding evidence that sex hormones such as progesterone and estrogen have target tissues. The evidence presented implies that the target tissue may also involve the accessory fat depots. In contrast, the adipose depot that appears most responsive to insulin appears to be the depot with the smallest fat cells. This will be discussed in more detail in the following section.

ADIPOCYTE SIZE AND INTERMEDIARY METABOLISM

In studies reported before the mid-1960s, the cellular composition of adipose tissue in relation to metabolism was rarely considered. Data were derived from *in vitro* studies of whole pads or tissue minces and expressed per wet weight of tissue or per lipid content. Since the introduction of the method for the preparation of isolated adipocytes (Rodbell, 1964), numerous investigators have focused their attention on the response of the individual adipocyte. In animal studies, the favored depot of study is the epididymal pad; in humans, it is the subcutaneous depot. No doubt these tissues have been favored by investigators for their ease of access. We have presented substantial evidence in this discussion of adipose cellularity that adipose tissue cannot be considered as a single entity, since the various depots react in a site-specific manner. It is likely that the morphological differences between various sites reflect basic metabolic differences.

Adipose cell size influences adipose tissue metabolism; however, the exact nature of the relationship varies with the particular facet of metabolism one is monitoring. For example, several investigators have reported that incorporation of labeled glucose into triglyceride increases with fat cell size. The greater the cell size, the more glucose is incorporated into glyceride glycerol and fatty acids (Smith, 1971; Bjorntorp and Sjostrom, 1972; Salans and Cushman, 1973; Hansen et al., 1974). Similarly, basal lipolysis, epinephrine-stimulated lipolysis, and fatty acid reesterification are also increased in larger fat cells (Bjorntorp and Sjostrom, 1972; Reardon et al., 1973; Hansen et al., 1974). Others report that fat cells of different sizes metabolize glucose to CO_2 and triglyceride at similar rates (Salans and Dougherty, 1971).

The response of adipocytes to insulin decreases with increased adipose cell size (Salans et al., 1968; Salans and Dougherty, 1971; Czech, 1976). When one measures glucose conversion to CO_2, adipocytes from obese subjects are less responsive to insulin than smaller adipocytes isolated from the same subjects after weight loss (Salans et al., 1968). In contrast, larger fat cells are more sensitive to the antilipolytic effect of insulin than smaller fat cells (Ostman et al., 1975; Jacobsson et al., 1976). The concentrations of insulin necessary to inhibit lipolysis are much less than those needed to stimulate glucose incorporation.

It has been hypothesized that decreased insulin sensitivity of adipocytes seen in obesity may reflect decreased binding of insulin to the fat cell membrane. However, the association between adipose cell size and number of insulin receptors and its physiological meaning have been a source of much debate, with much of the debate focusing on differences in methodology (e.g., Katzen and Vlahakas, 1973).

Olefsky (1976a) has reported a decrease in number of insulin receptors in large epididymal adipocytes from old, fatter rats (12 months) compared to adipocytes isolated from young, leaner rats (4-5 wk). Olefsky (1976b) has also reported a decrease in number of insulin receptors in subcutaneous adipocytes isolated from obese humans. Hyperglycemic obese (*obob*) mice show a decrease in insulin binding in epididymal adipocytes over a wide range of insulin concentrations added *in vitro* (Freychet et al., 1972; Kahn et al., 1973). There appears to be no correlation of age and the receptor defect, with young *obob* mice (6½ wk) and older *obob* mice showing a similar defect. In contrast, other investigators found no decrease in insulin binding when comparing larger and smaller fat cells (Livingston et al., 1972; Bennett and Cuatrecasas, 1972; Amatruda et al., 1975). In two of these studies (Livingston et al., 1972; Amatruda et al., 1975) results were expressed per microgram of adipocyte DNA. That these investigators did not find a decrease in insulin binding in large fat cells may merely reflect differences in contamination of adipocyte DNA with DNA from stromal vascular cells in the two different preparations. The physiological meaning of number of insulin receptors of adipocytes is unclear. However, recent work by Czech (1976) would indicate that the blunted insulin response of large adipocytes is not due to a decreased number of receptors but may be related to one or more intracellular enzymes involved in glucose metabolism.

While it is evident that cell size can significantly influence adipose tissue metabolism and its response to various stimuli, not all investigators report correlations of cell size with the various parameters discussed. Other factors such as age of the animal, diet composition, periodicity of eating, and even the composition of the incubation medium must be considered. For example, at a given fat cell size, basal lipolysis, lipolytic effects of hormones such as glucagon and norepinephrine, rate of glucose incorporation into triglyceride, and effect of insulin on glucose metabolism are all increased in similarly sized cells isolated from young rats (4 wk) compared to older rats (15 wk) (Holm et al., 1975). Because fat cell size increases with age, some differences attributed to cell size may merely reflect the age differences (Romsos and Leveille, 1972).

High-carbohydrate feeding enhances glucose conversion to CO_2 and the effects of insulin (Salans et al., 1974; Ogundipe and Bray, 1974; Stern et al., 1975). In rats fed diets high in fat, fat cell sizes and rates of lipolysis and glucose incorporation into triglyceride are not correlated (Smith et al., 1974).

Lipogenesis is enhanced in adipocytes isolated from animals that eat relatively few meals per day compared to animals that eat a large number of meals per day (Leveille, 1970). Finally, the stimulatory effect of insulin on glucose metabolism is greater in small adipocytes than in large adipocytes when the level of glucose in the incubation medium is high (5 mM) (Czech, 1976). When the level of glucose in the incubation medium is low (0.2 mM) and hexose transport is more rate-limiting, large cells utilize more glucose than small cells in the presence of insulin. The percentage stimulation by insulin, however, is still less in the large cells.

In conclusion, correlations have been reported between fat cell size and fasting plasma levels of triglyceride and insulin, and 2 hr levels of plasma insulin after an oral glucose challenge (Johnson et al., 1977; M. P. Stern et al., 1973; J. S. Stern et al., 1972a; Bjorntorp and Sjostrom, 1971). Increases or decreases in body weight result in similar changes in adipose cell size and triglyceride values, while cell number is unchanged. These correlations point to a possible direct relationship between enlargement of adipose cell size (seen in obesity) and pancreatic function and turnover of metabolites such as triglycerides. Data from *in vitro* studies suggest that the formerly obese individual with a large number of fat cells of smaller than normal size may be particularly sensitive to the lipogenic effects of hormones such as insulin and thus particularly vulnerable to regaining of lost weight.

CONCLUSIONS

Over the past 20 yr our concept of the role of adipose tissue in the energy economy of the mammal has altered in a fundamental way. Adipose tissue mass is no longer conceived to be the passive recipient of stored calories, but rather an active participant in the regulation of energy balance. All investigators would agree that adipose tissue is partially responsible for and involved in the daily flux of intermediary metabolites as it responds to signals instituted by the periodicity of eating, along with other varied hormonal and neural stimuli. Whether adipose tissue in turn produces its own metabolic signals, which are "read out" and responded to by other tissues and organs, is a more controversial but plausible hypothesis. In any case, this tissue is unique in its capacity to experience more than 1,000-fold changes in mass without the variations immediately becoming life-threatening to the organism. No other tissue of the mammal has this capacity, which is due in large measure to the ability of the white adipocyte to expand and shrink its size. Thus cell size is a major variable of extreme importance in all considerations of the tissue's responsiveness.

The cell number of adipose tissue appears to be subject to the same type of regulation during growth and development that is found in most tissues and organs of the mammal. Adult cell number is reached at a programmed time during organismal development and ordinarily varies little thereafter. It follows, then, that cell number may be manipulated to a larger degree before that critical developmental time, and much less after it. Cell size, on the other hand, is variable over a wide range and may be manipulated over the life span. There is some evidence to suggest, however, that cell size is not infinitely expandable but that a maximum size may be reached and, moreover, that an optimal size for a given species, strain, or individual may exist. We may hypothesize that the attainment of maximal or optimal cell size serves as a restraint on food intake and thus cell size itself becomes regulatory. On the other hand, it is possible that when maximum size is attained in a situation of continual substrate availability a response to proliferate may be triggered, cell numbers may increase, and thus regulation may fail. Such a failure in regulation may lead to obesity.

The importance of adipose cell number as a primary determinant of human obesity is still being debated. Individuals with the highest cell numbers are often the most obese, and there appears to be a limit to fat cell size.

Morbidly obese children, who are for the most part hypercellular, tend to become obese adults and do not appear to "lose their baby fat." Although it appears as if adipose tissue in the adult can respond to some stimuli by an increase in cell number, it does not respond to weight loss by the loss of fat cells.

In addition to the cell number hypothesis, there are a variety of other hypotheses that are addressed to the causes of excessive accumulation of adipose tissue as seen in obesity. The validation of any of these hypotheses must await the time when we can delineate the process of differentiation of the white adipocyte. A number of investigators have speculated that a precursor cell must appear at some point in the development of adipose tissue deposits and that it must be triggered by some stimulus or set of stimuli to differentiate into a lipid-laden mature adipocyte. However there are no functional markers or histochemical assays for such an adipoblast. Thus the time course of the appearance, proliferation, and differentiation of precursor into fat cell has only been elucidated by indirect methods—that is, cell counting and thymidine incorporation into adipocyte DNA. Moreover, there is evidence to suggest that these processes of growth and differentiation may vary from site to site and that we may no longer consider adipose tissue as a single uniform entity.

REFERENCES

Amatruda, J. M., Livingston, J. N. and Lockwood, D. H. 1975. Insulin receptor: Role in resistance of human obesity to insulin. *Science* 188:264.

Angel, J. L. 1949. Constitution in female obesity. *Am. J. Phys. Anthropol.* 7:433.

Ashwell, M. and Garrow, J. S. 1973. Full and empty fat cells. *Lancet* 2:1036.

Ashwell, M. A., Priest, P. and Sowter, C. 1975. Importance of fixed sections in the study of adipose tissue cellularity. *Nature (Lond.)* 256:724.

Babirek, S. P., Dowell, R. T. and Oscai, L. B. 1974. Total fasting and total fasting plus exercise: Effects of body composition of the rat. *J. Nutr.* 104:452.

Batchelor, B. R. and Stern, J. S. 1973. The effect of growth hormone upon glucose metabolism and cellularity in rat adipose tissue. *Horm. Metab. Res.* 5:37.

Batchelor, B. R., Stern, J. S., Johnson, P. R. and Mahler, R. J. 1975. Effects of streptozotocin on glucose metabolism, insulin response and adiposity in ob/ob mice. *Metabolism* 24:77.

Bennett, G. V. and Cuatrecasas, P. 1972. Insulin receptor of fat cells in insulin-resistant metabolic states. *Science* 176:805.

Bickman, L. 1975. The rate of weight loss after intestinal bypass operations for obesity. An analysis of factors of significance. *Acta Chir. Scand.* 141:424.

Bjorntorp, P. and Martinsson, A. 1966. The composition of human subcutaneous adipose tissue in relation to its morphology. *Acta Med. Scand.* 179:475.

Bjorntorp, P. and Sjostrom, L. 1971. Number and size of adipose tissue fat cells in relation to metabolism in human obesity. *Metabolism* 20:703.

Bjorntorp, P. and Sjostrom, L. 1972. The composition and metabolism in vitro of adipose tissue fat cells of different sizes. *Eur. J. Clin. Invest.* 2:78.

Bjorntorp, P., Gustafson, A. and Persson, B. 1971. Adipose tissue fat cell size and number in relation to metabolism in endogenous hypertriglyceridemia. *Acta Med. Scand.* 190:363.

Braun, T., Kazdova, K., Fabry, P., Lojda, A. and Hromadkova, V. 1968. "Meal eating" and refeeding after a single fast as a stimulus for increasing the number of fat cells in abdominal adipose tissue of rats. *Metabolism* 17:825.

Bray, G. A. 1970. Measurements of subcutaneous fat cells from obese patients. *Ann. Intern. Med.* 73:565.

Bray, G. A. and York, D. A. 1971. Genetically transmitted obesity in rodents. *Physiol. Rev.* 51:598.

Brill, A. B., Sandstedt, S. H., Price, R., Johnston, R. E., Law, D. H. and Scott, H. W., Jr. 1972. Changes in body composition after jejunoileal bypass in morbidly obese patients. *Am. J. Surg.* 123:49.

Brook, C. G. D. 1972. Evidence for a sensitive period in adipose cell replication in man. *Lancet* ii:624.

Challoner, D. R. 1969. A direct effect of triiodothyronine on the oxygen consumption of rat adipocytes. *Am. J. Physiol.* 216:905.

Cleary, M. P., Greenwood, M. R. C. and Brasel, J. A. 1975. Thymidine kinase as a measure of adipocyte proliferation in normal and obese rats. *Fed. Proc.* 34:908.

Cleary, M. P., Klein, B. E., Greenwood, M. R. C. and Brasel, J. A. 1976. Proliferative enzymes in adipose tissue of normal and obese rats. *Fed. Proc.* 35:502.

Coleman, D. L. and Hummel, K. P. 1967. Studies with the mutation diabetes in the mouse. *Diabetologia* 3:238.

Crews, E. L., Fuge, K. W., Oscai, L. B., Holloszy, J. O. and Shank, R. E. 1969. Weight, food intake and body composition. Effects of exercise and of protein deficiency. *Am. J. Physiol.* 216:351.

Czech, M. P. 1976. Cellular basis of insulin insensitivity in large rat adipocytes. *J. Clin. Invest.* 57:1523.

DiGirolamo, M. and Mendlinger, S. 1971. Role of fat cell size and number in enlargement of epididymal fat pads in three species. *Am. J. Physiol.* 221:859.

Enesco, M. and LeBlond, C. P. 1962. Increase in cell number as a factor in the growth of the organs and tissues of the young male rat. *J. Embryol. Exp. Morphol.* 10:530.

Fain, J. N. and Scow, R. O. 1965. Effect of hypophysectomy on lipid metabolism in pancreatectomized rats. *Endocrinology* 77:547.

Fain, J. N., Kovacev, V. P. and Scow, R. O. 1965. Effect of growth hormone and dexamethasone on lipolysis and metabolism in isolated fat cells of the rat. *J. Biol. Chem.* 240:3522.

Faust, I. M., Johnson, P. R. and Hirsch, J. 1976. Noncompensation of adipose mass in partially lipectomized mice and rats. *Am. J. Physiol.* 231:538.

Faust, I. M., Johnson, P. R. and Hirsch, J. 1977a. Surgical removal of adipose tissue alters feeding behavior and the development of obesity in rats. *Science* 197:293.

Faust, I. M., Johnson, P. R. and Hirsch, J. 1977b. Adipose tissue regeneration following lipectomy. *Science* 197:391.

Faust, I. M., Johnson, P. R., Stern, J. S. and Hirsch, J. 1977c. Dietary induction of adipocyte number increase in adult rats. Manuscript in preparation.

Freychet, P., Laudat, M. H., Laudat, P., Rosselin, G., Kahn, C. R., Gorden, P. and Roth, J. 1972. Impairment of insulin binding to the fat cell membrane in the obese hyperglycemic mouse. *FEBS Lett.* 25:339.

Garn, S. M., Clark, D. C. and Ullman, B. M. 1975. Does obesity have a genetic basis in man? *Ecol. Food Nutr.* 4:57.

Garrow, J. S. 1974. *Energy balance and obesity in man.* New York: American Elsevier.

Goldrick, R. B. and McLoughlin, G. M. 1970. Lipolysis and lipogenesis from glucose in human fat cells of different sizes. *J. Clin. Invest.* 49:1213.

Greenwood, M. R. C. and Hirsch, J. 1974. Postnatal development of adipocyte cellularity in the normal rat. *J. Lipid Res.* 15:474.

Greenwood, M. R. C., Johnson, P. R., Stern, J. S. and Hirsch, J. 1977. Postnatal development of adipose cellularity in obese and lean Zucker rats. In preparation.

Gurney, R. 1936. Hereditary factor in obesity. *Arch. Intern. Med.* 57:557.

Hansen, F. M., Nielsen, J. H. and Gliemann, J. 1974. The influence of body weight and cell size on lipogenesis and lipolysis of isolated rat fat cells. *Eur. J. Clin. Invest.* 4:411.

Hellman, B., Taljedal, I. B. and Westman, S. 1962. Morphological characteristics of the epididymal adipose tissue in normal and obese-hyperglycemic mice. *Acta Morphol. Neerl. Scand.* 5:182.

Herberg, L., Major, E., Hennings, U., Gruneklee, D., Freytag, G. and Gries, F. A. 1970. Differences in the development of the obese-hyperglycemic syndrome in obob and NZO mice. *Diabetologia* 6:292.

Herberg, L., Doppen, W., Major, E. and Gries, F. A. 1974. Dietary-induced hypertrophic-hyperplastic obesity in mice. *J. Lipid Res.* 15:580.

Hill, D. E., Hirsch, J. and Cheek, D. B. 1972. The noncollagen protein in adipose tissue as an index of cell number. *Proc. Soc. Exp. Biol. Med.* 140:782.

Hirsch, J. and Batchelor, B. R. 1976. Adipose tissue cellularity in human obesity. *Clin. Endocrinol. Metab.* 5:299.

Hirsch, J. and Gallian, E. 1968. Methods for the determination of adipose cell size in man and animals. *J. Lipid Res.* 9:110.

Hirsch, J. and Han, P. W. 1969. Cellularity of rat adipose tissue: Effects of growth, starvation and obesity. *J. Lipid Res.* 10:77.

Hirsch, J. and Knittle, J. L. 1970. Cellularity of obese and non-obese adipose tissue. *Fed. Proc.* 29:1516.

Hollenberg, C. H. and Vost, A. 1968. Regulation of DNA synthesis in fat cells and stromal elements from rat adipose tissue. *J. Clin. Invest.* 47:2485.

Holm, G., Jacobsson, B., Bjorntorp, P. and Smith, U. 1975. Effect of age and cell size on rat adipose tissue metabolism. *J. Lipid Res.* 16:461.

Jacobsson, B., Holm, G., Bjorntorp, P. and Smith, U. 1976. Influence of cell size and the effects of insulin and noradrenaline on human adipose tissue. *Diabetologia* 12:69.

Johnson, P. R. and Hirsch, J. 1972. Cellularity of adipose depots in six strains of genetically obese mice. *J. Lipid Res.* 13:2.

Johnson, P. R., Zucker, L. M., Cruce, J. A. F. and Hirsch, J. 1971. Cellularity of adipose depots in the genetically obese Zucker rat. *J. Lipid Res.* 12:706.

Johnson, P. R., Stern, J. S., Greenwood, M. R. C., Zucker, L. M. and Hirsch, J. 1973. Effect of early nutrition on adipose cellularity and pancreatic insulin release in the Zucker rat. *J. Nutr.* 103:738.

Johnson, P. R., Faust, I. M., Monahan, J. and Hirsch, J. 1976. Does high fat feeding or pregnancy increase adipocyte number in the adult rat? *J. Nutr.* 106:xxiv.

Johnson, P. R., Stern, J. S., Greenwood, M. R. C. and Hirsch, J. 1977. Adipose tissue hyperplasia and hyperinsulinemia in Zucker obese female rats—A developmental study. In preparation.

Kahn, C. R., Soll, A. H., Neville, D. M., Jr., Goldfine, I. D., Archer, J. A., Gorden, P. and Roth, J. 1973. The insulin receptor in obesity and other states of altered insulin sensitivity. In *Obesity in perspective*, ed. G. Bray. DHEW Publ. No (NIH) 75-708, p. 301.

Kamper, M. J., Galloway, D. V. and Ashley, F. 1972. Abdominal panniculectomy after massive weight loss. *Plast. Reconstr. Surg.* 50:441.

Katzen, H. M. and Vlahakas, G. J. 1973. Biological activity of insulin-Sepharose. *Science* 179:1142.

Kazdova, L., Fabry, P. and Vrana, A. 1974. Effect of small doses of insulin in vivo on the proliferation and cellularity of adipose tissue. *Diabetologia* 10:77.

Kennedy, G. C. 1950. The hypothalamic control of food intake in rats. *Proc. R. Soc. Lond. (Biol.)* 137:535.

Kirtland, J., Gurr, M. I. and Saville, G. 1975. Occurrence of "packets" of very small cells in adipose tissue of the guinea pig. *Nature (Lond.)* 256:723.

Knittle, J. L. 1972. Maternal diet as a factor in adipose tissue cellularity and metabolism in the young rat. *J. Nutr.* 102:427.

Knittle, J. L. 1973. Influences on development of adipose tissue. In *Obesity in perspective*, ed. G. Bray. DHEW Publ. No. (NIH) 75-708, p. 241.

Knittle, J. L. 1976. In *Nutrient requirements in adolescence*, eds. J. I. McKigney and H. N. Munro, p. 77. Cambridge, Mass.: M.I.T. Press.

Knittle, J. L. and Ginsberg-Fellner, F. 1972. Effect of weight reduction on *in vitro* adipose tissue lipolysis and cellularity in obese adolescents and adults. *Diabetes* 21:754.

Knittle, J. L. and Hirsch, J. 1968. Effect of early nutrition on the development of rat epididymal fat pads: Cellularity and metabolism. *J. Clin. Invest.* 47:2091.

Knittle, J. L., Sussman, L., Collip, P. J. and Gertner, M. 1972. The effect of treatment with human growth hormone on glucose tolerance and adipose tissue cellularity in ateliotic dwarfism. *Diabetes* 21:366.

Kral, J. G. 1975. Surgical reduction of adipose tissue hypercellularity in man. *Scand. J. Plast. Reconstr. Surg.* 9:140.

Kral, J. G. 1976. Surgical reduction of adipose tissue in the male Sprague-Dawley rat: Effects on body composition, adipose tissue cellularity and lipid and carbohydrate metabolism. *Am. J. Physiol.* 231:1090.

Kral, J. G. and Tisell, L. E. 1976. The effects of castration on body composition, adipose tissue cellularity and lipid and carbohydrate metabolism in adult male rats. *Acta Endocrinol.* 81:644.

Kral, J. G., Bjorntorp, P., Schersten, T. and Sjostrom, L. 1976. Body composition and adipose tissue cellularity before and after jejunoileostomy in severely obese subjects. *Am. J. Physiol.*, in press.

Krotkiewski, M. 1976. The effects of estrogens on regional adipose tissue cellularity in the rat. *Acta Physiol. Scand.* 96:128.

Krotkiewski, M. and Bjorntorp, P. 1975. The effects of dexamethasone and starvation on body composition and regional adipose tissue cellularity in the rat. *Acta Endocrinol.* 80:667.

Krotkiewski, M. and Bjorntorp, P. 1976. The effect of progesterone and of insulin administration on regional adipose tissue cellularity in the rat. *Acta Physiol. Scand.* 96:122.

Lau, H. C., Flaim, E. and Ritchey, S. J. 1976. Changes in body weight gain and adipose tissue cellularity in protein restricted and rehabilitated rats. *Nutr. Rep. Int.* 14:33.

Lemonnier, D. 1972. Effect of age, sex and site on the cellularity of the adipose tissue in mice and rats rendered obese by a high-fat diet. *J. Clin. Invest.* 51:2907.

Lemonnier, D. and Alexiu, A. 1974. Nutritional, genetic and hormonal aspects of adipose tissue cellularity. In *The regulation of adipose tissue mass,* eds. J. Vague and J. Boyer, p. 158. Amsterdam: Excerpta Medica.

Leveille, G. A. 1970. Adipose tissue metabolism: Influence of periodocity of eating and diet composition. *Fed. Proc.* 29:1294.

Livingston, J. N., Cuatrecasas, P. and Lockwood, D. 1972. Insulin insensitivity of large rat cells. *Science* 177:626.

Ljunggren, H. 1965. In *Human body composition,* ed. J. Brozek, p. 129. Oxford: Pergamon.

Masson, J. K. 1962. Lipectomy: The surgical removal of excess fat. *Postgrad. Med.* 32:481.

May, K. K. and Beaton, J. R. 1968. Hyperphagia in the insulin-treated rat. *Proc. Soc. Exp. Biol. Med.* 127:1201.

Mayer, J., Marshall, N. B., Vitale, J. J., Christensen, J. H., Mashayeki, M. B. and Stare, F. J. 1954. Exercise, food intake and body weight in normal rats and genetically obese adult mice. *Am. J. Physiol.* 177:544.

Mickelsen, O., Takahishi, S. and Craig, C. J. 1955. Experimental obesity. I. Production of obesity in rats by feeding high-fat diets. *J. Nutr.* 57:541.

Mohr, W. and Beneke, G. 1969. Histochemische Untersuchungen der Entstehung von Fettzellen. *Virchows Arch. B* 3:13.

Ogundipe, O. and Bray, G. 1974. The influence of diet and fat cell size on glucose metabolism, lipogenesis and lipolysis in the rat. *Horm. Metab. Res.* 6:351.

Olefsky, J. M. 1976a. The effects of spontaneous obesity on insulin binding, glucose transport, and glucose oxidation of isolated rat adipocytes. *J. Clin. Invest.* 57:842.

Olefsky, J. M. 1976b. Decreased insulin binding to adipocytes and circulating monocytes from obese subjects. *J. Clin. Invest.* 57:1165.

Oscai, L. B. 1973. The role of exercise in weight control. *Exercise Sport Sci. Rev.* 1:103.

Oscai, L. B. and Holloszy, J. O. 1969. Effects of weight changes produced by exercise, food restriction or overeating on body composition. *J. Clin. Invest.* 48:2124.

Oscai, L. B., Spirakes, C. N., Wolf, C. A. and Beck, R. J. 1972. Effects of exercise and of food restriction on adipose tissue cellularity. *J. Lipid Res.* 13:588.

Ostman, J., Backman, L. and Hallberg, D. 1975. Cell size and the antilipolytic effect of insulin in human subcutaneous adipose tissue. *Diabetologia* 11:159.

Panksepp, J., Pollack, A., Krost, K., Meeker, R. and Ritter, M. 1975. Feeding in response to repeated protamine zinc insulin injections. *Physiol. Behav.* 14:487.

Pitanguy, I. 1967. Abdominal lipectomy: An approach to it through an analysis of 300 consecutive cases. *Plast. Reconstr. Surg.* 40:384.

Rakow, L., Beneke, G., Mohr, W. and Brauchle, I. 1971a. Investigations on cell proliferation in white adipose tissue of albino mice obesified by administration of aurothioglucose. *Pathol. Microbiol.* 37:261.

Rakow, L., Beneke, G. and Vogt, C. 1971b. Changes in collagen content of white adipose tissue in starved-refed and obese mice. *Beitr. Pathol.* 144:377.

Reardon, M. F., Goldrick, R. B. and Fidge, N. H. 1973. Dependence of rates of lipolysis, esterification and free acid release in isolated fat cells on age, cell size and nutritional state. *J. Lipid Res.* 14:319.

Rehfield, J. F., Johl, E. and Quaade, F. 1970. Effect of jejunoileostomy on glucose and insulin metabolism in ten obese patients: *Metabolism* 19:529.

Rizack, M. A. 1961. An epinephrine sensitive lipolytic activity in adipose tissue. *J. Biol. Chem.* 236:657.

Robertson, R. P., Batchelor, B. R., Johnson, P. R. and Stern, J. S. 1974. Adipocyte cellularity in the desert sand rat (Psammomys obesus). *Proc. Soc. Exp. Biol. Med.* 147:134.

Rodbell, M. 1964. Metabolism of isolated fat cells. I. Effects of hormones on glucose metabolism and lipolysis. *J. Biol. Chem.* 239:375.

Romsos, D. and Leveille, G. 1972. Effect of cell size on in vitro fatty acid and glyceride-glycerol biosynthesis in rat adipose tissue. *Proc. Soc. Exp. Biol. Med.* 141:649.

Salans, L. B. and Cushman, S. W. 1973. Cellular consequences of obesity. In *Obesity in perspective,* ed. G. Bray. DHEW Publ. No. (NIH) 75-708, p. 245.

Salans, L. B. and Dougherty, J. W. 1971. The effect of insulin upon glucose metabolism by adipose cells of different sizes. *J. Clin. Invest.* 50:1399.

Salans, L. B., Knittle, J. L. and Hirsch, J. 1968. The role of adipose cell size and adipose tissue insulin sensitivity in the carbohydrate intolerance of human obesity. *J. Clin. Invest.* 47:153.

Salans, L. B., Horton, E. S. and Sims, E. A. H. 1971. Experimental obesity in man: The cellular character of the adipose tissue. *J. Clin. Invest.* 50:1005.

Salans, L. B., Zarrowski, M. J. and Segal, R. 1972. Effect of insulin upon the cellular character of rat adipose tissue. *J. Lipid Res.* 13:616.

Salans, L. B., Cushman, S. W. and Weismann, R. E. 1973. Studies of human adipose tissue, adipose cell size and number in nonobese and obese patients. *J. Clin. Invest.* 52:929.

Salans, L. B., Bray, G. A., Cushman, S. W., Danforth, E., Jr., Glennon, J. A., Horton, E. S. and Sims, E. A. H. 1974. Glucose metabolism and the response to insulin by human adipose tissue in spontaneous and experimental obesity. Effects of dietary composition and adipose cell size. *J. Clin. Invest.* 53:848.

Schemmel, R., Mickelsen, O. and Tolgay, Z. 1969. Dietary obesity in rats: Influence of diet, weight, age, and sex on body composition. *Am. J. Physiol.* 216:273.

Seltzer, C. C. and Mayer, J. 1965. A simple criterion of obesity. *Postgrad. Med.* 38:101.

Sims, E. A. H., Goldman, R. F., Gluck, C. M., Horton, E. S., Kelleher, P. C. and Rowe, D. W. 1968. Experimental obesity in man. *Trans. Assoc. Am. Physicians* 81:153.

Sjostrom, L. and Bjorntorp, P. 1974. Body composition and adipose tissue cellularity in human obesity. *Acta Med. Scand.* 195:201.

Sjostrom, L., Bjorntorp, P. and Vrana, J. 1971. Microscopic fat cell size measurements on frozen-cut adipose tissue in comparison with automatic determinations of osmium-fixed fat cells. *J. Lipid Res.* 12:521.

Sjostrom, L., Smith, U., Krotkiewski, M. and Bjorntorp, P. 1972. Cellularity in different regions of adipose tissue in young men and women. *Metabolism* 21:1143.

Smith, U. 1971. Effect of cell size on lipid synthesis by human adipose tissue in vitro. *J. Lipid Res.* 12:65.

Smith, U., Kral, J. and Bjorntorp, P. 1974. Influence of dietary fat and carbohydrate on the metabolism of adipocytes of different sizes in the rat. *Biochim. Biophys. Acta* 337:278.

Sneyd, J. G. T. 1964. Pancreatic and serum insulin in the New Zealand strain of obese mice. *J. Endocrinol.* 28:163.

Steffens, A. B. 1969. The influence of insulin injections and infusions on eating and blood glucose level in the rat. *Physiol. Behav.* 4:823.

Stern, J. S. and Greenwood, M. R. C. 1974. A review of development of adipose cellularity in man and animals. *Fed. Proc.* 33:1952.

Stern, J. S. and Hirsch, J. 1971. Obesity and pancreatic function. In *Handbook of physiology*, Sect. 1: *Endocrinology*, Vol. 1: *The endocrine pancreas*, eds. D. Steiner and N. Freinkel, p. 641. Washington, D.C.: American Physiological Society.

Stern, J. S. and Johnson, P. R. 1977. Spontaneous activity and adipose cellularity on the genetically obese Zucker rat (fafa). *Metabolism* 26:371.

Stern, J. S., Batchelor, B. R., Hollander, N., Cohn, C. K. and Hirsch, J. 1972a. Adipose cell size and immunoreactive insulin levels in obese and normal weight adults. *Lancet* 2:948.

Stern, J. S., Johnson, P. R., Greenwood, M. R. C., Zucker, L. M. and Hirsch, J. 1972b. Insulin resistance and pancreatic insulin release in the genetically obese Zucker rat. *Proc. Soc. Exp. Biol. Med.* 139:66.

Stern, J. S., Johnson, P. R., Batchelor, B. R., Zucker, L. M. and Hirsch, J. 1975. Pancreatic insulin release and peripheral tissue resistance in Zucker obese rats fed high- and low-carbohydrate diets. *Am. J. Physiol.* 228:543.

Stern, J. S., Levinson, M., Batchelor, B. R. and Johnson, P. R. 1976. The effect of forced exercise on the development of adipose cellularity in obese and lean Zucker rats. In preparation.

Stern, M. P., Olefsky, J., Farquhar, J. W. and Reaven, G. M. 1973. Relationship between fasting plasma lipid levels and adipose tissue morphology. *Metabolism* 22:1311.

Stiles, J. W., Francendese, A. A. and Masoro, J. 1976. Influence of age on the size and number of fat cells in the epididymal depot. *Am. J. Physiol.* 229:1561.

Tepperman, J., Brobeck, J. R. and Long, C. N. H. 1943. The effects of hypothalamic hyperphagia and of alterations in feeding habits on the metabolism of the albino rat. *Yale J. Biol. Med.* 15:875.

Therriault, D. G. and Mellin, D. B. 1971. Cellularity of adipose tissue in cold exposed rats and the calorigenic effect of norepinephrine. *Lipids* 6:486.

Vaughan, M. 1960. Effect of hormones on phosphorylase activity in adipose tissue. *J. Biol. Chem.* 235:3049.

Wertheimer, E. and Shafrir, E. 1960. Influence of hormones on adipose tissue as a center of fat metabolism. *Recent Prog. Horm. Res.* 16:467.

White, J. E. and Engel, F. L. 1958. Lipolytic action of corticotropin on rat adipose tissue "in vitro." *J. Clin. Invest.* 37:1556.

Widdowson, E. M. and Shaw, W. T. 1973. Full and empty fat cells. *Lancet* 2:906.

Winegrad, A. 1962. Endocrine effects on adipose tissue metabolism. *Vitam. Horm.* 20:141.

Winegrad, A. I. and Renold, A. E. 1958. Studies on rat adipose tissue *in vitro*. I. Effects of insulin on the metabolism of glucose, pyruvate and acetate. *J. Biol. Chem.* 233:267.

Winick, M. 1974. Childhood obesity. *Nutr. Today* 9:6.

Young, T. K. and Liu, A. C. 1965. Hyperphagia, insulin and obesity. *Chin. J. Physiol.* 19:247.

Zinder, O., Arad, R. and Shapiro, B. 1967. Effect of cell size on the metabolism of isolated fat cells. *Isr. J. Med. Sci.* 3:787.

Zingg, W., Angel, A. and Steinberg, M. D. 1962. Studies on the number and volume of fat cells in adipose tissue. *Can. J. Biochem. Physiol.* 40:437.

Zucker, L. M. and Antoniades, H. N. 1972. Insulin and obesity in the Zucker genetically obese rat "fatty." *Endocrinology* 90:1320.

Chapter 10

MODULATION AND IMPLICATIONS OF THE COUNTERREGULATORY HORMONES: GLUCAGON, CATECHOLAMINES, CORTISOL, AND GROWTH HORMONE

R. Philip Eaton and David S. Schade
University of New Mexico School of Medicine
Albuquerque, New Mexico

INTRODUCTION

As discussed in detail in several other chapters in this volume, insulin has evolved to assume central importance as the major anabolic hormone in humans, in the metabolism of both exogenous and endogenous substrates for caloric utilization. In this role, insulin guides the assimilation of calories ingested, limits the mobilization of both lipid and carbohydrate body stores of available calories, and participates in the peripheral disposal of circulating substrates.

This function assumes pathophysiological significance in the diabetic patient, in whom disordered insulin secretion is characteristic; in the obese patient, in whom "resistance" to many of the actions of insulin is characteristic; and in premature atherosclerosis, in which alterations in the peripheral disposal of the insulin-sensitive substrates—glucose, free fatty acids, and triglycerides—may be characteristic.

Several lines of investigation concerning these actions of insulin have led to the conclusion that a delicate counterregulatory hormonal system is present in humans, which may modulate caloric substrate metabolism. Thus, attention to insulin secretion and activity alone is insufficient to describe lipid and carbohydrate caloric mobilization during food deprivation, pregnancy, physical exercise, hibernation, and stress states, or to describe the altered substrate pathophysiology leading to hyperlipemia, hyperglycemia, or hyperketonemia in the various situations in which they occur.

In recent years, four such counterregulatory hormones have emerged in this role of modulating the activities of insulin, viz., glucagon, catecholamines, cortisol, and growth hormone. The normal human may be in a delicate balance between insulin and counterregulatory hormone activity, as visualized in Fig. 1. Disbalance is readily demonstrated by the observation that an excess of insulin leads to a compensatory rise in all counterregulatory hormone secretion. Similarly, an excess of any of these counterregulatory hormones commonly results in a compensatory rise in insulin secretion. When the compensatory insulin secretory response is inadequate to the degree of counterregulatory hormone excess, then deterioration of carbohydrate-lipid metabolism ensues—for example, diabetes mellitus, pheochromocytoma, Cushing's disease, acromegaly, and so on. Similarly, when the counterregulatory hormone secretory response is deficient, then consequences of insulin excess are expressed—for example, obesity, hyperlipemia, and hypoglycemia. It will be the objective of this review to examine the evolving understanding of the participation of these hormones in the normal and pathologic states in which data have been gathered.

GLUCAGON

Modulation of Energy Substrates in Humans

The hyperglycemic potential of glucagon has been recognized since 1923 from investigation of "contaminants" in partially purified insulin extracted from porcine pancreas (Collip, 1923). As reviewed extensively by Park and Exton (1972), this hyperglycemic effect is largely mediated by a 2- to 3-fold stimulation of hepatic glycogenolysis and a 1.5- to 2-fold stimulation of hepatic gluconeogenesis, as demonstrated by liver perfusion investigations. In addition to these actions on carbohydrate metabolism, glucagon is known to act on lipid metabolism at multiple regulatory sites. As recently reviewed in detail by LeFebvre (1972), glucagon is a lipolytic hormone recognized to enhance the *in vitro* release of glycerol and free fatty acids (FFA) in isolated adipose tissue. The net increased availability of FFA for hepatic metabolism may be expected to result in augmented hepatic ketone production, as has

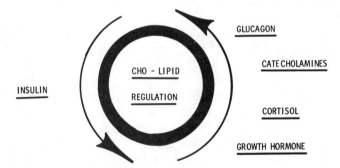

FIGURE 1   Hormonal balance involved in carbohydrate and lipid physiology.

been demonstrated in the perfused liver (Heimberg et al., 1969), and by arteriovenous difference studies in intact dogs (Basso and Havel, 1970).

In addition to an action of glucagon to make free fatty acid substrate available for hepatic ketogenesis, a direct stimulation of ketogenesis by glucagon has been demonstrated in the perfused liver (Heimberg et al., 1969). *In vivo* in humans, a similar augmentation of ketone concentration, which may be dissociated from the lipolytic response to glucagon, has also been reported (Schade and Eaton, 1975a, 1975b; Liljenquist et al., 1974). With a plasma half-life of 4–7 min (Alford et al., 1976), glucagon thus has the potential of participating in moment-to-moment substrate regulation in humans, in concert with growth hormone, catecholamines, and cortisol in counterregulation to the actions of insulin.

In addition to an independent action of glucagon on substrate regulation, glucagon derived from the gut ("gut-glucagon") is an insulinotropic hormone. In this capacity it serves with pancreozymin secretion as an early stimulus to insulin secretion in response to the presence of food in the bowel and before any significant elevation in blood glucose concentration. Samols et al. (1972) recently reviewed the concept that glucagon may thus have a role in the regulation of insulin secretion, in addition to its parallel role as a counterregulatory hormone at the level of substrate regulation (Mackrell and Sokal, 1969). Difficulty in interpreting plasma immunoassay data concerning glucagon is related to the several molecular species of this hormone circulating in the blood, which may be indistinguishable from each other by the usual immunoassay, and to the discrepancy between portal and peripheral vein hormone concentrations (Blackard et al., 1974).

While radioimmunoassay of glucagon has been focused on pancreatic extractable glucagon of molecular weight 3,500, it is known that at least three distinct molecular forms of the hormone circulate in human plasma. In normal subjects, most of the immunoreactive hormone is in a high-molecular-weight form greater than 15,000 (Valverde et al., 1974; Weir et al., 1975; Kuku et al., 1976). However, with alpha-cell stimulation by arginine, the 3,500 dalton form exhibits the greatest change in concentration (Valverde et al., 1974). In ketoacidosis, the predominant circulating form of glucagon has a molecular weight of 3,500, while in chronic renal failure the predominant molecular species has a molecular weight of 9,000 (Kuku et al., 1976; Bilbrey et al., 1974).

Evidence That Excess May Participate in the Diabetic State

The development of a radioimmunoassay for glucagon by Unger et al. (1961) provided the methodological techniques necessary for intensive investigation into the potential role of glucagon in the diabetic state. Basal plasma glucagon concentration was variously reported to be elevated in poorly controlled diabetics (Unger et al., 1970; Assan et al., 1969) and to return to the normal range with improved diabetic control (Beck et al., 1976; Sherwin et al., 1976). A similar state of hyperglucagonemia was reported in a variety of acquired hyperglycemic "stress-diabetic" states, similarly supporting a role for glucagon in the deterioration of carbohydrate tolerance—that is, in severely burned patients (Shuck et al., 1975), hyperosmolar coma (Lindsey et al., 1974), bacterial sepsis (Rocha et al., 1973), glucocorticoid excess (Marco et al., 1973), catecholamine excess (Lorenzi et al., 1975), and glucagon secretory tumors (Leichter et al., 1975; Lightman and Bloom, 1974). In addition, the hyperglycemic glucose tolerance and/or response to meal ingestion character-istic of juvenile diabetic patients was noted to be associated with abnormal elevations of pancreatic glucagon secretion (Muller et al., 1970; Gerich et al., 1975b; Buchanan, 1973), in addition to abnormal elevations in growth hormone secretion (Gerich et al., 1975b), suggesting participation of both hormones in this hyperglycemia.

Infusion of somatostatin to inhibit the postprandial rise in both glucagon and growth hormone was associated with correction of the hyper-glycemia (Gerich et al., 1975b), strongly implicating both counterregulatory hormones in the abnormal glucose tolerance of diabetes. The correction of the hyperglycemia with somatostatin induced inhibition of glucagon and growth hormone secretion without the addition of insulin in this and earlier reports (Gerich et al., 1975a; Alford et al., 1974) suggested a major regulatory role of these hormones on the dynamics of blood glucose regulation. Moreover, availability of insulin in normal subjects, or administration of insulin in diabetic subjects, effectively counterbalanced the glycemic response to gluca-gon and growth hormone.

In several investigations, a close relationship between glucagon and insulin levels in relation to blood glucose concentration has not been demonstrable (Barnes et al., 1975; Tasake et al., 1975). It seems reasonable that the failure to consider the additional interplay of growth hormone, cortisol, and catecholamines as other participating counterregulatory hor-mones, in addition to the immunoassay difficulties discussed above and the venous dilution of pancreatic glucagon secreted into the portal system, may be sufficient to explain the problem.

Infusion of physiological levels of glucagon into insulin-dependent juvenile diabetic human subjects during somatostatin suppression of endoge-nous insulin, glucagon, and growth hormone secretion has led to a rise in plasma glucose, FFA, and ketones, confirming the expected effects of the hormone in the absence of a normal insulin response (Gerich et al., 1976). The degree to which endogenous insulin secretion may modify the lipolytic and ketogenic response to glucagon has been examined by several investigators (Gerich et al., 1976; Schade and Eaton, 1975a–1975e). These investigations demonstrated that glucagon has a potent lipolytic effect in humans, which is modified by simultaneous endogenous insulin secretion in the normal human and unopposed in the insulin-deficient diabetic human. In addition, glucagon has a direct action to augment FFA conversion to ketones, independent of FFA availability. This action is also markedly modulated by simultaneous endogenous insulin secretion.

Much of the difficulty in demonstrating a direct ketogenic effect of glucagon is related to the failure of the investigator to make adequate FFA substrate available for ketogenesis. In the studies of McGarry et al. (1975) and Schade and Eaton (1975a-1975e), Intralipid (exogenous triglyceride[1]) and/or heparin-activated lipolysis has been utilized to avoid this problem. Figure 2 shows the effect of physiological infusion (3 ng/kg-min) of glucagon into diabetic humans. The rise in plasma FFA substrate is similar for both the control and the glucagon infusion study. The rise in plasma ketone bodies during glucagon infusion is statistically greater than that observed in the control study. Figure 2 emphasizes the fact that glucagon exerts a ketogenic action independent of its lipolytic activity.

Another location at which glucagon may regulate plasma substrate concentration is sites of peripheral disposal. Uptake of glucose and ketone bodies by peripheral tissues is augmented by insulin (Issekutz et al., 1974; Balasse and Havel, 1971) and inhibited by glucagon (Schneider et al., 1976). Regulation of substrate utilization by glucagon is currently under investigation

[1] Obtained from Cutter Laboratories.

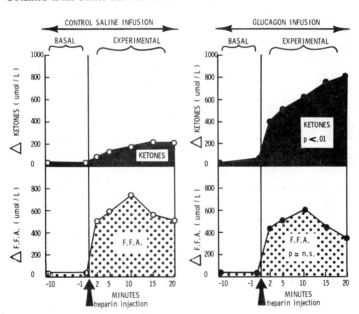

FIGURE 2 Ketogenic response to glucagon infusion in five insulin-dependent diabetic subjects. The FFA rise stimulated by heparin was utilized to provide adequate substrate availability for hepatic ketone generation in the control and hormone infusion studies.

at several laboratories, and conflicting observations have been reported (Schneider et al., 1976; Pozefsky et al., 1976).

Evidence That Deficiency May Participate in the Obese State

In contrast to the insulin-deficient diabetic state, where "normal" levels of plasma glucagon may be exerting an unopposed action on substrate regulation, the normal obese subject has elevated levels of plasma insulin (Bagdade et al., 1971; Kreisberg et al., 1967) so that normal levels of plasma glucagon may be unable to exert the expected catabolic effects on substrate metabolism. In fact, direct radioimmunoassay studies have shown the basal plasma glucagon concentration and secretory response in normal, nondiabetic obese subjects to be either reduced (Schade and Eaton, 1974; Wise et al., 1973) or indistinguishable from those in thin patients, suggesting a relative deficiency of net catabolic activity (Kalkhoff et al., 1973). Not only is a state of glucagon deficiency reported in obesity, but an altered tissue response to at least two of the catabolic actions of glucagon has been observed. Thus, FFA mobilization and elevation in plasma ketone body concentration are reduced in response to glucagon injection in this state (Schade and Eaton, 1975c, 1975f). This is documented in Fig. 3, in which the normal response to 1.0 μg/kg intravenous glucagon is depicted. In contrast, the obese state is characterized by an exaggerated insulin secretory response in concert with a "negative" change in the plasma concentrations of ketone bodies and FFA. Thus, like the loss of the counterregulatory actions of growth hormones in obesity, glucagon deficiency and/or resistance must be added to the hormonal imbalance that favors insulin excess in the area of substrate regulation.

Evidence for Participation in Lipid-Lipoprotein Regulation

The potent effect of glucagon in reducing plasma triglyceride concentration was first described by Amatuzio et al. (1962) and was confirmed by Paloyan et al. (1962). While the mechanism of this hypolipemic response has not been established, it has been reported that glucagon acts both at the liver to limit triglyceride (TG) and lipoprotein synthesis and release (Eaton, 1973b; Fallon and Kemp, 1968) and at the periphery to enhance disposal (Caren and Corbo, 1970). To the extent that insulin excess may oppose the actions of glucagon on hepatic lipogenesis, this lipid-lowering action of glucagon represents a counterregulatory hormonal process similar to that described for growth hormone in reducing cholesterol concentration.

It has been suggested by Eaton et al. (1974a) that a net loss of glucagon activity in reducing serum lipids could contribute to the genesis and/or maintenance of endogenous hyperlipemia (see Fig. 4). In the animal investigation of this hypothesis, it has been reported that a deficiency of immunoassayable glucagon or of glucagon activity, either in the basal state or in

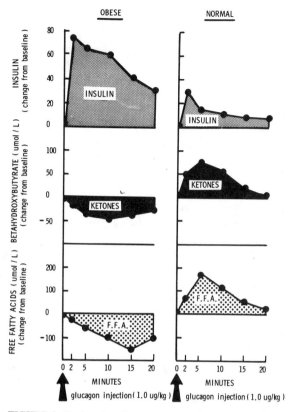

FIGURE 3 Lack of a ketogenic or lipolytic response to glucagon in five obese versus five normal weight subjects.

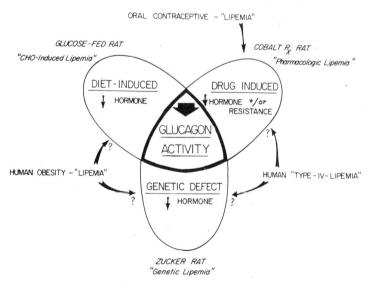

FIGURE 4 Decreased glucagon activity—a final common pathway for endogenous hyperlipemia in the human and the rat.

response to arginine stimulation, represents a common hormonal abnormality in genetic hyperlipemia (Zucker rat) (Eaton et al., 1976a), diet-induced hyperlipemia (glucose-fed rat) (Eaton et al., 1974b), and drug-induced hyperlipemia (cobalt-treated rat) (Eaton, 1973a). Moreover, treatment of hyperlipemia in the rat with the hypolipemic drug halofenate (Eaton et al., 1976b) or clofibrate (Eaton, 1973c) is associated with a reduction in insulin secretion and augmentation of glucagon secretion in synchrony with a fall in serum lipoprotein concentration. Since exercise (Felig et al., 1972) and fasting (Aguilar-Parada et al., 1969) are also associated with an elevation in glucagon secretion and a coincident fall in serum lipid concentration, these data concerning the lipid-lowering actions of drugs, exercise, and diet all support an active role for this hormone in lipoprotein metabolism.

Extrapolation to human hyperlipemia has been less extensively examined. However, as illustrated in Fig. 4, three clinical hyperlipemic states have been reported that demonstrate deficient glucagon secretion and/or activity. As described by Beck et al. (1975), estradiol administration in women is associated with a reduction in aminogenic glucagon secretion and a coincident elevation in serum lipids. The demonstration that plasma TG removal is unchanged has led to the suggestion that the estrogen activity may be mediated by a stimulation of endogenous TG synthesis and/or release into the plasma compartment (Hazzard et al., 1972; Rossner et al., 1971) due to the unopposed actions of insulin in the presence of glucagon deficiency. A similar situation occurs in the obese patient in whom an absolute and/or relative deficiency of glucagon is reported in relation to insulin secretion (see above). Such patients often demonstrate an increase in plasma lipoproteins. In response to clofibrate therapy, a reduction in insulin secretion is regularly observed in normal, obese, and hyperlipemic subjects (Tiengo et al., 1975; Eaton and Nye, 1973; Eaton and Schade, 1974a) with either unchanged or elevated glucagon secretion. This hormonal change in the direction of excess glucagon relative to insulin is associated with a reduction in plasma TG and/or very low density lipoprotein, consistent with an increase in the effective hypolipemic response to glucagon in these patients.

Patients with endogenous hypertriglyceridemia unrelated to obesity, diabetes, or estrogen therapy (Fredrickson's type IV) have been reported to demonstrate elevated levels of plasma immunoreactive glucagon (Tiengo et al., 1975; Eaton, 1973a–1973c). If absence of the hypolipemic response to glucagon is to apply as a mechanism of lipemia in these patients, resistance to the action of glucagon must be postulated (Eaton, 1973a–1973c). Tiengo et al. (1975) observed that treatment of type IV lipemic subjects with clofibrate induces a TG reduction that is correlated with the reduction in the insulin/glucagon molar ratio, consistent with a role for glucagon deficiency and/or resistance in their 13 patients. While a contributory role for deficient glucagon in the etiology of endogenous hyperlipemia relative to excess insulin seems attractive, the quantitative role of this hormone must be evaluated in the context of growth hormone, cortisol, and catecholamines, which undoubtedly represent additional factors in this complex counterregulatory phenomenon.

CATECHOLAMINES

Modulation of Energy Substrates in Humans

Catecholamines, principally epinephrine and norepinephrine, are derived from the sympathetic nervous system, including the adrenal medulla (Axelrod and Weinshilbaum, 1972). They have numerous physiological effects in humans, ranging from positive ionotropic cardiac activity to inhibition of gut motility. In fact, the symptomatology that characterizes counterregulatory hormone response has classically been attributed to elevation in catecholamines (Bray and De Quattro, 1972). Indeed, this symptom complex of tachycardia, diaphoresis, anxiety, and peripheral vasoconstriction may be absent in patients treated with catecholamine blocking drugs such as propranolol (Bray and De Quattro, 1972).

Participation of catecholamines in the counterregulatory response is well documented, particularly in response to hypoglycemia (Callingham, 1975; Garber et al., 1976). This response has recently been reexamined by Garber et al. (1976), who demonstrated that within minutes of insulin-induced hypoglycemia, plasma concentrations of both epinephrine and norepinephrine rise three- to tenfold above basal concentrations and then return toward basal concentrations when euglycemia is restored. Plasma catecholamines are also elevated during other forms of stress. Wilmore and co-workers (1974) have directly attributed the hypermetabolic response observed following thermal injury to catecholamine excess. In addition, increased sympathetic activity has been reported during diabetic ketoacidosis (Christensen, 1974), major trauma (Franksson et al., 1954), infection (Groves et al., 1973), severe anxiety (Taggart et al., 1973), exposure to cold (Hsieh and Carson, 1957), hypoxia (Porte and Robertson, 1973), and myocardial infarction (Vetter et al., 1974). Apparently, stress in any form results in release of epinephrine and norepinephrine into the general circulation with consequent alterations in many metabolic processes, including catecholamine-induced changes in energy substrates and regulatory hormones.

Catecholamines have profound effects on both carbohydrate and lipid metabolism. In humans epinephrine has potent lipolytic effects (Steinberg, 1966). This lipolytic activity may be the major determinant of the elevated concentration of circulating FFA characteristic of major stress. In addition, *in vitro* experiments have demonstrated that catecholamines possess glycogenolytic (Sherline et al., 1972), ketogenic (Exton and Park, 1972), and triglyceride secretion-inhibiting (Heimberg et al., 1964) activity. Thus, secretion of catecholamines during stress provides the organism with an increased availability of energy-yielding substrates such as glucose, ketone bodies, and free fatty acids.

In addition to regulation of substrates, catecholamines serve an important role as modulators of other hormones. The classical studies of Porte and co-workers have convincingly demonstrated that catecholamines directly inhibit the secretion of endogenous insulin (Porte et al., 1966). This direct suppression of insulin at the beta-cell is counteracted by simultaneous stimulatory activity of the catecholamine-induced hyperglycemia. The net result of these two events is usually insulin secretion at a reduced rate. This inhibitory activity is in contrast to the insulinotropic activity of glucagon (Samols et al., 1966) and, theoretically, prevents insulin from negating much of the catabolic actions of catecholamines. Thus, in the severely burned patient with elevated catecholamine secretion (Wilmore et al., 1974), plasma insulin is suppressed relative to the characteristic hyperglycemia (Batstone et al., 1976). Finally, catecholamines also stimulate the secretion of other counterregulatory hormones, particularly glucagon (Gerich et al., 1972; Schade and Eaton, 1976a) and growth hormone (Blackard and Heidingsfelder, 1968). This activity is important in providing additional stimulation of lipolysis, ketogenesis, and glucogenesis to the stressed organism. In summary, catecholamines are major stress hormones, and abnormalities in their secretion or regulation may be expected to participate in disease states.

Evidence That Excess May Participate in the Diabetic State

Patients with pheochromocytoma are characterized by glucose intolerance and, in some cases, diabetes mellitus (Bray and De Quattro, 1972). This clinical observation suggested that catecholamine excess may participate in the diabetic state. This was pursued by numerous workers, including Christensen (1974), who documented that in diabetic ketoacidosis, plasma concentrations of catecholamines were markedly elevated. Of particular importance was his observation that the degree of catecholamine elevation paralleled the degree of metabolic derangement. In addition to the elevation during diabetic ketoacidosis, the plasma catecholamine concentration in ketotic diabetic subjects following exercise exhibits large increments compared with that in controls. These data suggest that elevations in catecholamines may be responsible for initiation and/or maintenance of the decompensated metabolic diabetic state. Willms and co-workers (1969) infused norepinephrine into diabetic and normal subjects and demonstrated that the diabetic subjects are characterized by enhanced hyperglycemia, hyperketonemia, and increased plasma FFA concentration compared to controls. These data suggest that pharmacological modulation of catecholamine secretion may result in improved "control" in diabetic humans. This intriguing possibility has been explored by Baker et al. (1969) in two "brittle" juvenile diabetics. Treatment of these patients with pharmacological beta-adrenergic blockade agents improved diabetic control and markedly decreased the need for hospitalization.

The mechanism by which catecholamines induce metabolic decompensation in diabetic humans is under active investigation. In a review by Exton and Park (1972), activation of cyclic AMP by catecholamines is thought to be the primary cellular mechanism by which these hormones induce their effects. At the tissue level, activation of lipolysis in the fat cell has been repeatedly demonstrated to result in an increase in circulating FFA concentration. According to the FFA-glucose cycle hypothesis of Randle et al. (1963), this increase in itself would lead to glucose intolerance. In addition to their utilization as energy substrates by muscle, plasma FFA serve as substrates for hepatic ketogenesis and triglyceride synthesis.

Several studies have reported that infusion of catecholamines into diabetic humans results in a greater rise in the plasma concentration of both FFA and ketone bodies (Willms et al., 1969; Blackard and Omori, 1964) than in normal subjects. This substrate-product relationship has recently been reinvestigated in insulin-dependent diabetic humans (Schade and Eaton, 1976a). As shown in Fig. 5, when an equivalent amount of FFA substrate is exposed to the diabetic liver *in vivo,* in which there are excess catecholamine levels, the liver exposed to catecholamines produces approximately twice the quantity of ketone bodies as the control. These experiments suggest that catecholamines have direct hepatic ketogenic stimulatory activity in addition to their lipolytic activity. However, these experiments may also reflect the ketogenic activity of glucagon, since the concentration of this hormone

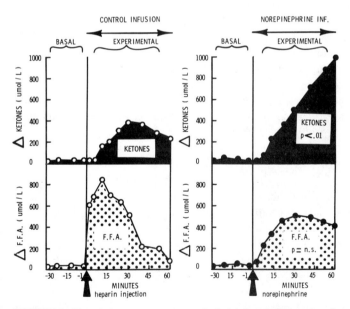

FIGURE 5 Ketogenic response to catecholamine infusion in six insulin-dependent diabetic subjects. FFA availability in the control study was provided by heparin injection in the absence of catecholamine.

increased during the infusion of norepinephrine. Additional liver infusion experiments employing catecholamines in the perfusate are needed to clarify the ketogenic activity of this hormone in diabetic humans.

The glucogenic activity of catecholamines is well established (Exton et al., 1971) and is related to stimulation of glycogenolysis and gluconeogenesis. However, this hyperglycemic activity is undoubtedly aided by the concurrent catecholamine-induced secretion of glucagon (Gerich et al., 1972) and growth hormone (Blackard and Heidingsfelder, 1968) and the peripheral resistance to glucose uptake resulting from the catecholamine-induced increase in plasma FFA concentration.

Evidence That Deficiency May Participate in the Obese State

Because obesity represents a state of lipid storage in excess of antici-pated need, it has been postulated that a metabolic defect in obesity could logically involve decreased responsiveness to the lipolytic activity of catechol-amines. This postulate has not been supported by experimental evidence. For example, when catecholamines were infused into obese humans (Willms et al., 1969), an exaggerated lipolytic response was observed. In addition, obese subjects are characterized by a normal (Bagdade et al., 1969) or increased (Opie and Walfish, 1963; Schade and Eaton, 1974) plasma concentrations of FFA. Metabolic turnover studies reported by Issekutz et al. (1968) have convincingly demonstrated that the obese human is not characterized by inhibition of FFA oxidation.

In addition to the data cited above, patients who have undergone adrenalectomy (thus removing the main source of epinephrine) are not characterized by obesity. Furthermore, obesity that follows destruction of the ventromedial nucleus of the hypothalamus of rats is unaffected by adrenal-ectomy (York and Bray, 1972). Thus, although the data are limited, a primary role for catecholamine deficiency in obesity is not apparent.

Evidence for Participation in Lipid-Lipoprotein Regulation

As reviewed above, catecholamines possess potent lipolytic activity at physiological concentrations in humans. Since circulating plasma FFA serve as the major substrate for hepatic lipogenesis and very low density lipoprotein production in postabsorptive humans, an increase in this substrate may result in increased hepatic triglyceride production. Such a relationship between increasing concentrations of plasma FFA and correspondingly increasing hepatic TG production has been demonstrated both *in vivo* in normal and hyperlipemic humans (Havel et al., 1970; Sailer et al., 1966) and *in vitro* in the perfused rat liver (Heimberg et al., 1969). However, when the hormonal state is altered, as with fasting, pregnancy, exercise, or drug therapy, this substrate-product relationship between FFA availability and hepatic TG

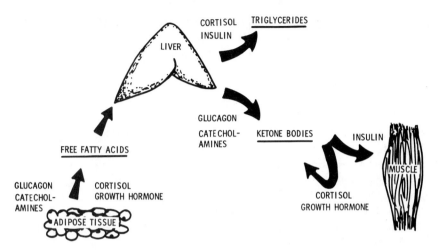

FIGURE 6 Multiple sites of counterregulatory hormone modulation of lipolysis, lipoprotein production, and ketone production and disposal in humans.

synthesis may be altered. Catecholamines have been shown to reduce the conversion of FFA to secreted TG in the perfused liver preparation (Heimberg et al., 1964) and to reduce the fractional rate of conversion of FFA to plasma TG *in vivo* in humans (Eaton et al., 1969). However, the marked lipolytic response occurring *in vivo* results in such a large rise in plasma FFA available to the liver, that the usual net observed response to catecholamine infusion is a rise in hepatic TG production and ultimate hyperlipemia in association with a fatty liver (Eaton et al., 1969; Dury and Treadwell, 1955; Boberg et al., 1974).

The catecholamine-induced reduction in hepatic conversion of FFA to TG is associated with a simultaneous rise in plasma ketone body concentration (Heimberg et al., 1964). This apparent "shift" of FFA metabolism into the beta-oxidative pathway of ketone formation and away from the synthetic pathway of TG formation is similar to the direct effect of glucagon on the liver (Heimberg et al., 1969). Thus, these two counterregulatory hormones share a similar action to promote lipolysis augmenting FFA availability to the liver, and to shift the hepatic conversion of FFA away from TG synthesis and into ketone production, as illustrated in Fig. 6. The net effect of these hormones on lipoprotein physiology will thus depend on the initial levels of substrates, the "set" of the liver at the time of hormone stimulation, and the simultaneous counterregulatory effects of insulin on these events.

CORTISOL

Glucocorticoid Regulation of Energy Substrates in Humans

Of the four counterregulatory hormones discussed in this chapter, the glucocorticoids (primarily cortisol in humans) are probably the most essential for the steady-state maintenance of the organism in its environment. For this reason, much scientific effort has been devoted to the definition of cortisol's effects and mechanism of action. Of particular interest are its effects on carbohydrate, lipid, and protein metabolism and its potential contribution to the pathogenesis of the diabetic state.

Cortisol is considered to be a stress hormone and is secreted in response to virtually all stressful stimuli. During insulin-induced hypoglycemia, for example (Garber et al., 1976; Donald, 1971), the plasma cortisol concentration begins to rise 10 min following the development of hypoglycemia. This delay has been attributed to the time necessary for pituitary secretion of ACTH and subsequent adrenal stimulation (Gallagher et al., 1973). Following the elevation of the plasma cortisol concentration, significant elevations of energy-yielding substrates are demonstrable in normal humans. These metabolic alterations include hyperglycemia, hyperketonemia, and increased FFA concentrations. All of these events emphasize the catabolic role of glucocorticoids in the counterregulatory hormone response to stress.

Although cortisol is properly considered a counterregulatory hormone, it differs from the other three hormones reviewed in this chapter in both the time course of its activity and its mechanism of action. As recently reviewed by O'Malley (1971), steroids alter metabolic activity by regulating both DNA and RNA synthesis within cells. This mechanism of action requires the entrance of the steroid molecule into the cell, with subsequent cytoplasmic and nuclear protein-specific binding. This mechanism of action differs markedly from that of glucagon and catecholamines, which do not enter cells but rather bind to cell surface receptors and activate cyclic AMP (Exton and Park, 1972). This difference in mechanism is in turn reflected in the onset and duration of action of the different counterregulatory hormones. Glucagon and catecholamines produce very rapid changes in cellular enzyme activity—that is, within minutes (Greene et al., 1974)—with a characteristically short duration of action on plasma substrate concentration (Schade and Eaton, 1975a). In contrast, steroids require at least one half-hour before their effect on enzymatic activity is evident, and this effect is apparently to increase the concentration of enzymes rather than the activity of specific preexisting enzymes (Exton et al., 1976). In addition, although there is a delay before the effects of glucocorticoids on carbohydrate metabolism are evident, the duration of action on plasma substrate concentrations, once established, is prolonged (Schade and Eaton, 1976b).

Evidence That Excess May Participate in the Diabetic State

The concept that cortisol may participate in the diabetic state is not new. In 1926, Unverricht first described a case of diabetes in which the insulin requirements decreased rapidly with the onset of adrenal insufficiency (Unverricht, 1926). In 1954, Baird and Munro reported a patient with adrenal insufficiency and diabetes mellitus, who developed diabetic ketoacidosis following the usual steroid replacement dosages. Following these and other similar case reports (Conn and Fajans, 1956), interest developed in the role of steroids in the pathogenesis of diabetes mellitus. Utilizing the urinary excretion of 17-OH corticosteroids as a measure of cortisol secretion, Jakobson (1958) clearly demonstrated that excessive cortisol secretion was characteristic of diabetic ketoacidosis. Following the development of the radioimmunoassay of cortisol, the observations of Jakobson were confirmed by many other investigators (Gerich et al., 1971; Garces et al., 1969). In addition, when cortisol secretory rates were measured during diabetic ketoacidosis, they were found to be two- to fourfold elevated and to return to normal with correction of the ketoacidotic state (Garces et al., 1969). These clinical observations support the concept that steroid excess may initiate or maintain the decompensated metabolic state of diabetes mellitus.

Important effects of glucocorticoids on carbohydrate homeostasis have been recognized since the description of hypoglycemia during adrenal insufficiency (Addison, 1855). Intensive investigations by many workers have established important metabolic effects of steroids at all sites of glucose metabolism. Administration of cortisone to hypopituitary children results in an increase in circulating concentrations of alanine and glutamine, which then serve as substrates for gluconeogenesis (Haymond et al., 1976). In addition, liver perfusion experiments have demonstrated that cortisol promotes not only glycogen synthesis, but also gluconeogenesis with subsequent net secretion of hepatic glucose (Exton et al., 1976). Glucocorticoids also have peripheral effects on carbohydrate metabolism. The recently reported studies of Olefsky (1975) have demonstrated that glucocorticoids not only inhibit insulin-mediated glucose transport but also directly inhibit transfer of glucose across cell membranes. Thus, these ubiquitous activities of glucocorticoids on carbohydrate metabolism all result in an increase in circulating plasma glucose concentration and a deterioration of diabetic "control."

Glucocorticoids probably have equally important effects on lipid metabolism in diabetes mellitus, but these effects have received less attention. The lipolytic activity of cortisol has been well documented *in vitro* (Fain et al., 1963). Infusion of cortisol into normal humans has resulted in an increase in plasma ketone body concentration, which has been attributed to its lipolytic effect (Mischke et al., 1974). Prolonged administration of glucocorticoids to insulin-dependent diabetic humans produces marked effects on plasma ketone body concentration, as shown in Fig. 7 (Schade and Eaton, 1976b). Although the hyperketonemia may have been secondary to the small increase in plasma FFA concentration, additional experiments (Schade and Eaton 1976b) suggested that the primary effect of steroids on inducing hyperketonemia are probably related to the inhibition of their utilization. There is indirect evidence to support this concept. In diabetic dogs, insulin has been reported to augment the peripheral utilization of ketone bodies (Balasse and Havel,

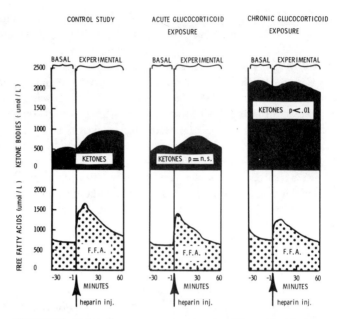

FIGURE 7 Ketogenic response to chronic glucocorticoid exposure (1 mg dexamethasone BID) but not to acute glucocorticoid injection (50 mg hydrocortisone iv) in six insulin-dependent diabetic subjects. FFA availability was provided by heparin injection in all studies. Inhibition of peripheral ketone body utilization is suggested as the mechanism for steroid ketonemia.

1971). Steroids, by decreasing the binding of insulin to cells (Olefsky et al., 1975), would be expected to inhibit this action of insulin. These data support the concept that excess glucocorticoid secretion during stress in the diabetic patient results in metabolic decompensation.

Evidence That Deficiency May Participate in the Obese State

Cortisol is a catabolic hormone and it would be anticipated that its deficiency might result in obesity. Although plasma cortisol concentrations may be low in obesity (Schteingart et al., 1963), this reduction is due to an increased turnover rate of cortisol rather than to a decrease in cortisol secretion (Migeon et al., 1963). In fact, in experimental obesity in humans, Sims et al. (1968) demonstrated that the absolute production rate of cortisol was increased during weight gain but was normal when related to body weight. In addition, the clinical observation that patients with adrenal insufficiency are lean and those with Cushing's disease are overweight does not support a role for glucocorticoid deficiency as an etiological factor in obesity.

Evidence for Participation in Lipid-Lipoprotein Regulation

The biological effects of administered corticosteroids in humans and animals appear to involve two phases. Initially, a depression of serum triglyceride concentration occurs, which lasts for a variable length of time depending on the species studied (Kyner et al., 1972). This phase is followed by a sustained elevation in serum TG concentration, which may be of considerable clinical significance in patients receiving anti-inflammatory corticosteroid therapy or steroid immunosuppressive therapy, particularly in renal transplant recipients (Bagdade et al., 1976a). In general, this phase of hyperlipemia represents an induced form of "endogenous" lipemia, composed of cholesterol-rich low-density lipoprotein (LDL) and/or triglyceride-rich very low density lipoprotein (VLDL) classes (Bagdade et al., 1976a, 1976b). These responses are both dosage- and drug-dependent, such that various synthetic steroids (prednisone, triamcinalone, dexamethasone, etc.) appear to differ in their specific effects.

In animal investigations, ultrastructural examination of the liver has demonstrated a close correlation between the appearance of the hepatocyte vesicles in the Golgi apparatus and the state of hepatic VLDL-TG production (Mahley et al., 1968; Reaven et al., 1974). During the phase of reduced serum lipid levels, typical Golgi apparatus are rare in the hepatocyte, and lysosomes containing VLDL particles appear. During the phase of elevated serum lipid levels, there is a disappearance of hepatocyte liposomes and a dramatic increase in Golgi apparatus containing numerous large particles clustered in secretory vesicles. During this time, large cytoplasmic lipid droplets characterize the fatty liver and probably reflect increased FFA uptake and VLDL synthesis. These ultrastructural changes in the second phase of steroid exposure suggest active lipid-lipoprotein synthesis and production. Direct evaluation of hepatic triglyceride production utilizing the Triton methodology (Bagdade et al., 1976a; Reaven et al., 1974) has confirmed increased hepatic VLDL production during prolonged steroid exposure (see Fig. 6).

The mechanisms mediating this second phase of increased hepatic VLDL production are not clear. Corticosteroids are known to increase plasma FFA by activation of adipose tissue lipase (Krotkiewski et al., 1970), and this increase in substrate availability for hepatic TG synthesis may explain the augmented VLDL production. In the perfused liver, hepatic TG production has been shown to be linearly related to perfusate FFA concentration (Klausner and Heimberg, 1967). However, Klausner and Heimberg (1967) have also shown that cortisone added to the perfusate will increase both FFA extraction by the hepatocyte and TG production. Moreover, livers from adrenalectomized rats demonstrated decreased FFA uptake, decreased TG production, and a reciprocal increased ketone production, which were all correctable with cortisol replacement and unrelated to perfusate FFA availability. These data suggest a direct hepatic action of corticosteroids to augment TG production and depress ketone production independent of any action to modulate FFA availability to the liver. This action, if confirmed, is remarkably different from the evolving understanding of glucagon, growth hormone, and catecholamines. In general, the latter three counterregulatory hormones either do not act at the liver directly, or appear to augment ketogenesis with a reciprocal depression of TG production. Thus, the actions of corticosteroids at the hepatocyte seem to be similar to those of insulin in promoting TG production (Reaven et al., 1974; Nikkila, 1974) and suppressing ketone production (Heimberg et al., 1964) as illustrated in Figs. 6 and 7.

Finally, Bagdade et al. (1976a) recently reported that cortisone also acts peripherally to inhibit the action of adipose tissue lipoprotein lipase. Such a blockade would lead to plasma TG accumulation and might be expected to contribute to the hyperlipemia of chronic corticosteroid administration. Thus, the lipemia of cortisol excess appears to be the result of three simultaneous mechanisms: (1) increased free fatty acid release, making more substrate available for hepatic lipogenesis; (2) direct hepatic shift of free fatty acid metabolism away from oxidation to ketones and into triglyceride synthesis; and (3) inhibition of peripheral disposal, leading to triglyceride accumulation in the blood.

GROWTH HORMONE

Modulation of Energy Substrates in Humans

Acute and profound hypoglycemia induced in humans by rapid intravenous injection of insulin results in a significant elevation of plasma growth hormone (Luft et al., 1966; Garber et al., 1976). This growth hormone rise may represent a response to the actual reduction in blood glucose concentration, or in part a response to the simultaneous rise in other counterregulatory hormones—plasma glucagon, corticosteroids, or catecholamines. Glick (1970) found that the threshold for release of growth hormone was a fall of blood glucose of 20-30 mg/100 ml, which was not associated with subjective manifestations of stress. Nevertheless, whether by a glucoprival mechanism or by a stress-induced mechanism (hormone or substrate), the basis for involvement of growth hormone in glucose physiology was established by these early investigations.

In addition to a role in the regulation of blood glucose homeostasis, growth hormone has been implicated in the regulation of body fat mobilization (Raben and Hollenberg, 1959), and subsequent ketogenesis (Felig et al., 1971; Merimee et al., 1971). With the administration of exogenous growth hormone to obese subjects during prolonged (5-6 wk) starvation, a 50% elevation in blood glucose was observed in association with a 50% rise in plasma FFA concentration and a marked associated elevation in plasma β-hydroxybutyrate and acetoacetate concentration (Felig et al., 1971). An absolute increase in ketogenesis was established by the demonstration of increased urinary ketone excretion, and the patients responded with the development of acidosis (arterial pH and total CO_2 reduction) including symptoms of nausea, mild vomiting, weakness, and myalgias. Although a direct insulinotropic effect of growth hormone was suggested by a rise in plasma insulin concentration preceding the altered glucose and lipid metabolism, it would appear that the counterregulatory response to growth hormone effectively overwhelmed the insulin response in this experimental situation. A similar mobilization of FFA and elevation in plasma and urine ketones has been reported in growth hormone-deficient dwarfs during exogenous growth hormone replacement (Merimee et al., 1971). It is important to note that growth hormone is not the exclusive counterregulatory hormone for ketogenesis, as evidenced by the observation of Merimee et al. (1971) that untreated growth hormone dwarfs demonstrate significantly greater plasma levels of FFA, β-hydroxybutyrate, and acetoacetate during fasting than are seen in normal control subjects. Thus, while growth hormone would appear to participate in glucose and lipid-ketone physiology in opposition to the actions of insulin, it cannot be the sole hormone responsible for normal and pathological counterregulatory events.

A consideration of growth hormone in the pathophysiology events surrounding human diabetes, obesity, and hyperlipemia (Cahill and Soeldner, 1974; Luft and Guillemin, 1974) may best be divided into three broad clinical categories: (1) data supporting a participation of growth hormone in the deterioration of glucose and lipid metabolism characteristic of the ketoacidotic state, (2) data supporting a role for reduction in growth hormone in the resistance to lipid catabolism characteristic of obesity, and (3) data concerning growth hormone relative to lipoprotein regulation.

Evidence That Excess May Participate in the Diabetic State

In 1930, Houssay and Biasotti demonstrated that the severity of diabetes decreases following extirpation of the hypophysis in animals and deteriorates after implantation or injection of the pars distalis. Young, in 1937, further demonstrated hyperglycemia in intact dogs by the administration of crude anterior pituitary extracts. Twelve years later it was demonstrated that growth hormone was the active substance in pituitary extracts that induced diabetes in these animals (Cotes et al., 1949; Houssay and Anderson, 1949). Extrapolation to human diabetes was initiated in 1960 with the demonstration that growth hormone administration to hypophysectomized nondiabetic patients induced a deterioration of carbohydrate tolerance (Ikkos and Luft, 1960a), and administration to hypophysectomized juvenile diabetics resulted in frank metabolic acidosis (Ikkos and Luft, 1960b). In contrast, growth hormone administration to normal subjects rarely results in significant deterioration of carbohydrate tolerance (Ikkos et al., 1962), and the diabetic complications of acromegalic patients rarely exceed mild glucose intolerance (Luft and Cerasi, 1968; Luft et al., 1967).

These historically important observations indicated a role for growth hormone in the regulation and/or caloric utilization of glucose and fatty acids, but suggested that this hormone was not the key to decompensation of the diabetic state. Further clarification of this point emerged from two routes of investigation—by immunoassay of plasma growth hormone in appropriate patients, and by pharmacological blockade of growth hormone secretion with somatostatin. By direct immunoassay, plasma levels of growth hormone have been reported by many investigators to be variably elevated in patients with diabetes (Knopf et al., 1973; Cryer and Daughaday, 1970; Alberti and Hockaday, 1973). Most of these observations were performed in the basal or overnight-fasted state, leading to the suggestion that more definitive information might be gained by examining growth hormone dynamics. Thus, studies of diurnal variation (Vazquez et al., 1973), suppression with glucose ingestion (Tchobroutsky, 1973), secretion in response to aminoacid stimulation (Genuth and Castro, 1974; Burday et al., 1968; Koncz et al., 1973), response to acute exercise (Passa et al., 1974; Lundbaek, 1973; Tchobroutsky et al., 1974; Hansen, 1973a), and serial response to therapy during ketoacidosis were performed (Alberti and Hockaday, 1973; Assan and Tchobroutsky, 1972; Cryer and Daughaday, 1970). This abundant literature may be summarized as indicating a marked tendency for fluctuating but elevated growth hormone levels in poorly controlled diabetic patients, which approach normal with improved management toward normoglycemia and correction of acidosis (Corrall et al., 1974; Hanssen, 1974). This conclusion is clearly shown by the work of Hansen (1971, 1973a) in the investigation of exercise-induced growth hormone secretion. These data demonstrated that hypersecretion of growth hormone in response to exercise in juvenile diabetics could be completely normalized after a period of exceedingly strict metabolic control of the diabetes. Management to attain normal growth hormone secretion required diurnal blood sugar levels in the normal range from 80–120 mg/100 ml. Progressive lowering of the mean blood sugar level resulted in growth hormone responses to exercise that were more delayed and showed lower maximum values, until finally no rise in serum growth hormone occurred when the blood sugar level was completely normal.

Additional confusion in the understanding of the fluctuating and elevated levels of growth hormone in juvenile diabetic patients stems from the investigation of arginine-stimulated growth hormone secretion (Burday et al., 1968; Koncz et al., 1973). Apparently, hyperglycemia in both normal and diabetic subjects blunts the growth hormone response to infused arginine. Thus, if arginine were the physiologic stimulus for growth hormone secretion, diabetic patients with hyperglycemia would have reduced growth hormone secretion relative to normal subjects with euglycemia.

Another curious observation documented by several investigators is the rise in growth hormone within 2 hr of initiation of insulin and fluid therapy in ketoacidosis (Corrall et al., 1974; Hanssen, 1974), suggesting superimposition of an acute alteration in growth hormone dynamics on the background issue of elevated basal growth hormone levels. The observation that relatively normal growth hormone values were often seen initially in the presence of diabetic ketoacidosis, with a rise during therapy, has led most investigators to conclude that growth hormone is probably of little importance as an insulin antagonist in the evolution and/or etiology of hyperglycemia and ketosis in diabetic subjects.

Further investigation into the role of growth hormone in the metabolic decompensation of diabetes mellitus has progressed with the use of somatostatin infusion to block the release of growth hormone (Gerich et al., 1975a, 1976; Lundbaek et al., 1976). Interpretation of these data is difficult since this polypeptide also blocks the secretion of glucagon, another counterregulatory hormone in the same category as growth hormone. Plasma glucose levels as well as plasma ketones are clearly reduced during somatostatin infusion in diabetic subjects. However, the reinfusion of either growth hormone or glucagon reverses the effect, although the onset of the effect is more delayed after growth hormone infusion (Gerich et al., 1976). Nevertheless, a clear role for growth hormone is again suggested by these studies, although it still seems more likely to be involved as a participating hormone rather than the sole counterregulatory hormone. This suggestion is supported by the report that somatostatin infusion in a hypophysectomized juvenile diabetic subject with no endogenous growth hormone secretion also results in a marked reduction in blood glucose level (Gerich et al., 1974). This clearly indicates an effect mediated by other hormones in addition to growth hormone. Finally, attempts to correct frank diabetic ketoacidosis with somatostatin infusion have been generally unsuccessful (Gerich et al., 1975a; Lundbaek et al., 1976), suggesting participation by growth hormone in this state, although not as the determining factor exclusive of other counterregulatory hormones and events.

The mechanism of action and time of onset of growth hormone's ketogenic activity have recently been examined in insulin-dependent diabetics (Schade and Eaton, 1977). This study is summarized in Fig. 8. Compared to a control study, no effect on the concentration of FFA or ketone bodies of acute (60 min) growth hormone infusion was observed. In contrast, when growth hormone was administered by subcutaneous injection 12 hr before the study (18 μg/kg), a marked ketotic effect was observed. This increase was probably greater than could be accounted for by the slight lipolytic effect of growth hormones. Administration of heparin to augment plasma FFA availability indicated that growth hormone also either directly stimulates the hepatic conversion of FFA to ketone bodies or inhibits the peripheral utilization of ketone bodies by peripheral tissue.

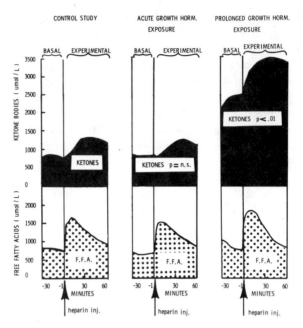

FIGURE 8 Ketogenic response to chronic growth hormone injection (im) (18 ng/kg, 12 hr prior to study) but not to acute growth hormone injection (4 μg/kg-hr by iv constant infusion) in six insulin-dependent diabetic subjects. Fatty acid availability was provided by heparin injection in all studies. Both inhibition of peripheral utilization and augmented hepatic production may mediate the ketonemia.

Evidence That Deficiency May Participate in the Obese State

During prolonged fasting, obese patients are less prone to develop ketosis than are normal subjects, although they appear to metabolize a comparable amount of adipose tissue (Schwarz et al., 1966). In contrast to normal-weight subjects, they also demonstrate a subnormal rise in plasma growth hormone with fasting (Schwarz et al., 1966; Beck et al., 1964; Roth et al., 1963; Ball et al., 1972; Danowski et al., 1969; El-Khodary et al., 1971). This failure to augment growth hormone secretion with fasting is also demonstrable in response to a variety of stimuli that produce growth hormone release in normal subjects; for example, hypoglycemia (Carnelutti et al., 1970; Beck et al., 1964), arginine infusion (Burday et al., 1968; Merimee et al., 1969; Carnelutti et al., 1970), exercise (Hansen, 1973b; Roth et al., 1963), glucose ingestion (Roth et al., 1963), sleep (Quabbe et al., 1971), and L-Dopa (Fingerhut and Krieger, 1974).

One might expect the effects of insulin on anabolic processes to be exaggerated in the presence of this relatively subnormal counterregulatory growth hormone secretion in the obese patient. Such an expectation is certainly not realized for glucose disposal, which is commonly delayed in obesity, but it may be partially realized in the reduced ketosis with starvation common in obesity. The oversimplicity of this hypothesis is indicated by the failure of growth hormone-deficient dwarfs to exhibit obesity or resistance to ketosis. Thus, while a reduction in availability of this single counterregulatory hormone may participate in the stability of the metabolic state and tendency for adipose tissue accumulation in obesity, involvement of the other counterregulatory hormones and altered insulin responsiveness must be carefully considered to complete the hormone status.

Evidence for Participation in Lipid-Lipoprotein Regulation

The modulation by insulin of hepatic lipoprotein production and secretion and of peripheral lipid disposal has been reviewed elsewhere in this volume (see Chaps. 5 and 4 by Bierman and Brunzell, and Wilson and Brown, respectively). It should be sufficient to recall that excess insulin may have the potential to augment both hepatic lipoprotein production leading to hyperlipemia, and lipoprotein lipase-mediated peripheral disposal of lipoproteins leading to hypolipemia. Which of these two responses will predominate may depend on the simultaneous activity and concentration of the counterregulatory hormones, including growth hormone. In the growth hormone-deficient state of ateliotic dwarfs (Merimee et al., 1972), marked hypercholesterolemia is characteristic of an increase in the pre-beta lipoprotein fraction by lipoprotein electrophoresis. Similarly, in the obese patient with relative growth hormone deficiency (see above) a type IV hyperlipemia with excess pre-beta lipoprotein by electrophoresis is a frequent observation. Conversely, the state of growth hormone excess in acromegaly is associated with a reduced plasma cholesterol concentration (Nikkila and Pelkonen, 1975), and administration of exogenous growth hormone to normal and hypercholesterolemic patients is reported to result in a reduction in plasma cholesterol concentration (Azizi et al., 1973; Aloia et al., 1975; Friedman et al., 1974), consistent with a restraining action by growth hormone on net cholesterol metabolism. It should be noted that a reciprocal elevation in plasma triglyceride concentration is also reported in acromegaly (Nikkila and Pelkonen, 1975) and during growth hormone administration in growth hormone-deficient dwarfs (Friedman et al., 1974), which has been attributed to the additional insulin secretion in response to this beta-cell secretagogue.

While the molecular biology of these growth hormone effects on lipid metabolism remains to be examined, it should be noted that growth hormone pretreatment results in augmented glucagon secretion in normal subjects (Pek et al., 1973). This could mediate part of the lipid-lowering response of growth hormone. Thus, a counterregulatory role for growth hormone in hormonal balance with insulin must be considered in the evaluation of lipid metabolism of diabetes, obesity, and all conditions in which growth hormone regulation may be altered.

HORMONAL REGULATION OF KETOSIS IN HUMANS— UNRESOLVED ASPECTS

During the last 50 yr, many workers have contributed to our understanding of ketosis both at the clinical and at the metabolic level. These workers have established that ketone bodies are both a major source of oxidizable fuel and, when not adequately regulated, a pathogenic substrate that could induce acidosis. Excessive plasma levels of ketones have been shown to be the consequence of either excessive FFA availability, augmented hepatic conversion of fatty acid to ketones, or reduced peripheral utilization of ketones as depicted in Figs. 6 and 7.

In 1974, Garber and co-workers demonstrated that plasma ketone body concentration in humans is regulated at multiple sites. Utilizing hepatic catheters in fasting humans, they observed that within 72 hr of initiating a fast, maximal hepatic production of ketone bodies was obtained. In spite of maximal production, plasma ketone body concentration did not attain maximal concentration until 17 days after initiation of the fast. These observations strongly support the concept that plasma ketone body concentration is regulated at both the source of production and the site of utilization. This regulation of plasma ketone body concentration is complex, but the factors involved may be categorized into two groups: intermediary substrates and regulatory hormones. *In vivo* studies have demonstrated that glucose enhances uptake of ketone bodies by peripheral tissues (Soling et al., 1965), and both lactate and pyruvate have been shown to inhibit hepatic ketogenesis (McGarry and Foster, 1971). More pertinent to the present chapter is the regulation of plasma ketone body concentration by insulin and the four counterregulatory hormones.

Insulin was the first hormone whose ketone body regulatory properties were demonstrable. It is generally agreed that insulin exerts an important antiketogenic action by limiting the release of FFA substrate from adipose tissue (Cahill et al., 1966). Since hepatic production of ketone bodies is dependent on the availability of plasma FFA (Woodside and Heimberg, 1972), the antilipolytic action of insulin is also antiketogenic. Insulin may also inhibit the hepatic β-oxidation pathway of ketogenesis, as demonstrated by both *in vitro* (Woodside and Heimberg, 1976) and *in vivo* (Bieberdorf et al., 1970) investigations. In contrast, there are both *in vitro* (Beatty et al., 1959) and *in vivo* (Balasse and Havel, 1971) data suggesting that insulin enhances peripheral utilization of ketone bodies. Thus, in insulin-deficient diabetic ketoacidotic dogs, peripheral utilization of ketone bodies is significantly decreased (Balasse and Havel, 1971). In fact, it has been stated that severe ketoacidosis would not occur if peripheral utilization of ketone bodies were not decreased. When these dogs were treated with insulin, peripheral utilization of ketones returned toward normal and the plasma ketone body concentration declined. From these data, it is probable that insulin plays a major role in the reduction of plasma ketone body concentration. This would imply that relative insulin deficiency is a necessary concomitant for the development of severe keto-acidosis.

Although relative insulin deficiency may be necessary for ketoacidosis to develop, clinical observations would suggest that it is not sufficient to result in severe decompensation of the metabolic state. In fact, plasma insulin concentration in diabetic ketoacidosis may actually be within the normal range for overnight-fasted nondiabetic subjects (Muller et al., 1973; Kitabchi et al., 1976). As schematized in Fig. 9, counterregulatory hormone excess may be equally as important as relative insulin deficiency in the pathogenesis of ketoacidosis.

The role of counterregulatory hormones in plasma ketone body regulation has only recently begun to emerge, in spite of the fact that all four of these hormones (glucagon, catecholamines, cortisol, and growth hormone) have definitely been shown to possess ketogenic activity at physiological concentrations (Schade and Eaton, 1975d; Mischke et al., 1974; Gerich et al., 1976). Both glucagon and norepinephrine may be considered to have an acute onset of ketogenic activity (within minutes), both on the fat cell to enhance release of FFA substrate (Pozza et al., 1971; Grosso et al., 1964) and on the liver to enhance the conversion of FFA to ketone bodies (Exton et al., 1971; Schade and Eaton, 1975d). A similarity in time of onset between these two hormones would be expected since the ketogenic activities of both hormones

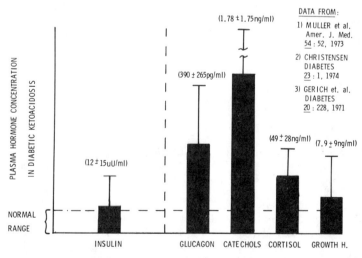

FIGURE 9 Plasma insulin and counterregulatory hormone excess in a diabetic ketoacidotic man. Values are means ± SE.

are believed to be mediated by cyclic AMP production (Exton and Park, 1972). However, their ketogenic potencies are not equal. Catecholamines are very potent lipolytic hormones, in contrast to glucagon, in which the lipolytic activity is occasionally not demonstrable at physiological concentration (Schade and Eaton, 1975d). In contrast, on the liver, glucagon is far more potent that catecholamines at enhancing the ketogenic β-oxidation pathway (Exton et al., 1971). Whether these two counterregulatory hormones also modulate the plasma ketone body concentration by inhibiting peripheral utilization of ketones has not been established (Pozefsky et al., 1976; Schneider et al., 1976).

In contrast to the two acutely acting counterregulatory hormones discussed above, cortisol and growth hormone require a more prolonged exposure before their ketogenic effects are evident. This has been documented by *in vivo* (Schade and Eaton, 1976b, 1977; Gerich et al., 1976) and *in vitro* liver perfusion experiments (Chernick et al., 1972) in which no acute effects of these two hormones on hepatic ketogenesis were evident. With prolonged exposure (more than 60 min) these two hormones have potent effects on plasma ketone body concentrations. However, the mechanism by which these hormones induce ketosis is now known. Both hormones have weak lipolytic activity, which is probably not sufficient to account for their total ketogenic activities. More likely is an action to inhibit utilization of ketone bodies by peripheral tissues.

From these data has emerged the concept of two counterregulatory hormones acting from minute to minute to increase plasma ketone concentration, and two counterregulatory hormones acting only after prolonged exposure to elevated plasma ketone concentrations. The physiological and pathological implications of this time-related hormonal regulatory system may form the basis of the evolving therapeutic approach to the metabolic aberrations of diabetes, obesity, pregnancy, and cachectic states.

REFERENCES

Addison, T. 1855. *On the constitutional and local effects of disease of the suprarenal capsules.* London: Highley.

Aguilar-Parada, E., Eisentraut, A. M. and Unger, R. H. 1969. *Diabetes* 18:717–723.

Alberti, K. G. and Hockaday, T. D. 1973. *Diabetologia* 9:13–19.

Alford, F. P., Bloom, S. R., Hall, R., Besser, G. M., Coy, D. H., Kastin, A. J. and Schally, A. V. 1974. *Lancet* 2(Oct 26):974–977.

Alford, F. P., Bloom, S. R. and Nabarro, J. D. N. 1976. *J. Clin. Endocrinol. Metab.* 42:830–838.

Aloia, J. F., Zanzi, I. and Cohn, S. H. 1975. *Metabolism* 24:795–798.

Amatuzio, D. S., Grande, F. and Wada, S. 1962. *Metabolism* 11:1240–1246.

Assan, R. and Tchobroutsky, G. 1972. *Horm. Metab. Res.* 4:317–321.

Assan, R., Hautecouverture, G., Buillemant, S., Dauchy, R., Protin, P. and Derot, M. 1969. *Pathol. Biol.* 17:1095–1105.

Axelrod, J. and Weinshilbaum, R. 1972. *N. Engl. J. Med.* 287:237.

Azizi, F., Castelli, P., Raben, M. S. and Mitchell, M. L. 1973. *Proc. Soc. Biol. Med.* 143:1187–1190.

Bagdade, J. D., Porte, D. and Bierman, E. L. 1969. *Diabetes* 18:759.

Bagdade, J. D., Bierman, E. L. and Porte, D., Jr. 1971. *Diabetes* 20:664.

Bagdade, J. D., Yee, E., Alberts, J. and Pykalisto, O. J. 1976a. *Metabolism* 25:533–542.

Bagdade, J. D., Casaretto, A. and Alberts, J. 1976b. *J. Lab. Clin. Med.* 87:37–48.

Baird, I. M. and Munro, D. S. 1954. *Lancet* 1:962.

Baker, L., Barcai, A., Kaye, R. and Haque, N. 1969. *J. Pediatr.* 75:19.

Balasse, E. O. and Havel, R. J. 1971. *J. Clin. Invest.* 50:801–813.

Ball, M. F., El-Khodary, A. Z. and Canary, J. J. 1972. *J. Clin. Endocrinol.* 34:498.

Barnes, A. J., Bloom, A., Crowley, M. F., et al. 1975. *Lancet* 2:734–737.

Basso, L. V. and Havel, R. J. 1970. *J. Clin. Invest.* 49:537–547.

Batstone, G. F., Alberti, M. M., Hinks, L., Smythe, P., et al. 1976. *Burns* 2:207.

Beatty, C. H., Peterson, R. D., Bocek, R. M. and West, E. S. 1959. *J. Biol. Chem.* 234:11.

Beck, J., Koumans, J. H. T., Winterling, C. A., Stein, M. D. and Daughaday, W. H. 1964. *J. Lab. Clin. Med.* 64:654.

Beck, P., Eaton, R. P., Arnett, D. M. and Alsever, R. N. 1975. *Metabolism* 24:1055–1065.

Beck, P., Arnett, D. M., Alsever, R. N. and Eaton, R. P. 1976. *Metabolism* 25:23–31.

Bieberdorf, F. A., Chernick, S. S. and Scow, R. D. 1970. *J. Clin. Invest.*49:1685.

Bilbrey, G. L., Faloona, G. R., White, M. C. and Knochel, J. P. 1974. *J. Clin. Invest.* 53:841–846.

Blackard, W. G. and Heidingsfelder, S. A. 1968. *J. Clin. Invest.* 47:1407.

Blackard, W. G. and Omori, Y. 1964. *Diabetes* 13:518–526.

Blackard, W. G. and Orcori, Y. 1975. *Diabetes* 13:518.

Blackard, W. G., Nelson, N. C. and Andrews, S. S. 1974. *Diabetes* 23:199–202.

Boberg, J., Freysehuss, F., Lassers, B. W. and Wahlquist, M. L. 1974. *Horm. Metab. Res. Suppl.* Series 4:34–37.

Bray, G. A. and De Quattro, V. 1972. *Calif. Med.* 117:32.

Buchanan, K. D. 1973. *Postgrad. Med. J. Suppl.* 49:604–606.

Burday, S. Z., Fine, P. H. and Schalch, D. S. 1968. *J. Lab. Clin. Med.* 71:897–911.

Cahill, G. F., Jr. and Soeldner, J. S. 1974. *N. Engl. J. Med.* 291:577–579.

Cahill, G. F., Jr., Herrera, M. G., Morgan, A. P., Soeldner, J. S. and Steinke, J. 1966. *J. Clin. Invest.* 44:1751.

Callingham, B. A. 1975. In *Handbook of physiology*, Sect. 7: *Endocrinology*, vol. 6, p. 427. Washington, D.C.: American Physiological Society.

Caren, R. and Corbo, L. 1970. *Metabolism* 19:598–607.

Carnelutti, M., del Guercio, M. J. and Chiumello, G. 1970. *J. Pediatr.* 77:285.

Chernick, S. S., Clark, C. M., Gardiner, R. J. and Scow, R. O. 1972. *Diabetes* 21:946.

Christensen, N. J. 1974. *Diabetes* 23:1.

Collip, J. B. 1923. *Am. J. Physiol.* 63:391–392.

Conn, J. W. and Fajans, S. S. 1956. *Metabolism* 5:114.

Corrall, R. J., Hunter, W. M., Campbell, I. W., Harrower, A. D., Duncan, L. J. and Clarke, B. F. 1974. *Acta Endocrinol.* 77:115–121.

Cotes, P. M., Reid, E. and Young, F. G. 1949. *Nature (Lond.)* 164:209.

Cryer, P. E. and Daughaday, W. H. 1970. *Diabetes* 19:519–523.

Danowski, T. S., Tsai, C. T., Morgan, C. R., Sieracki, J. C., Alley, R. A., Robbins, T. J., Sabeh, G. and Sunder, J. H. 1969. *Metabolism* 18:811.

Donald, R. A. 1971. *J. Clin. Endocrinol.* 32:225.

Dury, A. and Treadwell, C. R. 1955. *J. Clin. Endocrinol. Metab.* 15:818–821.

Eaton, R. P. 1973a. *J. Lipid Res.* 14:312–318.

Eaton, R. P. 1973b. *Am. J. Physiol.* 225:67–73.

Eaton, R. P. 1973c. *Metabolism* 22:763–767.

Eaton, R. P. and Nye, W. H. R. 1973. *J. Lab. Clin. Med.* 81:682–695.

Eaton, R. P. and Schade, D. S. 1974a. *Metabolism* 23:445–454.

Eaton, R. P. and Schade, D. S. 1974b. *Lancet* 1(May 5):973–974.

Eaton, R. P., Berman, M. and Steinberg, D. 1969. *J. Clin. Invest.* 48:1560–1579.

Eaton, R. P., Schade, D. S. and Conway, M. 1974a. *Lancet* 2(Dec. 28):1545–1549.

Eaton, R. P., Kipnis, D. M., Karl, I. and Eisenstein, A. B. 1974b. *Am. J. Physiol.* 227:101–104.

Eaton, R. P., Conway, M. and Schade, D. S. 1976a. *Am. J. Physiol.* 230:1336–1341.

Eaton, R. P., Schade, D. S. and Oase, R. 1976b. *Metabolism* 25:245–249.

El-Khodary, A. Z., Ball, M. F., Stein, B. and Canary, J. J. 1971. *J. Clin. Endocrinol.* 23:42.

Exton, J. H. and Park, C. R. 1972. In *Handbook of physiology,* Sect. 7: *Endocrinology,* vol. 1, p. 437. Washington, D.C.: American Physiological Society.

Exton, J. H., Lewis, S. B., Ho, R. J., Robison, G. A. and Park, C. R. 1971. *Ann. N.Y. Acad. Sci.* 185:85.

Exton, J. H., Miller, T. B., Harper, S. C. and Park, C. R. 1976. *Am. J. Physiol.* 230:163.

Fain, S. N., Scow, R. O. and Chernick, S. S. 1963. *J. Biol. Chem.* 238:54.

Fallon, H. J. and Kemp, E. L. 1968. *J. Clin. Invest.* 47:712–719.

Felig, P., Marliss, E. B. and Cahill, G. F., Jr. 1971. *J. Clin. Invest.* 50:411–421.

Felig, P., Wahren, J., Hendler, R. and Ahlborg, G. 1972. *N. Engl. J. Med.* 287:184–185.

Fingerhut, M. and Krieger, D. R. 1974. *Metabolism* 23:267–271.

Franksson, C., Gemzell, C. A. and Von Euler, U. S. 1954. *J. Clin. Endocrinol.* 14:608.

Friedman, M., Byers, S. O., Rosenman, R. H., Li, C. G. and Neuman, R. 1974. *Metabolism* 23:905–911.

Gallagher, T. G., Yoshida, K., Roffwarg, H. D., Fukushima, D. K., Weitzman, E. A. and Hellman, L. 1973. *J. Clin. Endocrinol. Metab.* 36:1058.

Garber, A. J., Manzel, P. H., Boden, G. and Owen, O. E. 1974. *J. Clin. Invest.* 54:981.

Garber, A. J., Cryer, P. E., Santiago, J. V., Haumond, M. W., Pagliara, A. S. and Kipnis, D. M. 1976. *J. Clin. Invest.* 58:7–15.

Garces, L. Y., Kenny, F. M. and Drash, A. 1969. *J. Pediatr.* 74:517.

Genuth, S. M. and Castro, J. 1974. *Metabolism* 23:375–386.

Gerich, J. E., Martin, M. M. and Recant, L. 1971. *Diabetes* 20:228.

Gerich, J. E., Karam, J. H. and Forsham, P. H. 1972. *Diabetes* 21(Suppl. 1):332.

Gerich, J. E., Lorenzi, M., Schneider, V., Karam, J. H., Rivier, J., Guillemin, R. and Forsham, P. 1974. *N. Engl. J. Med.* 29:544–547.

Gerich, J. E., Lorenzi, M., Bier, D. M., Schneider, V., Tsalikian, E., Karam, J. H. and Forsham, P. H. 1975a. *N. Engl. J. Med.* 292:985–989.

Gerich, J. E., Lorenzi, M., Karam, J. H., Schneider, V. and Forsham, P. H. 1975b. *J. Am. Med. Assoc.* 234:159–165.

Gerich, J. E., Lorenzi, M., Bier, D. M., Tsalikian, E., Schneider, V., Karam, J. H. and Forsham, P. H. 1976. *J. Clin. Invest.* 57:875–884.

Glick, S. M. 1970. *J. Clin. Endocrinol.* 30:619–623.

Greene, H. L., Taunton, O. D., Stifel, F. B. and Herman, R. H. 1974. *J. Clin. Invest.* 53:44.

Grosso, S., Michaels, G. D. and Kinsell, L. W. 1964. *Diabetes* 13:1333.

Groves, A. C., Griffiths, J., Leung, F. and Meek, R. N. 1973. *Ann Surg.* 178:102.

Hansen, A. P. 1971. *J. Clin. Invest.* 50:1806–1811.

Hansen, A. P. 1973a. *Diabetes* 22:619.

Hansen, A. P. 1973b. *Scand. J. Clin. Lab. Invest.* 31:175–178.

Hanssen, K. F. 1974. *Acta Endocrinol.* 75:50–63.

Havel, R. J., Kane, J. P., Balasse, E. O., Segel, N. and Basso, L. V. 1970. *J. Clin. Invest.* 49:2017.

Haymond, M. W., Karl, I. and Weldon, V. V. 1976. *J. Clin. Endocrinol. Metab.* 42:846.

Hazzard, W. R., Notter, D. R., Spiger, M. J. and Bierman, E. L. 1972. *J. Clin. Endocrinol. Metab.* 35:425–432.

Heimberg, M., Fizette, N. B. and Klausner, H. 1964. *J. Am. Oil Chem. Soc.* 41:774–779.

Heimberg, M., Weinstein, I. and Kohout, M. 1969. *J. Biol. Chem.* 244:4131–4139.

Houssay, B. A. and Anderson, E. 1949. *Endocrinology* 45:627.

Houssay, B. A. and Biasotti, A. 1930. *Rev. Soc. Argent. Biol.* 6:251.

Hsieh, A. C. L. and Carson, L. D. 1957. *Am. J. Physiol.* 190:243.

Ikkos, D. and Luft, R. 1960a. *Lancet* II:897.

Ikkos, D. and Luft, R. 1960b. *Ciba Found. Colloq. Endocrinol.* 13:106.

Ikkos, D., Luft, R., Gemzell, A. and Almquist, S. 1962. *Acta Endocrinol.* 39:547.

Issekutz, B., Paul, P., Miller, H. I. and Bortz, W. M. 1968. *Metabolism* 17:62.

Issekutz, B., Issekutz, T. B., Elahi, D. and Borkow, I. 1974. *Diabetologia* 10:323–328.

Jakobson, T. 1958. *Acta Endocrinol.* 29 (Suppl. 41):7.

Johansen, K., Soeldner, J. S. and Gleason, R. E. 1974. *Metabolism* 23:1185–1199.

Kalkhoff, R. K., Gossain, V. V. and Matute, M. L. 1973. *N. Engl. J. Med.* 289:465–467.

Kitabchi, A. E., Ayagari, V., Guerra, S. M. D., et al. 1976. *Ann. Intern. Med.* 84:633.

Klausner, H., and Heimberg, M. 1967. *Am. J. Physiol.* 212:1236–1246.

Knopf, R. F., Fajans, S. S., Pek, S., Floyd, J. C., Jr., Prehkov, V. D. and Conn, J. W. 1973. *Adv. Metab. Disord.* 2(Suppl 2):215–225.

Koncz, L., Soeldner, J. S., Balodimos, M. D., Boden, G., Gleason, R. E. and Younger, D. 1973. *Diabetes* 22:694–705.

Kreisberg, R. A., Boshell, B. R., Di Placidos, J. and Roddam, R. F. 1967. *N. Engl. J. Med.* 276:314–319.

Krotkiewski, M., Krotkiewska, J. and Bjorntorp, P. 1970. *Acta Endocrinol.* 63:185–192.

Kuku, S. F., Zeidler, D. S., Emmanouel, A. I., Katz, A. I. and Rubenstein, A. H. 1976. *J. Clin. Endocrinol. Metab.* 42:173–176.

Kyner, J. L., Levy, R. I., Soeldner, J. S., Gleason, R. E. and Fredrickson, D. S. 1972. *Metabolism* 21:329–336.

LeFebvre, P. J. 1972. In *Glucagon, molecular physiology, clinical and therapeutic implications,* eds. P. J. Lefebvre and R. H. Unger, pp. 109–123. Elmsford, N.Y.: Pergamon.

Leichter, S. B., Pagliara, A. S., Greider, M. H., Pohl, S., Rosai, J. and Kipnis, D. M. 1975. *Am. J. Med.* 58:285–293.

Lightman, S. L. and Bloom, S. R. 1974. *Br. Med. J.* 1:367–368.

Liljenquist, J. E., Bomboy, J. D., Lewis, S. B., Sinclair-Smith, B. C., Felts, P. W., Lacy, W. W., Crofford, O. B. and Liddle, G. W. 1974. *J. Clin. Invest.* 53:190–197.

Lindsey, C. A., Faloona, G. R. and Unger, R. H. 1974. *J. Am. Med. Assoc.* 229:1771–1773.

Lorenzi, M., Karam, J. H., Schneider, V., Gustafson, G., Horita, S. and Gerich, J. E. 1975. *Clin. Res.* 23:112A (abstract).

Luft, R. and Cerasi, E. 1968. *Diabetologia* 4:1.

Luft, R. and Guillemin, R. 1974. *Diabetes* 23:783–787.

Luft, R., Cerasi, E., Madison, L. L., Von Euler, U. S., Casa, L. D. and Roovete, A. 1966. *Lancet* 1:254–257.

Luft, R., Cerasi, E. and Hamberger, C. A. 1967. *Acta Endocrinol.* 56:593.

Lundbaek, K. 1973. In *Proceedings of the International Diabetes Federation, 7th Congress, Brussels,* eds. W. J. Malaisse, J. Pirart, and J. Vallance-Owen, pp. 657–666. New York: American Elsevier.

Lundbaek, K., Hansen, A. P., Orskov, H., Christensen, S. E., Iversen, J. and Seyer-Hansen, K. 1976. *Lancet* 1:215–218.

Mackrell, D. J. and Sokal, J. E. 1969. *Diabetes* 18:724–732.

Mahley, R. W., Gray, M. E., Hamilton, R. L. and SeQuire, V. S. 1968. *Lab. Invest.* 19:358–369.

Marco, J., Calle, C., Roman, D., Diaz-Fierros, M., Villanueva, M. L. and Valverde, I. 1973. *N. Engl. J. Med.* 288:128–132.

McGarry, J. D. and Foster, D. S. 1971. *J. Biol. Chem.* 246:6247.

McGarry, J. D., Wright, P. H. and Foster, D. W. 1975. *J. Clin. Invest.* 55:1202–1209.

Merimee, T. J., Rabinowitz, D. and Fineberg, S. E. 1969. *N. Engl. J. Med.* 280:1434.

Merimee, T. J., Felig, P., Marliss, E., Fineberg, S. E. and Cahill, G. F., Jr. 1971. *J. Clin. Invest.* 50:574–582.

Merimee, T. J., Hollander, W. and Fineberg, S. E. 1972. *Metabolism* 21:1053.

Migeon, C. J., Green, O. C. and Eckert, J. P. 1963. *Metabolism* 12:718.

Mischke, W. G., Ebers, S. and Boisch, K. H. 1974. *Acta Endocrinol.* 75(Suppl. 186):1.

Muller, W. A., Faloona, G. T., Aguilar-Parada, E., et al., 1970. *N. Engl. J. Med.* 283:109–115.

Muller, W. A., Faloona, G. R. and Unger, R. H. 1973. *Am. J. Med.* 54:52.

Nikkila, E. A. 1974. *Proc. R. Soc. Med.* 67:662–665.

Nikkila, E. A. and Pelkonen, R. 1975. *Metabolism* 24:829–838.

Olefsky, J. M. 1975. *J. Clin. Invest.* 56:1499.

Olefsky, J. M., Johnson, J., Lin, F., et al. 1975. *Metabolism* 24:517.

O'Malley, B. 1971. *N. Engl. J. Med.* 284:370.

Opie, L. H. and Walfish, P. G. 1963. *N. Engl. J. Med.* 268:757.

Paloyan, E., Dimboys, N., Gallagher, T. F., Rogers, R. E. and Harper, P. V. 1962. *Fed. Proc.* 21:200–204.

Park, C. R. and Exton, J. H. 1972. In *Glucagon, molecular physiology, clinical and therapeutic implications.* Eds. P. J. Lefebvre and R. H. Unger, pp. 77–109. Elmsford, N.Y.: Pergamon.

Passa, P., Gauville, C. and Canivet, J. 1974. *Lancet* 2:72–74.

Pek, S., Fajans, S. S., Floyd, J. C., Jr. and Knopf, R. F. 1973. In *Proceedings of the International Diabetes Federation, 8th Congress,* eds. W. V. Malaisse and J. Pirart, p. 209. New York: American Elsevier.

Porte, D., Jr. and Robertson, R. P. 1973. *Fed. Proc.* 32:1792.

Porte, D., Jr., Graber, A. L., Kuzuya, T. and Williams, R. H. 1966. *J. Clin. Invest.* 45:228.

Pozefsky, T., Tancredi, R. G., Maxley, R. T., Dupre, J. and Tobin, J. D. 1976. *Diabetes* 25:128–135.

Pozza, G., Pappalettera, A. and Malogli, O. 1971. *Horm. Metab. Res.* 3:291.

Quabbe, H. J., Helge, H. and Kubicki, S. 1971. *Acta Endocrinol.* 67:767.

Raben, M. S. and Hollenberg, C. H. 1959. *J. Clin. Invest.* 38:484.

Randle, P. J., Garland, P. B., Hales, C. N. and Newsholme, E. A. 1963. *Lancet* 1:785.

Reaven, E. P., Kilterman, O. G. and Reaven, G. M. 1974. *J. Lipid Res.* 15:74–83.

Rocha, D. M., Santeusanio, F., Faloona, G. R. and Unger, R. H. 1973. *N. Engl. J. Med.* 288:700–703.

Rossner, S., Larsson-Cohn, U., Carlson, A. and Boberg, J. 1971. *Acta Med. Scand.* 190:301–309.

Roth, J., Glick, S. M., Yalow, R. S. and Berson, S. 1963. *Metabolism* 12:577.

Sailer, S., Sandhofer, F. and Braunsteiner, H. 1966. *Klin. Wochenschr.* 44:1032–1036.

Samols, E., Marri, G. and Marks, V. 1966. *Diabetes* 15:855.

Samols, E., Tyler, J. M. and Marks, V. 1972. In *Glucagon, molecular physiology, clinical and therapeutic implications,* eds. P. J. Lefebvre and R. H. Unger, pp. 151–173. Elmsford, N.Y.: Pergamon.

Schade, D. S. and Eaton, R. P. 1974. *Diabetes* 23:657–661.

Schade, D. S. and Eaton, R. P. 1975a. *Diabetes* 24:502–509.

Schade, D. S. and Eaton, R. P. 1975b. *Diabetes* 24:510–515.

Schade, D. S. and Eaton, R. P. 1975c. *Diabetologia* 11:555–559.

Schade, D. S. and Eaton, R. P. 1975d. *J. Clin. Invest.* 56:1340–1344.

Schade, D. S. and Eaton, R. P. 1975e. *Diabetes* 24:1020–1026.

Schade, D. S. and Eaton, R. P. 1975f. *J. Clin. Endocrinol. Metab.* 40:732–735.

Schade, D. S. and Eaton, R. P. 1976a. *Clin. Res.* 24:531A.

Schade, D. S. and Eaton, R. P. 1976b. *Diabetes* 25 (Suppl. 1):330.

Schade, D. S. and Eaton, R. P. 1977. *Clin. Res.* 25:33A.

Schneider, S. H., Fineberg, S. E. and Blackburn, G. 1976. *Diabetes* 25 (Suppl. 1):341a.

Schteingart, D. E., Gregerman, R. I. and Conn, J. W. 1963. *Metabolism* 12:484.

Schwarz, F., van Riet, H. G. and Schopman, W. 1966. *Metabolism* 15:194.

Sherline, P., Lynch, A. and Glinsmann, W. H. 1972. *Endocrinology* 91:680.

Sherwin, R. S., Fisher, M., Hendler, R. and Felig, P. 1976. *N. Engl. J. Med.* 294:455–461.

Shuck, L. W., Eaton, R. P. and Shuck, J. M. 1975. *Surg. Forum* 26:39–42.

Sims, E. A. H., Goldman, R. F., Gluck, C. M., et al. 1968. *Trans. Assoc. Am. Physicians* 81:153.

Soling, H. D., Garlepp, H. J. and Creutzfeldt. 1965. *Biochim. Biophys. Acta* 100:530.

Steinberg, D. 1966. *Pharmacol. Rev.* 18:217.

Taggart, P., Carruthers, M. and Somerville, W. 1973. *Lancet* 2:341.

Tasake, Y., Sekine, M., Wakatsuki, M., et al. 1975. *Horm. Metab. Res.* 7:205–206.

Tchobroutsky, G. 1973. *Acta Endocrinol.* 74:67–78.

Tchobroutsky, G., Lenormand, M. E., Michel, G. and Assan, R. 1974. *Horm. Metab. Res.* 6:184–187.

Tiengo, A., Muggeo, M., Assan, R. Fedele, D. and Crepaldi, G. 1975. *Metabolism* 24:901–914.

Unger, R. H., Eisentraut, H. M., McCall, M. S. and Madison, L. L. 1961. *J. Clin. Invest.* 40:1280–1289.

Unger, R. H., Aguilar-Parada, E., Muller, W. A. and Eisentraut, A. M. 1970. *J. Clin. Invest.* 49:837–848.

Unverricht, A. 1926. *Dtsch, Med. Wochenschr.* 52:1298.

Valverde, I., Villanueva, M. L., Lorano, I. and Marco, J. 1974. *J. Clin. Endocrinol. Metab.* 39:1090–1098.

Vazquez, A. M., Schutt-aine, J., Drash, A. L. and Kenny, F. M. 1973. *J. Pediatr.* 83:578–586.

Vetter, N. J., Strange, R. C., Adams, W. and Oliver, M. F. 1974. *Lancet* 1:284.

Weir, G. C., Knowlton, S. D. and Martin, D. B. 1975. *J. Clin. Endocrinol. Metab.* 40:296–302.

Willms, B., Bottcher, M., Wolters, V., Sakamoto, N. and Soling, H. D. 1969. *Diabetologia* 5:88–96.

Wilmore, D. W., Long, J. M., Mason, A. D., Skreen, R. W. and Pruitt, B. A. 1974. *Ann. Surg.* 180:653.

Wise, J. K., Hendler, R. and Felig, P. 1973. *N. Engl. J. Med.* 288:487–490.

Woodside, W. F. and Heimberg, M. 1972. *Isr. J. Med. Sci.* 8:309–316.

Woodside, W. F. and Heimberg, M. 1976. *J. Biol. Chem.* 251:13.

York, D. A. and Bray, G. A. 1972. *Endocrinology* 90:885.

Young, F. G. 1937. *Lancet* 2:373.

AUTHOR INDEX

SUBJECT INDEX